'Sethness's excellent book is a wide-ranging and erudite examination of Tolstoy through the lenses of queerness and anarchism, and what is remarkable is how many contradictions and mysteries in Tolstoy's life and work get clarified by this double focus. It is as if he had suddenly popped into three dimensions. The close reading of *War and Peace* is full of startling new insights, and the study as a whole brings Tolstoy into our time in a new and important way. Wonderful to see!'

Kim Stanley Robinson, *author of* The Ministry for the Future, *USA*

'This passionate, ground breaking study of Tolstoy's bisexuality, politics and art offers fascinating new insights into our understanding of the Russian writer's life. By detailing Tolstoy's relationships, experiences and creative process, the author reveals Tolstoy's far sighted literary support for what we would now call LGBT+ liberation, his resistance to war and oppression, and his support for egalitarian social change. Bravo!'

Peter Tatchell, *human rights campaigner and Director, Peter Tatchell Foundation, UK*

QUEER TOLSTOY

Queer Tolstoy is a multidimensional work combining psychoanalysis, political history, LGBTQ+ studies, sexology, ethics, and theology to explore the life and art of Count Lev Nikolaevich Tolstoy.

Using a psychobiographical framework, Sethness Castro uncovers profoundly queer dimensions in Tolstoy's life experiences and art. Deftly contributing to the progressive and radical analysis of gender and sexuality, this book examines how Tolstoy's erotic dissidence informed his anarchist politics, anti-militarist ideals, and voluminous literary production. Sethness Castro analyzes the influence of Buddha, Socrates, Jesus, Cervantes, Rousseau, Kant, Herzen, Proudhon, Chernyshevsky, and his mother Marya Volkonskaya on the artist's writings. Furthermore, he details Tolstoy's emblematic linking of LGBTQ+ desire with moral and erotic self-determination and resistance to Tsarist despotism—especially in *War and Peace*.

This book is vital reading for those interested in the intersection of literature, psychoanalysis, queer studies, and Russian history.

Javier Sethness Castro is a primary-care provider, and the author and editor of four other volumes on a range of topics, from critical theory and social ecology to the work of Herbert Marcuse and Praxedis G. Guerrero.

QUEER TOLSTOY

A Psychobiography

Javier Sethness Castro

Routledge
Taylor & Francis Group
LONDON AND NEW YORK

Designed cover image: Alamy. Ilya Repin, *Tolstoy in the Forest* (1891)

First published 2023
by Routledge
4 Park Square, Milton Park, Abingdon, Oxon OX14 4RN

and by Routledge
605 Third Avenue, New York, NY 10158

Routledge is an imprint of the Taylor & Francis Group, an informa business

British Library Cataloguing-in-Publication Data
A catalogue record for this book is available from the British Library

ISBN: 978-1-032-35850-5 (hbk)
ISBN: 978-1-032-34255-9 (pbk)
ISBN: 978-1-003-32896-4 (ebk)

DOI: 10.4324/9781003328964

Typeset in Bembo
by Taylor & Francis Books

CONTENTS

ILLUSTRATIONS

Maps

Figures

DEDICATION AND ACKNOWLEDGMENTS

Queer Tolstoy is dedicated to my comrade Alexander V., who inspired me to write it. I am very grateful for my sources and the Routledge editorial board. Moreover, I am indebted to Mark Mola, with whom I consulted on the history, geography, and politics of the Caucasus; to Dave Zeglen, Andrew Smolski, and my parents for help in locating sources; to my mother María Castro for our illuminating conversations about Tolstoy and Pasternak, and her help locating paintings; to Liz Lopez, Elena Castro (†), Danish Sheikh, and Chris Sethness for their support; to Paul Murufas for recommending Isaac Babel; to Samuel Clarke for help with a citation; to Hari Prasad for suggestions on map-making; to Siobhán Hearne for her counsel; to Elaine Leeder for a tip about Emma Goldman's sexual history; and to my fellow organizers, panelists, and moderators at "Kronstadt as Revolutionary Utopia, 1921–2021," particularly Joe Scheip. Special thanks are due to Peter Wright (†), David Goldfrank, Tatiana Alexeevna Olbrich, John P. Clark, Jana Craddock, Zoe Meyer, Tom Bedford, Alison Macfarlane, my anonymous fellow nurse, and two anonymous reviewers. Dates are rendered in the Julian calendar, otherwise known as "Old Style," unless otherwise stated. I follow the Russian practice of employing the first name and patronymic as an alternative to using first or last names when discussing particular persons and characters. All errors are my own.

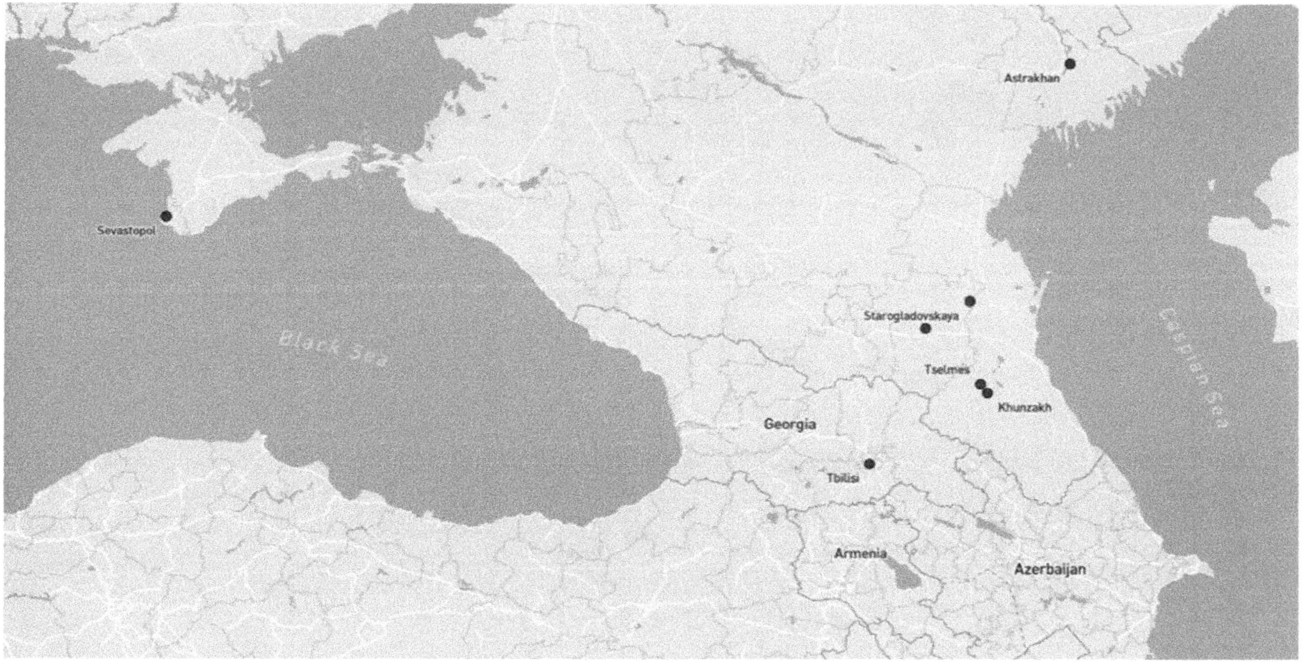

MAP 1 Transcaucasia, referencing cities and villages mentioned in "The Sevastopol Sketches," *The Cossacks* and *Hadji Murat* (using current State borders)

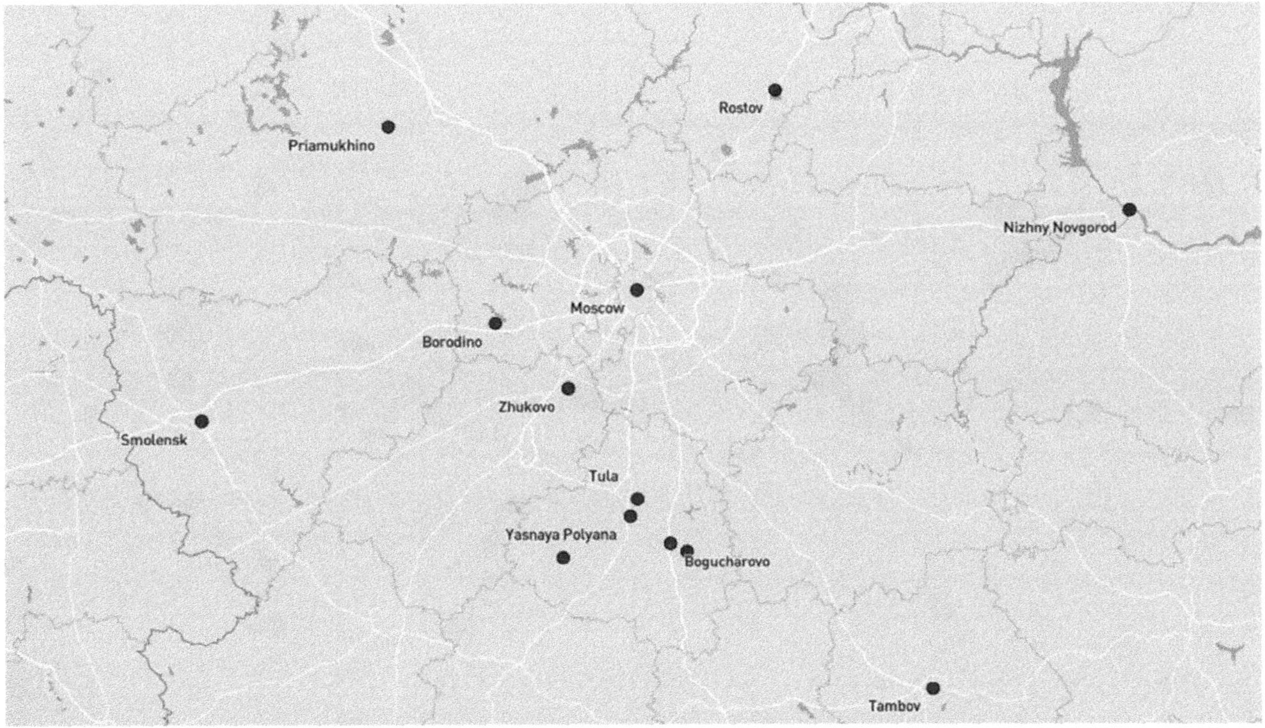

MAP 2 Central Russia, marking important cities and villages from Russian history, literature, and Tolstoy's life

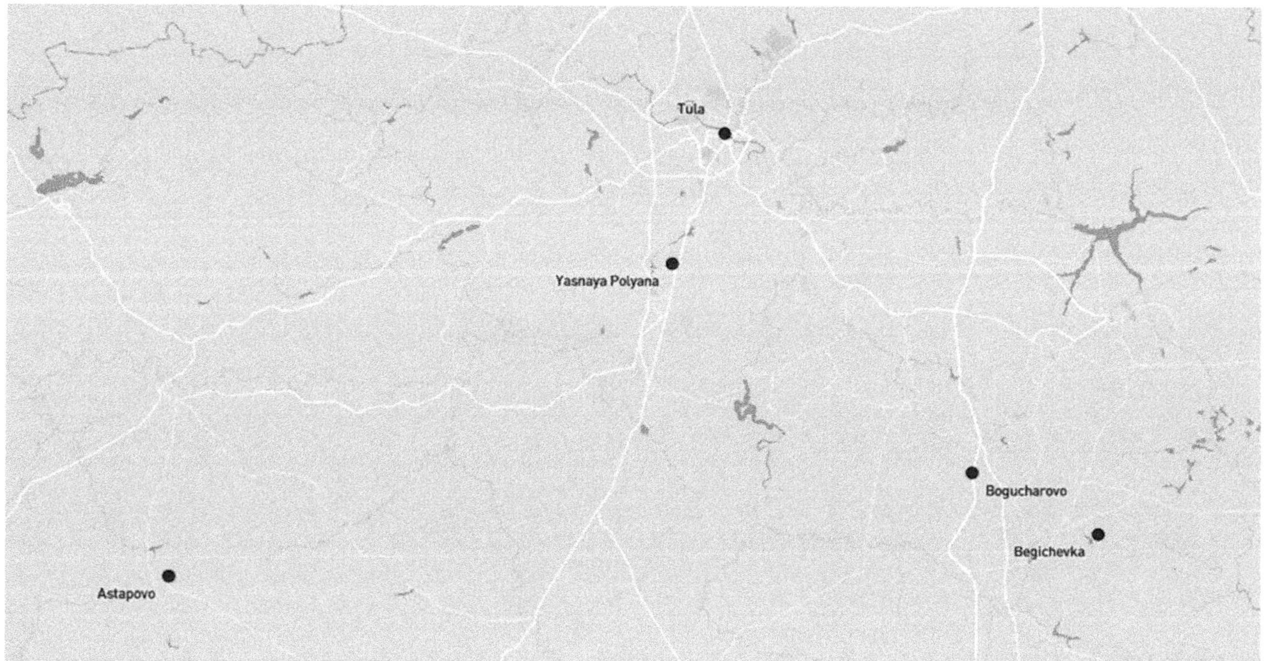

MAP 3 Tula and Yasnaya Polyana, Tolstoy's home

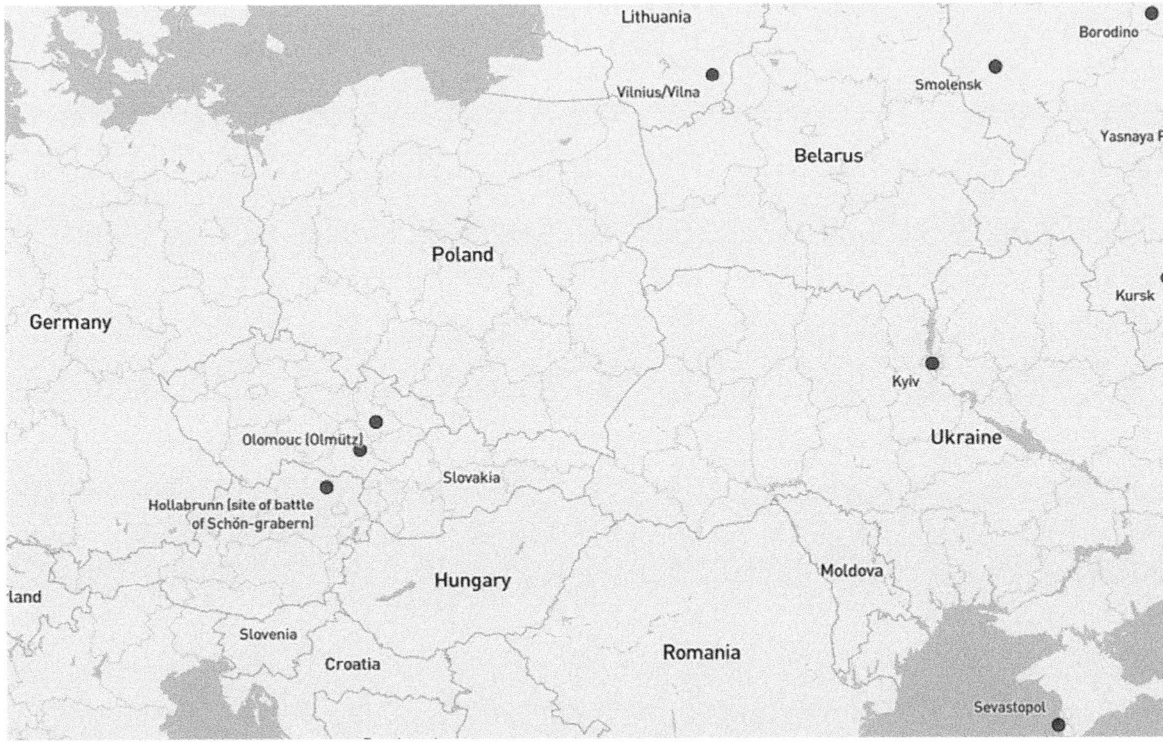

MAP 4 Central and Eastern Europe, referencing cities and battle-sites mentioned in *War and Peace* (using current State borders)

1

THEORETICAL PREFACE ON QUEER ANARCHISM

Queer Tolstoy is a psychobiographical, historical, and sexological study of Count Lev Nikolaevich Tolstoy (1828–1910), a White-Russian Christian anarchist who had become the world's most famous living novelist by the late 1880s.[1] This book investigates the underappreciated queer anarchism of Tolstoy's life and art-works, using psychoanalytic and feminist lenses. Specifically, we analyze Tolstoy according to the frameworks and findings of Sigmund Freud, Otto Gross, Erich Fromm, Herbert Marcuse, Ernest Becker, Nancy Chodorow, Lynn S. Chancer, and Jessica Benjamin.

Broadly speaking, we uncover a powerful attraction to sexual anarchy, otherwise known as free love, in Tolstoy's biography and artistic creativity. This subversiveness of Eros—one of the divine patrons of homoeroticism in classical Greece—was as equally feared by Plato in *The Republic* (c. 375 BCE), who banned poets from his utopia due to its disruptive potential, as it was welcomed by the anarchist psychiatrist Gross (1877–1922), champion of the "sexual revolution," and the critical theorist Marcuse (1898–1979), author of *Eros and Civilization* (1955). Gross saw this life force as superseding the patriarchal will to power and stimulating the egalitarian "will to relatedness," whereas Marcuse envisioned a future non-repressive and post-capitalist civilization.[2] Likewise, the Black lesbian feminist Audre Lorde (1934–1992) saw Eros as "opening up an entire realm of human understanding otherwise unavailable."[3] In *War and Peace* (1869), in parallel, Tolstoy celebrates queer desire as a passionate urge to relate socially and contest violence, exploitation, and despotism.

However, human sexuality is more complicated than that. While *Queer Tolstoy* is about exploring the intersections between erotic dissidence and radical politics, tracing the continued relevance of the "ancient association of same-sex eroticism with the hatred of tyranny," the idea is not to essentialize LGBTQ+ desire as necessarily linked to any theory of emancipation.[4] After all, in *Three Essays on the Theory of Sexuality* (1905), Freud (1856–1939) argues that "[h]uman cultural history

DOI: 10.4324/9781003328964-1

shows beyond any doubt that there is an integral connection between cruelty and the sexual drive," adding that sexual sadism of any orientation is a "relic of cannibalistic pleasures."[5] Historically speaking, "bad gays" from Alexander the Great to King James, Ernst Röhm, Roy Cohn, and J. Edgar Hoover have promoted social hierarchies and the abuse of power.[6] In Chapter 6, we analyze Tolstoy's depiction of a Russian troop-review before Tsar Alexander I at Olmütz (now the Czech Republic), as a prominent example of the mobilization of same-sex desire for authoritarian political ends. We also examine the phenomenon whereby the Nazis encouraged homoeroticism in their ranks during the Weimar Republic, only to criminalize and persecute suspected homosexuals after seizing power. We speculate that Stalin and Hitler had a platonic gay bond, despite the General Secretary's ban on homosexuality, which followed the *Führer*'s own, and regardless of the Soviet regime's official medicalization of lesbians and bisexuals.

Evidently, homophobia in the Soviet Union conveyed a hostility to eroticism as an autonomous realm, impenetrable to State control.[7] While this bias surely reflects the power of heterosexism in hegemonic Russian culture, Marxism—being the Soviet Union's official ideology—bears some of the blame. After all, the private correspondence between Karl Marx (1818–1883) and Friedrich Engels (1820–1895) reveals heterosexist revulsion over the gay-friendly findings of the German sexologist Karl Heinrich Ulrichs (1825–1895), as well as contempt for their political rival, Johann Baptist von Schweitzer (1833–1875), who was the first explicit Social Democrat to be elected in Europe. In 1862, despite a lack of evidence, Schweitzer was convicted and imprisoned for public indecency over having supposedly propositioned an adolescent boy in a Mannheim park. Just as Marx, Engels, and their allies circulated baseless rumors for decades that the Russian anarchist revolutionary Mikhail Bakunin (1814–1876) was a Tsarist agent, with an eye to weakening the libertarian wing of the International Workingmen's Association (IWMA), or First International, Marx instructed Engels to humiliate Schweitzer in the newspapers.[8]

In 1868, bristling at the call for the equalization of the sexes in the program of the International Alliance for Socialist Democracy, which Bakunin had founded the same year, Marx underlined this demand in his reading of the text, and wrote with amused contempt, "Hermaphrodite man! Just like the Russian Commune!"[9] Later, at the IWMA's September 1872 Hague Congress, Marx notoriously employed a threatening letter written by Bakunin's junior partner, Sergei Nechaev (1847–1882), as key evidence to expel Bakunin and the Swiss anarchist James Guillaume (1844–1916) from the organization. By so eliminating his rivals in a bid to consolidate power, Marx utterly wrecked the IWMA.[10] This tragic historical episode reflects psychological and political distinctions between Marxists and anarchists in terms of what might be called a "power-distance orientation," or a tolerance for hierarchy, with anarchists typically tolerating this less than Marxists.[11]

Theorizing *Queer Tolstoy*

Theoretically speaking, we integrate aspects of Freudian and Frommian psycho-socioanalysis into *Queer Tolstoy*. We concur with Freud and Fromm about the importance of both pre-Oedipal (or infantile/early childhood) and Oedipal (or adolescent-adult) attachments in the development of the human personality. In other words, both sexual satisfaction and existential meaning are important for well-being, whether or not they coincide. We agree with Freud that humans are innately bisexual and gender fluid, having a "polymorphously perverse disposition" from birth, and that the growing boy's identification with the mother, both early and later in life, is decisive for the development of consciously homosexual object-choice.[12]

Indeed, in the *Symposium* (c. 385 BCE)—which Tolstoy had first read in French translation as a young adult in 1851—Plato records the physician Eryximachos as declaring that Eros resides "in the bodies of all living creatures," and that the pull of Eros and Heavenly Aphrodite (Aphrodite Urania) reflects man's instinctual desire to reunite with the (male) Other.[13] Likewise, Charles Darwin held that "every man & woman is hermaphrodite," in an echo of "some extremely remote progenitor of the whole vertebrate kingdom [that] appears to have been hermaphrodite or androgynous."[14] Lesbian feminist theorists such as Adrienne Rich (1929–2012) assert the existence of a "lesbian continuum," meaning that lesbian Eros underpins many intimate relationships among women.[15] Plus, Tolstoy's life and art provide strong evidence for the importance of maternal attachment in the development not only of male homosexuality, but also of anarchist and anti-militarist principles.

In parallel, Freud describes how the love between Leonardo da Vinci (1452–1519) and his mother Caterina inspired both his same-sex desires and his best art, including *The Virgin and Child with St. Anne* (c. 1501) and *The Mona Lisa* (c. 1503). Chancer adds that a "pre-oedipal" concern with relatedness underpins Fromm's humanistic psychology.[16] In the same vein, Tolstoy's memory of early prosocial emotions with his mother, Princess Marya Volkonskaya (1790–1830), and "allomothers" such as his aunts Aline Tolstaya and Tatiana Ergolskaya, likely inspired *War and Peace*.[17]

In contrast to the tendency toward "desexualized psychoanalysis" present in Fromm's work, we assert, with Marcuse and Jean Laplanche (1924–2012), the value to be found in Freud's findings about ubiquitous polymorphous perversity.[18] Echoing the postulated lesbian continuum, Tolstoy's art gives voice to a "gay continuum," even if gay and lesbian identities are not exactly interchangeable.[19] At the same time, we cannot ignore that psychoanalytic practice considered homosexuality a mental illness for much of the twentieth century. To an extent, this may reflect the marginalization of Gross's radical psychoanalytic approach, which appears to have been LGBTQ+-friendly.[20] Although Freud disagreed with and fought against the psychiatric classifications of same-sex attachment, it is undeniable that his psychosexual theory is heteronormative, and that his treatment of erotic "inversion" as an "aberration" may have legitimized the subsequent psychological abuse of queer people. Similar criticism could be made of Fromm's view of the "homosexual deviation" and endorsement of the gender binary—ironically, in spite of this theorist's reliance on homoerotic and gender-queer sources.[21]

Critique of the hyper-masculinity encoding misogyny, heteronormativity, and transphobia are especially needed, in light of the criminalization of abortion with the overturning of *Roe v. Wade*; the scourge of so-called conversion therapy, which persists to this day; and the hateful "Don't Say Gay" laws being passed in Republican-controlled states.[22] The psychiatrist Terry Kupers defines toxic masculinity as "the constellation of socially regressive male traits that serve to foster domination, the devaluation of women, homophobia, and wanton violence."[23] In this sense, it is striking indeed to contemplate just how closely the US far-right's promotion of "traditional values" has both influenced *and* borrowed from Vladimir Putin's reactionary reign, which banned "propaganda of non-traditional sexual relations" in 2013, intervened militarily to prop up Bashar al-Assad's ghastly regime in 2015, decriminalized domestic violence in 2018, and now carries out horrifying war crimes in neighboring Ukraine.[24] Putin has rationalized his institutionalized homophobia, which has encouraged ultraviolence against the LGBTQ+ community in Chechnya, as a reassertion of Eastern tradition against Western liberalism.[25] Now, the Republican Party joins suit, by systematically stifling any discussion of gender or sexual diversity in schools.

However, against the claims of heterosexists of all stripes, there is no question that same-sex desire is a "frequently occurring phenomenon."[26] Beyond exploring the role of male courtesans in ancient Syrian-Canaanite religions, the gay English anarchist Edward Carpenter (1844–1929) lists the androgynous-queer presentation of Shiva, Brahm, Buddha, Dionysus, Apollo, and Jesus, and the prevalence of comrade-love among Samurai, as evidence for this claim.[27] To these, we can add the Persian and Urdu *ghazals* performed in Sufi *qawwali* music, which are amorous poems typically written by older males as lamentations over lost love with idealized junior partners. Moreover, "men's houses" have been documented among the Sedang-Moi of Vietnam; the Batak of Sumatra; and the Marind Anim, Kaluli, Sambia, and Keraki of New Guinea.[28] The late Christopher Chitty (1983–2015) summarizes: "the behavior appears universal, more or less common to all social forms, modified here and there by various institutional, cultural, and economic contexts."[29]

That being said, Eric de Kuyper channels Laplanche in asserting that homosexual desire is also a fundamental aspect of ostensible straightness: that is, in choosing heterosexuality, the son both identifies with, and expresses love for, the father.[30] Intimate care among women and the breastfeeding of infant girls are arguably part of a lesbian continuum.[31] Plus, in his study of da Vinci, the evidently bisexual Freud himself admits to having "succumbed to the attraction of this great and mysterious man"![32]

In a similar vein, research on relationships among gay males supports the Freudian hypothesis that homosexual men (un)consciously follow the sexual preferences of their (presumably straight) mothers, in that they tend to select fit, masculine men as partners.[33] The unfortunate tendency among certain gay men to compensate for their marginalization and abuse by affirming toxic masculinity admittedly challenges the emancipatory potential of LGBTQ+ liberation. In place of destituent power and the alternatives of mutual relation and recognition offered by Gross and Benjamin, much less Lorde's lesbian Eros, we confront a situation that could merit Marcuse's critique of "repressive desublimation," whereby strict sexual attitudes are progressively relaxed, but only to shore up the existing system of domination.[34]

Hence, the importance of the intersection between queerness and anarchism. Indeed, along these lines, the sexual researcher Hubert Kennedy remarks on the widespread perception, in late nineteenth-century Europe, that "a disproportionately large number of anarchists was homosexual."[35]

Defining *Queer Tolstoy*

In this section, we will define some of the most important terms used in this book using italics.

Though "*queer*" is often considered an amorphous and ambivalent term, it can be distinguished from strictly lesbian, gay, bisexual, or transgender (LGBTQ+) experience or identities with reference to political radicalism, especially as crystallized in opposition to the idea of assimilation or integration into mainstream society.[36] At the same time, queer can also be synonymous with *libidinal*, or sexual, deviance and freely chosen LGBTQ+ desire and experience. It can even anticipate the abolition of sexual identity altogether.[37] The term *hermaphrodite*, which is admittedly dated, refers to the more current term intersex, and has some overlap with being transgender. The adjective "queer" and its corresponding noun are used to denote both its political and erotic meanings in this volume.

When describing gay male relationships, we use the terms *homosocial*, or platonic; *homophilic*, or sexual-emotional in nature, whether genital *or* platonic; and *homosexual*, meaning a specifically genital attachment.

Camp is a queer form of communication centering subversion and *double entendre*, connoting the Greek god Dionysus' androgynous, gay, and intoxicated dimensions.[38]

The Russian *intelligentsia* refer to oppositional artists and intellectuals under Tsarist rule. Some well-known figures include Vissarion Belinsky (1811–1848), Alexander Herzen (1812–1870), Ivan Turgenev (1818–1883), Peter Lavrov (1823–1900), Nikolai Chernyshevsky (1828–1889), Vera Zasulich (1849–1919), Sofia Perovskaya (1853–1881), Bakunin, and Tolstoy himself, among others. According to the late historian Richard Stites, the utopias sought by these radicals "did not diverge greatly from the European enlightenment tradition."[39]

After years of participation in revolutions, political imprisonment, and struggles against Marx and his followers in the First International, Bakunin formulated six fundamental *anarchist* political principles. These include anti-authoritarianism, anti-statism, anti-parliamentarism, federalism, libertarianism, and social revolution.[40] To this list, Jeff Shantz and Dana Williams add solidarity, mutual aid, cooperation, egalitarianism, and direct action.[41] In keeping with these principles, anarchists disavow the centralist and vertical strategies endorsed by Marxists as residues of the bourgeois world. They favor *social revolution*, or the abolition of class hierarchy and State power through workers' control, over any seizure of the State apparatus or political revolution. In this sense, Bakunin aptly predicted the tragedy of the Russian Revolution, as the stunning popular uprising of February 1917 against Tsarism, landlordism, and militarism descended into a state-capitalist nightmare, once it had been appropriated by the Bolshevik Party.

Although Tolstoy also criticized Marxism for its statism and economic determinism, his *Christian anarchism* took inspiration from the Gospels.[42] In contrast to the rituals, mysteries, and dogmas advanced by the various churches of the past two millennia, which Lev Nikolaevich considered mere distractions that have served to perpetuate class domination and enslave humanity, he echoed the literary critic Belinsky in distinguishing between the institutionalized opportunism of the churches and the "liberty, equality, and fraternity" preached by Jesus the Galilean.[43]

The *Narod* is Russian for "People." A *Narodnik* is a Populist. By *Populism*, we refer not only to discourses that seek to unify the "People" against given "elites," but specifically, to the nineteenth-century Russian revolutionary tradition (Народничество) that aimed to overthrow Tsarism by organizing the peasantry and urban workers.[44] *Anarcho-Populism*, then, refers to specifically anarchist expressions of this radical current.

The critical theorist Axel Honneth (b. 1949) defines *socialism* well: namely, as the political project to cooperatively expand social freedom through the overcoming of coercion and domination in the economy, polity, and personal relationships.[45] While socialism can be reformist and statist, anarchism shows that it does not have to be. *Humanism*, for its part, refers to the "idea of the perfectibility of the individual and of the unity of the human race."[46]

According to Freud, *Eros* is the "preserver of all things."[47] As the presumptive life force, Eros "*extend[s]*" sexual sensibility "anatomically beyond the regions of the body designed for genital union," and "tends to involve all sensations emanating from it."[48] For the psychoutopian Gross, Eros meant "not only sexuality but relatedness in a psychological and anthropological sense"; it refers to the combination of "innate morality" and "innate sexuality" that recalls the hypothesized memory of ancestral matriarchal communism. As such, Eros is "an 'anarchistic' destabilizer of the bourgeois order, a troublemaker and a destroyer of social control."[49] In fact, Lorde points out that Eros was "born of Chaos."[50] Arrayed against Thanatos, otherwise known as the death-drive, Eros upholds the will to live by ensuring love, union, libidinal satisfaction, and survival. As Marcuse stressed, under prevailing conditions of oppression, it requires social revolution to flourish—just as revolution needs Eros to succeed.[51]

Applying psychoanalytic categories, we can appreciate the robust processes of *transference* ("prism[s]" of meaning), *introjection* (internalization/identification), and *projection* (externalization) involved in Tolstoy's artistic process, which amounted to a prolonged process of *sublimation*—or diversion of psychosexual energies into culture and creativity—that yielded over 80 volumes.[52] In creating his art, Lev Nikolaevich provided outlets for not only his sexual fantasies, but also his political, historical, and sociological ones.[53] Through transference, the prose poet unconsciously used past experiences and ongoing dreams and feelings to give meaning to his life and literary production.[54]

Tolstoy and the Oedipus Complex

The controversial Freudian concepts of the Oedipus and Electra complexes propose that all boys and girls desire sexual union with their opposite-sex parents, and resent their same-sex parents for the same reason. Admittedly, supporting evidence for these ideas is lacking from anthropological, biological, and psychological research, and feminists have rightly criticized them for its male bias.[55] Still, according to Freud, boys normally resolve this ostensibly unconscious conflict through identifying with their fathers and choosing heterosexual partners as vicarious mothers, while girls end up choosing boys and men to replace their fathers, while identifying with their mothers. However, "deviations" are certainly possible from the contours of this thought experiment.

For instance, da Vinci identified with his mother, rather than his father, and Gross envisioned the future revolution being matriarchal, just as he raged against the significance of the father in human destiny—a theme that the psychiatrist Carl Jung (1875–1961), Gross's "twin brother," would appropriate from him after destroying his career.[56] Similarly, Tolstoy rejected the conventional, hyper-masculine idea that men must not be compassionate, tender, or nurturing, but rather, "aggressive [...] and menacing."[57]

Developmentally speaking, to a great extent, Tolstoy's art can be considered a sustained endeavor to get in touch again with the emotional attunement, cooperation, and "sharing [of] states of mind" experienced with his mother, Marya Nikolaevna, in pre-individuated, infantile life.[58] This psychical space held by the writer connected his vital sense of goodness with the sacred memory of his mother, to whom he would appeal in prayer during difficult times in both middle and old age.[59] Two years before passing, Tolstoy recalled, "[w]hat a good feeling I have toward her [Princess Marya]. How I would like to have that feeling toward all, women and men."[60] In turn, the writer's concerns for sharing, connection, and communion all suggest a persistent identification with the mother, a desire for recognition, and resistance to toxic male socialization processes.[61]

Like Tolstoy, da Vinci declined to eat meat and "condemned war and bloodshed," signaling a critique of hyper-masculinity. Taking into account Freud's remarks about the Italian polymath's work engineering weapons of war for Cesare Borgia, though, he cannot be considered as consistent an anti-militarist as Lev Nikolaevich.[62] Freud believed that the novelist Fëdor Mikhailovich Dostoevsky (1821–1881) had a "double attitude" toward Oedipal conflict, in that the artist supported the political father-figure while harboring repressed urges to kill him. Politically, this translated into Dostoevsky "land[ing] in the retrograde position [...] of veneration both for the Tsar [...] and of a narrow Russian nationalism," while Tolstoy applied concepts of Christian love to blossom into an anarchist internationalist, and become one of the greatest critics of Tsarism. Whereas Fëdor Mikhailovich "made himself one with [humanity's] gaolers," Lev Nikolaevich became an anarchist prophet. Building on Freud's analysis, and notwithstanding the "extraordinary intensity" of both their "emotional li[ves]," Tolstoy was less gripped by the "filial guilt" that evidently fettered his compatriot to the State.[63]

Instead, Tolstoy's queer-humanist and anti-militarist ideals—as featured, above all, in *War and Peace*—convey a simultaneous rejection of the repressive reality principle imposed by despotic men, on the one hand, and an approximation to feminist approaches centering care, mutual recognition, and inter-subjectivity, on the other. Plus, as with the "sublimated" homosexual da Vinci, Tolstoy's artistic contributions were based on an almost-monastic sublimation of the "greater part of his libido into an urge for research"—that is to say, when either one was not "surrounded [by] handsome boys and youth whom he took as pupils."[64] In this light, Freud likely would have viewed Tolstoy's approach to the hypothesized Oedipus complex as "abnormal"—as he did da Vinci's.[65]

Even so, like Dostoevsky, Tolstoy too had a "double attitude" toward the conflict. The recurrent sadism and misogyny that Lev Nikolaevich expressed in his life and art affirm the Oedipal internalization of male identity and hegemonic masculinity, which base themselves on the repudiation of mothers and femininity.[66] While day-dreaming about matriarchal and anarchical pasts and futures, freed from authority, exploitation, and violence, Tolstoy paradoxically also re-entrenched the patriarchal fixation on men and masculinity exhibited in many homoerotic contexts, at least since classical Greece.[67] His infamous repudiation of women's liberation, as conveyed in *Anna Karenina* (1875–1877) and "The Kreutzer Sonata" (1889), is consistent with Freud's comment that "the most complete psychical masculinity is perfectly compatible with [homosexuality]" in men.[68]

Eros and Authority, Part I: Androphilia and Queer Revolution

There is a risk, then, that focusing on homophilia could paradoxically strengthen the patriarchal status quo, instead of contributing to social revolution as an insurgent, destituent force. Taking an historical view, Chitty links the "near-universal homosexuality" of Mediterranean men in antiquity to the forms of labor and servitude established in the Iron Age (c. 1200 BCE), which persist even in late capitalism. In this sense, we appreciate the Italian Enlightenment thinker Cesare Beccaria (1738–1794) for condemning the predominantly pederastic form of homosexuality of his time, which he found to affirm the archaic forces of hierarchy and domination, inherited from ancient civilizations.[69]

To clarify this point is in no way to lend support to Marx and Engels's equating of homosexuality with pederasty, as seen during their struggle against Schweitzer, much less to Putin, Viktor Orbán, or Ron DeSantis's contemporary mobilization of delusions about the LGBTQ+ community being inherently predatory toward minors. After all, such campaigns overlook the sex crimes perpetrated by the Russian military against children in Ukraine since its February 2022 full-scale invasion, not to mention those committed by Jeffrey Epstein and his cronies. As the Russian psychologist Vladimir Shakhizhanian notes, "[a]ny exploitation of children is always wrong."[70]

That being said, Tolstoy's life and art combine queerness and anarchism to show that androphilic bonds developed among men, based in mutual recognition, a commitment to social freedom, and rebellion against authority, are a crucial dimension of liberation. The same, of course, is true of lesbian, bisexual, and transgender union and self-determination. Along these lines, the Slavist Jennifer Wilson writes that Tolstoy's imaginative depictions of "sexual alterity [...] allo[w] for a critical rethinking of those institutions that are based on strict gender roles, such as the military and marriage, war and peace [...]."[71] Anti-authoritarian LGBTQ+ themes feature in Tolstoy's fiction, whether in *The Cossacks* (1863), *War and Peace* (1869), *Resurrection* (1899), "The Death of Ivan Ilych" (1886), or "Master and Man" (1895); in Herman Melville and J. R. R. Tolkien's novels; and in many pirate tales.[72]

Seen in such light, Lev Nikolaevich's surreal experience of an anti-clerical, anti-militarist epiphany during the siege of Sevastopol in 1855, which revealed to him his vocation of founding a new religion, together with his stated desire to be a "literary general"; his recurrent artistic critique of marriage; his childhood nickname of *Leva-reva* ("Lev, the crybaby"); and the indelible link between affect and utopianism all point to a hitherto underappreciated sexual dissidence that permeated Tolstoy's life and art.[73] In reality, as we shall see in the following nine chapters, the poet was a partisan of "beautiful, non-violent, anarchist, *queer* revolution."[74]

Notes

1 Dynes 1990f; Zorin 137. "White-Russian" is equivalent to "Great Russian."
2 Pietikainen 65, 73, 84; Marcuse 1955.
3 Ginzberg 73–4, 84.
4 Chitty 59.
5 Freud 2016: 72.
6 Staples.
7 Mole 4–5.
8 Kennedy 69–87; Graham 173.
9 Leier 237.
10 Avrich; Graham; Goodwin; Kennedy.
11 Fischer et al.
12 Freud 2016: 91–2; Murphy.
13 Harris 85; Johansson 1990n; Orwin 2002b: 2.
14 Plato 2015: 87; Darwin 1987: 384; Darwin 1981: 207.
15 Ginberg 78–9.
16 Freud 1961b; Chancer 2020: 104.
17 Hrdy 7, 78.
18 Smith D 131; Marcuse 1955; de Lauretis.
19 Ginzberg 78–9.
20 Heuer 61–2.
21 Fromm 2006: 31; Bauer 1104–6.
22 Murphy; Bauer; Freud 2016: 58–9; Cornett and Hudson.
23 Salter.
24 Essig and Kondakov 89–95.
25 Merz; Mole 9–10.
26 Freud 2016: 60.
27 Carpenter 1919: 28–83, 147–160.
28 Rancour-Laferriere 1985: 348.

29 Chitty 30.
30 de Kuyper 138–42.
31 Ginzberg 78–9.
32 Freud 1961b: 97.
33 Lanzieri and Hildebrant 276.
34 Benjamin; Heuer 10; Ginzberg; Marcuse 1964.
35 Kennedy 89.
36 Kouri-Towe.
37 de Lauretis; Hájková 114–15.
38 Dynes 1990f; 1990h; Benjamin 147.
39 Stites 1989: 226.
40 Goodwin; Graham.
41 Shantz and Williams 159.
42 Gustafson 1986: 393.
43 Bulgakov 49n20.
44 Smolski et al.; Venturi; MacLaughlin.
45 Honneth 24–7, 89–106.
46 Sternhell 76.
47 Freud 1961b: 17.
48 Freud 2016: 67 (emphasis in original).
49 Pietikainen 66–9, 82–4.
50 Ginzberg 74.
51 Marcuse 1955; Marcuse 1980.
52 Benjamin 21–43; Freud 2016: 84.
53 Freud 1961a: 94, 98; Stites 1989.
54 Chodorow 1999: 14–41.
55 Kupfersmid.
56 Freud 1961b; Pietikainen 58–62, 68; Heuer 17, 91–5.
57 Lanzieri and Hildebrant 278.
58 Benjamin 16–27.
59 Zorin 10–11; Benjamin 163. In turn, Tolstoyan intellectuals and peasants would meditate on their inner strength and their love for Lev Nikolaevich as solace when imprisoned in the GULAG by the Stalinist regime in the 1930s and 1940s (Mazurin; Morgachëv).
60 Gustafson 1986: 29.
61 Benjamin 19–76, 126.
62 Freud 1961b: 15–16.
63 Freud 1961a: 177, 179, 187.
64 Freud 1961b: 9–11, 20, 30.
65 de Kuyper 140–2; Freud 1961b: 54–5.
66 Benjamin 167–85.
67 Lanzieri and Hildebrant 278–84.
68 Freud 2016: 63.
69 Chitty 83, 116–17.
70 Shakhidzhanian and Reiter.
71 Wilson J 2014: 30.
72 Johansson 1990h; Child B.
73 Zorin 81; Rancour-Laferriere 1998: 20; Maude 1987a: 111; Bulgakov 7; Stites 1989; Rubin.
74 Warfield et al. 122 (emphasis in original).

2

LEV NIKOLAEVICH TOLSTOY

A Queer, Christian-Anarchist Writer

As a prose poet, literary author, journalist, and ethicist, Lev Nikolaevich Tolstoy served as a radical critic of the instrumentalization of life, whether perpetrated through war, feudal-capitalist exploitation, or State oppression. In the estimation of Vladimir Vasilievich Stasov (1824–1906), head of the Imperial Academy Library in St. Petersburg, Tolstoy ranks not only among Russia's greatest writers. He also stands upright alongside the poet-ambassador Alexander Griboyedov (1795–1829) and the revolutionary Populist "father" of Russian socialism Alexander Herzen as one of the three "preeminently intellectual" Russian writers.[1] In parallel, the artist's fellow Christian anarchist Nikolai Berdyaev (1874–1948) lauds his predecessor for having exposed the "falsehood and injustice [that] lie at the very roots of civilization," revolted "against the false standards of greatness and the false sanctities of history," and "rebelled against history and civilization with unheard of radicalism."[2] Furthermore, according to the literary critic Inessa Medzhibovskaya (b. 1964), Lev Nikolaevich Tolstoy was Russia's "first modern man, the first defender of the autonomous freedom of conscience."[3]

In his commitment to liberative social ethics, which espouses human equality, liberty, and struggle, Tolstoy was related by creed to the radical Iranian intellectual Ali Shariati (1933–1977), who was "essentially a modern religious man," as well.[4] As Tolstoy posthumously inspired the Russian Revolution of 1917, so Shariati influenced the coming of the Iranian Revolution after his death. For the Russian novelist and prose poet, the "fundamental desire[s] of the human individual" are for freedom, free cooperation, sympathy, and unity, and love is both the "natural state of the soul" and the "natural form of interaction among people."[5] In consonance with the Russian existentialist Lev Shestov (1866–1938), his namesake remains "an important witness, to whom one not only can listen but to whom it is our duty to listen"—especially given that this preacher, "throughout all his life, stubbornly professed the conviction that outside the 'good' there is no salvation."[6]

DOI: 10.4324/9781003328964-2

In its edict of February 1901 excommunicating Tolstoy, the Most Holy Governing Synod, an arm of the Tsarist State founded by Peter I (the "Great"), referred to him as a "new false teacher […] seduc[ed by] his intellectual pride."[7] Such ideological disciplining functioned to punish the humanist prophet for the "pride" of confidently relying on his own powers, defying the masochistic passivity on which the parasitical existence of Church and State depend, and seeking the liberation of the *Narod* (Народ, "People") through an anarchistic universalization of his own aristocratic sense of personal dignity.[8] In light of the fundamental threat posed to every abuser by the freedom of the spirit, the Synod's depravity is unsurprising.[9] These representatives of State authority evidently felt threatened by Tolstoy's emblematic scorn for the father-figure, and thus also for the internalized aggression, unconscious guilt, and repression expected of those subjected to hierarchical social institutions.[10]

Arguing in better faith than the Synod, the anarchist's wife Sofia Andreevna Tolstaya (1844–1919) saw her partner "both [as] an artistic genius and a moral hypocrite," particularly in light of his sexist attitudes.[11] In like fashion, the Formalist literary critic Viktor Shklovsky (1893–1984) perceived that "[t]here lived at Yasnaya Polyana"—the main Volkonsky-Tolstoy estate—"an intemperate, unfulfilled and restless man."[12] In contrast, his friend, the liberal author Ivan Turgenev, wrote in 1882 that his counterpart was "a very queer fellow but undoubtedly a genius, and the kindliest of men," just as another colleague, the conservative literary critic Nikolai N. Strakhov (1828–1896), painted him as "a sensitive aesthete by nature."[13] Above all, the Symbolist poet Dmitri Sergeivich Merezhkovsky (1866–1941) welcomed the prose poet's 80th birthday in 1908 as a "celebration of the Russian revolution" against despotism, and the Polish Jewish Marxist Rosa Luxemburg (1871–1919) praised Tolstoy as a "vehement prophet" for tirelessly preaching the abolition of private property, militarism, and the State.[14] The two shared a common commitment to romance and freedom, as summarized by Luxemburg: "My ideal is a social system that allows one to love everybody with a clear conscience."[15]

One might add that, following his religious "conversion" in the late 1870s, the count semi-consciously repudiated heterosexuality and increasingly withdrew from his marriage, while hinting at his unsatisfied homosexual desires, which in reality had permeated his art from the beginning.[16] Historically, non-normative, alternate, or queer sexuality, particularly as expressed in revolutionism, has had a close relationship with Eastern-Christian monastic and ascetic traditions.[17] Along these lines, during the Russian Civil War (1918–1920), the Bolshevik authorities prosecuted numerous "class enemies," especially Orthodox clerics, for ostensibly "unnatural acts," thus anticipating Stalin's totalitarian mobilization of compulsory heterosexuality in the 1930s.[18]

Lev Nikolaevich Tolstoy's writings flourished as a subversive symbolic system in late Imperial Russia, both despite official preliminary censorship, and because the arts under Tsarism served as "an arena for political, philosophical and religious debate" and the development of social thought "in the absence of a parliament or a free press."[19] Pervasive in Tolstoy's work is the concept of "the natural love and unity immanent in [hu]man[ity]," in the formulation of philosopher Ludwig

Feuerbach (1804–1872), who likewise believed in the word's "power to redeem, to reconcile, to bless, to make free."[20] Thus, like the literary knight-errant Don Quixote, Lev Nikolaevich sought to "sustain the imaginary universe which captivate[d] him" by connecting with others in affective, sexual, creative, and political ways.[21] The writer believed the "mingl[ing of] souls with another" to be "the very essence of art," which at its best manifests successful human interrelatedness.[22] Those who—like Tolstoy—have a highly developed "Openness/Intellect" domain of personality often dream and engage in reverie and emotional subversion not just at night, but also during the day.[23] The writer did not fear his dreams or hide them from others. In political and erotic terms, he identified the need to "destro[y] the wall that separates us from the people, retur[n] what we have taken from them, dra[w] nearer to them and unit[e] with them as a natural result of abandoning our privileges."[24]

Through intercourse of many kinds, whether artistic, social, erotic, or political, we express that "[w]e all want to be together and at one."[25] One could say that the goal of the "One Big Union" animating the anarcho-syndicalist cause is the same. Yet, in Tolstoy's case, it is evident that, although the man sought to "merge with" the People, he was "equally a loner, a 'stranger'" in his relation to the human collective, for both economic and psychological reasons.[26] This thematic opposition between estrangement, or separation, and residence, or union, reverberates throughout Tolstoy's life and art. His insider-outsider status, his anarchist politics, his delayed marriage, and the precarity of his love bonds with other men, "outside the institutions of family, property, and couple form," all convey his queerness.[27] Reflecting a cultural introjection of Eastern-Christian concepts, some of which in turn may reflect the imprints of Daoism and Buddhism, the writer believed God could be readily accessed through experiences of residence and redemptive expressions of "anti-authoritarian unity" in the world. As he would declare emphatically, "[m]y anarchism is only an application of Christianity to human relationships." In contrast, Tolstoy held sin to be "dissociation among people," or the denial of our essential oneness.[28]

Whereas the "Stranger lives outside the bond of human relatedness," isolated, unloving, and awaiting death, the Resident affirms life and love, individual and communal, together with "unity in multiplicity and multiplicity in unity."[29] Given the tragic absence in death of Marya Nikolaevna Tolstaya (1790–1830), Lev's mother, who died weeks before he turned two, it was his paternal Aunt Tatiana Alexandrovna Ergolskaya—so "peaceful, sweet, [...] and loving," as he later recalled—who served as a surrogate mother.[30] Likewise, Tolstoy's father, Nikolai Ilych, about whom the artist wrote less than his mother, died suddenly before his youngest son's eighth birthday.[31] Thus, in effect, his orphancy constituted a serious psychological conflict to which the poet would frequently return through the "living past" of transference, both as a bottomless well of suffering, and as an inspiration for his highest ideals and art.[32] Historically speaking, we speculate that Tolstoy took up a psychoutopian "Redeemer phantasy" in committing himself to ascetic militancy, political rationalism, and horizontal collectivism, with the aim of healing the fragmentation rending Russian society and impelling a new age: namely, to overcome the seventeenth-century schism between the Orthodox Church and Old Believers, which echoed the eleventh-century split between the Roman Catholic and Eastern Orthodox Churches, together with Tsar Peter Romanov's despotic self-assertion.[33]

Even so, seeking to be the Resident in tune with the authentic collective, Tolstoy was a Stranger and a horizontal individualist who prioritized autonomy and justice over the conventions of his in-group.[34] In particular, the defiant Lev Nikolaevich appears to have felt an intense need to undo the damage wrought by his ancestor Peter Andreevich Tolstoy (1645–1729), who had served as Tsar Peter I's envoy to the self-exiled heir, Prince Alexis Petrovich Romanov (1690–1718). The *tsarevich* Alexei had rejected the Tsar's methods. Yet Peter Andreevich succeeded in convincing him to return to Imperial Russia, where he was duly murdered on his self-aggrandizing father's orders.[35] In contrast, Tolstoy's resignation from his commission as an artillery officer conveyed his loyalty to Jesus the Nazarene, who momentously repudiates Satan's temptation of sovereignty over humanity in the desert by proclaiming that we are called to serve the Kingdom of God instead.[36] The artist's focus on the Old Believer sect, the community from which hailed the pioneering poet Mikhail Alekseevich Kuzmin (1872–1936)—author of the modern world's first gay memoir—evinces Tolstoy's political *and* psychosexual interest in anarchism and revolutionary Populism.[37] Indeed, Lev Nikolaevich must have found the erotic dissidence and asceticism of non-conformist communities fascinating, for *Khlysty* ("flagellants") and *Skoptsy* ("castrators") reportedly practiced homosexuality and bisexuality openly, while *Postniki* ("fasters") would ritualistically fast, and *Skotpsy* would observe sexual abstinence and/or mutilate themselves.[38]

From the Loss of Maternal Love to Proselytizing the Kingdom of God

In turn working through the maternal love he missed, affirming motherly archetypes and the theory of primordial matriarchal communism, and lending credence to the philosopher John Dewey's belief that "'associational' or 'communal' behavior constitutes a basic feature of all things," Tolstoy retrospectively declared that he had felt the happiest in life on three occasions. This was when he was teaching at the rural peasant schools he had first founded at his Yasnaya Polyana estate in 1849, composing the *ABC* (Азбука, 1872/1875), and collaborating philanthropically with Countess Tolstaya and their daughters Tanya and Masha to provide famine relief to peasants in the Tula and Ryazan regions between 1891 and 1893.[39]

Integrating psychology, anthropology, history, Enlightenment philosophy, Eastern-Christian and Asian theology, and robust popular traditions, Count Tolstoy's extensive life-work seeks to establish a legacy of love, based on the ideal of (allo) maternal affection provided during infancy and early childhood, that will persist beyond the grave.[40] From this starting point follow his efforts to uncover and fight for what he calls the Kingdom of God, which is not to be deferred to any afterlife, but rather, to be realized through generations of struggle to combat finitude by creating a global utopia. In the words of the Eastern-Christian existentialist Berdyaev, who was expelled from the Soviet Union on the so-called "philosopher's ship" in 1922, rather than the cataphatic theology which celebrates, the Kingdom of God is intimately connected with the negativity of apophatic theology.[41]

> There is absolute truth in anarchism and it is to be seen in its attitude to the sovereignty of the state and to every form of state absolutism. It is an exposure of the wrongness of despotic centralization [...]. The religious truth of anarchism consists in this, that power over man [*sic*] is bound up with sin and evil, that a state of perfection is a state where there is no power of man over man [or woman], that is to say, anarchy. The Kingdom of God is freedom and the absence of such power [...]. The Kingdom of God is anarchy.[42]

Likewise, Tolstoy wrote the following in his diary in May 1890:

> I've been thinking all this time [...]. The anarchists are right about everything—the rejection of what exists and the assertion that anything worse than the oppression of authority, with its existing rights, would be impossible in the absence of that authority.[43]

For the artist, the point of life is to "assist in the creation of the Kingdom of God."[44] He avows self-help, self-perfection, self-determination (разумение), and fusion, or unity with others, toward this end.[45] In his fiction, Count Tolstoy uses defamiliarizing, deprovincializing, and estranging effects to call into question dominant social institutions, hegemonic lies, and learned helplessness, as through emblematic *Weltanschaaungkriegen*, or wars over worldviews.[46] His art poses questions, expresses truths, and suggests proposals through an iconic "theology in colors" that helps us both to "discern what is good and what is bad," and "to help the former and resist the latter."[47] His writings represent expressive therapy, or "social daydreaming," that explores "imagined solutions to real life problems" at the personal, interpersonal, and societal levels.[48] Politically, Lev Nikolaevich combines his reading of the German idealist Immanuel Kant (1724–1804) with the revolutionary Populism of his compatriots to champion an anarcho-Populist vision that seeks to overthrow the Church, State, and landlord class. He aimed to transform the condition of the *Narod* by means of "the establishment of social rights, redistributive policies, and self-government institutions," utilizing a blend of respect for popular institutions and customs with Enlightenment philosophy.[49] The "prophetic humanism" of Tolstoyan anarcho-Populism thus naturally appealed to conscious intellectuals and progressive peasants who sought "communit[ies] of cooperative subjects" in late Imperial and early post-revolutionary Russia.[50]

Arguably, Tolstoyans and insurgent *Narodniki* alike resembled subversive monastic orders in their cross-class organizing, embodying the Christian concept of *kenosis*, or renunciation, regarding past and future, as these activists knew they would face persecution and martyrdom for their organizing efforts.[51] Over a thousand radical young Russians suffered imprisonment and torment by the Tsarist State for having "gone to the people" in the 1870s, aiming to share their plight and exhort them to revolt and level society, while hundreds of Tolstoyans were killed by Lenin and Stalin's regimes.[52] Instead of the reactionary suicide of a living death serving authority, Populist and Tolstoyan youth, mirroring Jesus and Lev Nikolaevich himself, were prepared for revolutionary suicide: to serve and die for the People, as Huey P. Newton (1942–1989), co-founder of the Black Panther Party, would theorize in the 1970s.[53]

Despite greatly sympathizing with and advancing anarchism and human freedom, while grievously contradicting both causes through his misogyny, Tolstoy was not per se an organizer like his revolutionary compatriots Herzen, Bakunin, Nikolai Chaikovsky, Peter Kropotkin, Vera Zasulich, or Sofia Perovskaya. Perhaps this is all for the better, in the interest of avoiding the masochistic compulsion to repeat prior defeats and identify with the "Big" or "Dominant" Other.[54] Remarkably in this sense, Tolstoy's distant cousin, General Sergei Grigorievich Volkonsky (1788–1865), a revolutionary Decembrist leader, veteran of the war of 1812, and "peasant-prince," did not adequately prepare for the insurrection that his fellow constitutionalist and socialist mutineers had planned during Nicholas I's accession to power in December 1825. Crucially, he had avoided organizing with the rank-and-file soldiers.[55] Likewise, one could argue that the Paris Commune of March–May 1871 was doomed by its Central Committee's reluctance to use the Communards' initial overwhelming military advantage to march on the Versaillais government, which would soon thereafter crush them.[56] In his poem "The Insect," Turgenev emblematizes such defeatism by considering how a literary salon of idealists is disturbed by the sudden appearance of a bug—yet, no one acts to defend the collective against the insect, which promptly starts killing them.[57]

Nevertheless, we must not reduce Tolstoy to his erstwhile friend's caricature. Rather, let us look to Lev Nikolaevich's "writings, his personal example, and the stimulus and inspiration he gave," as a military officer who resigned his post, a Rousseauvist teacher of peasant children, a world-renowned novelist who renounced his previous art-work (искусство) as artificial (искусственное), and a wealthy landowning aristocrat who, imperfectly observing his wish to divest himself of his property through class suicide, became "a ploughman, a mower, a sower, a woodsman, a stovebuilder, a carpenter and a bootmaker" late in life.[58] As an atypical proprietor, Count Tolstoy decided to work the land he owned together with the peasants, to become vegetarian, and to adopt a simple manner of living.[59] Be that as it may, although he personally renounced his property late in life, swore off writing, and performed manual labor in the fields, Lev Nikolaevich paradoxically continued "liv[ing] off his property and writ [ing] literary works" until his final flight from home in October 1910.[60]

From Dionysianism to Asceticism

Like most others, Tolstoy's life provides evidence for the idea that the human being is a "freak of nature," whose sexuality is "polymorphously perverse."[61] Like

Frankenstein's Creature, as imagined by Mary Shelley (1797–1851), the subject is akin to a monster that conveys our deepest fears and desires.[62] We find ourselves "thrown" into a world not of our own choosing, confronting life and death. How we respond to this interplay of Eros and Thanatos, libido and *mortido*, shapes our character. In the case of that "strange being" Lev Nikolaevich, it is evident that almost "[e]verything [he] did in his life he did with intensity."[63] His biographer Richard F. Gustafson comments: "Few men, and especially men of such noble position and privilege as Count Tolstoy, have lived life thus on the brink" of existential crisis and suicide.[64] His friend Vasily P. Botkin (1812–1869), in reacting to a characteristic rift that had opened in the early 1860s between Tolstoy and Turgenev, writes that he "believe[s] that in reality Tolstoy has a passionately loving soul [...]. [But] his mind is in a chaos [...]. His soul burns with unquenchable thirst."[65]

Although his wife Countess Tolstaya found some of his ideas attractive, she believed that the prospects of their realization were often spoiled by her husband's recurrent lack of focus.[66] Her father, Dr. Andrei Behrs, who initially opposed the count's marriage proposal, similarly and knowingly observed that Tolstoy was "skilled at writing and talking, but not [...] when it came to practical things."[67] As if illustrating their point, a brick hut that Lev Nikolaevich, his daughters Tanya and Masha, and the painter Nikolai Gay had collectively built in 1885 for a widow at Yasnaya Polyana soon collapsed.[68] In psychoanalytic and psychiatric terms, such symptoms are consistent with intense sublimation, post-traumatic stress disorder, bipolar disorder, and the conversion of sexual frustration into depressive anxiety.[69]

Notably, in the wake of one of the most significant turning points of his life, after finishing *Anna Karenina* (1875–1877), Tolstoy began to idealize a monastic type of Christian social life.[70] Along these lines, he outlined what he considered the six cardinal sins perpetuating our individual and collective separation: "self-indulgence, sloth, acquisitiveness, love of power, lechery, and intoxication."[71] Evidently, the artist himself was steeped in all of these ostensible sins in his youth, and some—especially sexual temptation from potential male *and* female partners—continued to haunt him after his conversion to Christian asceticism, despite his conscious experiments in self-denial. In truth, Tolstoy's lifelong tormented relationship with sexuality is reminiscent of the struggles of Peter Ilych Tchaikovsky (1840–1893), the esteemed gay Russo-Ukrainian composer who died from cholera rather than suicide, as some have argued, in keeping with negative tropes about the suffering spiritual homosexual.[72]

Queer Tolstoy

Queer Tolstoy challenges the Russian State's aggressive homonegativity, the historians of Russia who re-entrench the dominant sex/gender system by overlooking erotic dissent in the country, the LGBTQ+ historians who ignore same-sex love in the region, and the overall heterosexist presumption that queer people should remain invisible.[73] The aim is to fulfill the Slavist Simon Karlinsky's wish, that a "special study [...] undoubtedly be written one day" about the "theme of homosexuality in the life of Leo Tolstoy."[74] In this study, seeking to contribute to the "radical" and "progressive" analysis of the "politics of sexuality," we argue that the Christian-anarchist and anarcho-Populist ideals guiding Lev Nikolaevich's art have profoundly queer psychosexual dimensions, reflecting the intimate link between interpersonal relationships and political philosophies.[75] As a reflective elder, in 1903, Tolstoy declared to his biographer Pavel Biryukov that he "owe[d] the brightest time in [his] life not to the love of woman but to love of people [...]."[76] Likewise, in his diary, the 23 year old Lev Nikolaevich confesses, "*I have never been in love with women* [...]. I have very often been in love with men."[77]

Tolstoy's admission of his gay impulses here may help to shed a new light on his art and politics, tying together his intellect, his altruism, and his infantile and mature identification with his mother.[78] Lev Nikolaevich's own anarchist desire to merge with the *Narod* and level feudalism by observing the kenotic "law of descent" involving voluntary subordination and joy in residence with the marginalized is conveyed by the artist's intense eroticization of male "peasant-Kantians."[79] The physician-writer Anton Chekhov (1860–1904), Tolstoy's friend, agrees with the count that war and judgment are social evils, but he clarifies that he could not follow his mentor's call to wear traditional peasant shoes and "sleep on the stove *with the worker and his wife*."[80] Along similar lines, Alan Forrest stops just short of explicitly identifying Tolstoy's queer yearnings in his remarks on how the author "admired the dash and daring of soldiers in battle, the strength and physical prowess that were the very essence of youth," and incorporated a "strong autobiographical aspect to [...] the feelings he attributed to his characters."[81]

In the groundbreaking 1948 article "Come Back to the Raft Ag'in, Huck Honey!" the literary critic Leslie Fiedler (1917–2003) places interracial homoerotic relationships among men and boys front and center within the canon of American literature. For this reason, the "Fiedler thesis" is highly relevant to Lev Nikolaevich's revolutionary-romantic idealization of "enlightened" officers bonding with "dark" serf-soldiers or indigenous warriors to annihilate caste, capital, and empire.[82] Fiedler finds the novels of James Fenimore Cooper, Nathaniel Hawthorne, Herman Melville, Mark Twain, Ernest Hemingway, and Henry James to have idealized "chaste male love as the ultimate emotional experience" and endorsed the subversive "sacred marriage of males."[83] By means of engaging with these same-sex literary relationships, both authors and audiences access the "childish, impossible [*sic*] dream" of homoerotic union and abolition of racial and class inequalities.[84] Similarly, Tolstoy's "patrician gayness" marries the gay love that arouses and ascends with the compassionate or kenotic love that descends.[85] In turn, the intersection of queerness and anarchism in Count Tolstoy's life and art confirms Amia Srinivasan's argument in *The Right to Sex: Feminism in the Twenty-First Century* (2021) that sexual desire is political and intimately related to the struggle against injustice.[86]

Politically speaking, same-sex union has plenty of subversive potential: as the infamous political consultant Niccolò Machiavelli (1469–1527), the Florentine rulers of early capitalist modernity, and late nineteenth-century French medical forensic writers were all too aware, cross-class mingling could threaten bourgeois and State authority. Chitty explains how, in the cities, armies, and navies of early-modern Europe, "interclass sexual contact" among men imparted resistance to bourgeois "sexual hegemony," hence threatening "social anarchy."[87] In the same vein, the French Trotskyist-turned-anarcho-syndicalist Daniel Guérin (1904–1988) would profess that cross-class gay bonding could promote revolutionary consciousness.[88] In a lyrical scene atop Moscow's Sparrow Hills in 1826, the noble teenage rebels Alexander Herzen and Nikolai Ogarëv (1813–1877), devastated by the Tsar's execution of most of the Decembrist leadership, embraced and swore to give their lives to struggling against "that throne, [...] that altar, [and] those cannon."[89]

Though the above scene in early nineteenth-century Moscow refers to the feudal, proto-capitalist world, several queer theorists have proposed a dialectical relationship between the emergence of global capitalism and the development of gay identities in historical modernity. On this account, young men, rent from their traditional peasant surroundings, jointly suffered abuses *and* experienced joys as workers, soldiers, and sailors in sex-segregated settings, leading to the emergence of gay love "at sea" and "on land."[90] This was true of the Mediterranean port-cities of Venice, Genoa, Florence, Barcelona, and Cairo, among others, as of such "caravan cities" as Petra and Kandahar.[91] Along similar lines, historian John D'Emilio traces the Stonewall uprising of 1969 in part to "same-sex intimacies enjoyed by soldiers in World War II."[92] A similar analysis might be made of the Decembrist mutineers of 1825; of the Red sailors who in 1921 declared the Kronstadt Commune in defiance of the Bolshevik autocracy; or of the peasant anarchists who fought in the Revolutionary Insurgent Army of Ukraine, led by the anarchist Nestor Makhno (1888–1934).

We know that lesbian and bisexual women played important roles in Ireland's ill-fated 1916 Easter Rising, a forerunner of the Irish Revolution against British rule.[93] During the 1871 Paris Commune, women analogously developed revolutionary "bonds of sisterhood" through a combination of friendship and fellow-feeling. Inspired by an at least sublimated lesbianism, they cared for the wounded and defended the communal experiment from its external Prussian and Versaillais enemies, and its internal misogynist foes, alike.[94] As of this writing, the Ukrainian LGBTQ+ community and anarchist collectives are resisting Russia's full-scale assault on the country, both by coordinating supplies and tending to the injured, and by fighting the invaders directly.[95]

Attesting to the radical power of Eros, Boris Pasternak's titular character from *Doctor Zhivago* (1957), a humanistic physician and poet, explains that in Tolstoyanism he has found "the dream of a dignified existence, which [had] filled my adolescence." In parallel, his foil Strelnikov perceptively notes that the causes of socialism and revolution have been impelled by "selfless young men mount[ing] the barricades" and risking their lives.[96] Indeed, the political cultures of both the Russian intelligentsia and the Soviet State encouraged sublimated devotion for the archetype of the male freedom fighter and revolutionary martyr, in keeping with such models as the Sacred Band of Thebes, a fearsome fighting unit from classical Greece that was comprised of 150 male warrior couples.[97] In parallel, virility and the male and female nude permeated the art—and therefore, psychical reality—of twentieth-century Spanish anarcho-syndicalists.[98]

Considering the intimate associations between anarchism and free love, Freud's point that "the repressed is a foreign territory," and the "exotic becomes erotic" theory of sexuality, we speculate that Tolstoy had a youthful gay interest in the Chechen Sado Miserbiyev during his time in the Eastern Caucasus, and that this bond both influenced and reflected his burgeoning cosmopolitan internationalism.[99] In Chechnya, on the edge of what the British Orientalist explorer Richard Burton (1821–1890) termed the "Sotadic Zone"—which refers to a proposed erotic social geography found in the Mediterranean region, Central and East Asia, and among the indigenous peoples of the Americas, where homosexuality, pederasty, and gender fluidity are practiced and observed more openly, so the argument goes, than in northern Europe—Lev Nikolaevich feels liberated to explore his politics and sexuality.[100] In fact, the only time Tolstoy mentions Sado in his diary is within the context of confessing to hyper-sexual mania for women *and* men in Transcaucasia.[101] Likewise, many English, French, and Russian explorers and military officers wrote romantically about the Arab, Circassian, and Afghan men they met, even those they were ordered to fight and kill.[102] Along similar lines, Joseph Massad cites the example of André Gide's novel *L'immoraliste* (1902) as a "prominent example of the new Western fiction of homosexual self-discovery in the Orient."[103] We believe that *The Cossacks* could be read as a less overt, earlier entry in the same genre (see Chapter 4 below).

In light of the humanistic and anti-authoritarian dimensions of Tolstoyan art, the weight placed by the artist on the rationalist concept of self-determination (разумение) can be fruitfully compared with the intimate relationship that exists between Malcolm X's transgressive racial politics and his erotic non-conformism.[104] In other words, alongside Malcolm X (1925–1965), who was persecuted and even martyred by the State—in his case, by the Federal Bureau of Investigation (FBI) and New York Police Department (NYPD)—Tolstoy was a kindred spirit to Virginia Woolf (1882–1941), who also "drew emotional sustenance from her intense [same-sex] relationships," and in her literature likewise centers the individual's search for meaning and identification.[105] With his closest male friends, Lev Nikolaevich sought what the poet Alexander Pushkin (1799–1837), Tolstoy's third cousin once removed, calls in Orientalist fashion the "Imitation of the Arabic": namely, the sharing of a "sole insurgent fire" and "boundless brotherhood."[106]

Russian and Ukrainian LGBTQ+ History and the International Homosexual Conspiracy

Now, let us turn to the numerous antecedents for non-traditional sexualities in Russian and Ukrainian history. The medieval Rus' *Legend of Boris and Gleb* features a same-sex couple, Boris and George, who are killed together with Boris' half-brother Gleb, once the power-hungry Sviatoslav the Accursed (c. 978–1019) decides to eliminate them as rivals. In turn, this tragedy echoes the tyrannical Hippias' execution of the Athenian rebel-couple Harmodius and Aristogeiton, following their assassination of the ruler's despotic brother, Hipparchus, in 514 BCE.[107] Likewise, the *Life of*

St. Moses the Hungarian features a male slave, brother of the martyred George, who is mutilated by his owner Predslava, a daughter of Great Prince Vladimir I (r. 980–1015), over his preference for male partners and attendant lack of interest in a conventional marriage. Ultimately, Moses retires to a monastery—as Tolstoy will dramatically seek to do, at life's end. For his part, Grand Prince Vasili II of Moscow (r. 1505–1533), sire to Tsar Ivan IV ("the Terrible"), was nearly exclusively homosexual, and Tsar Peter I was reportedly bisexual. Foreign and domestic observers alike would remark on the open male homosexuality practiced among all social classes, but especially the peasantry, during the Muscovite period which predated the rise of the Romanov Tsarist dynasty.[108]

Many historians find the Russian Orthodox Church to have been relatively less heterosexist, compared to the Roman Catholic Church, at least prior to the Russian Revolution. Be that as it may, Eastern Orthodoxy struggled long to suppress pagan gay practices, including orgies, and Peter I banned same-sex relations in the armed forces in 1716, on the advice of his German advisers. The ban on sodomy, imposed in the interest of "mental or sexual hygiene," followed the example set by the European "military revolution" of the sixteenth and seventeenth centuries—and anticipated Stalin's reimposition of this ban, beginning in 1933, after his predecessors had suspended it after seizing power. Stalin recriminalized homosexuality using the pretext of protecting young soldiers, sailors, students, and Party members from would-be male seducers, foreign agents, and/or seditionists. In parallel, his predecessor Vladimir Lenin considered psychoanalysis, homosexuality, and free love to be bourgeois.[109] However, as Tolstoy's *War and Peace* clarifies, spontaneous same-sex attachment played a crucial role in the early nineteenth-century Russian military struggle against the *Grand Armée* led by Napoleon Bonaparte.

Although Nicholas I would promulgate a new criminal code extending the ban on homosexual relations to civilians in 1835, even the Grand Duke Constantin Romanov (1858–1915), cousin to Nicholas II, could not resist indulging at the bathhouses of St. Petersburg. Remarkably, Vladimir D. Nabokov (1870–1922), father of the renowned poet and novelist of the same name, openly avowed the decriminalization of same-sex relations in Imperial Russia. Karlinsky discloses that there were "at least seven gay grand dukes"—meaning uncles, nephews, or cousins, related to Tsars Alexander III and Nicholas II.[110]

The truth is that several well-known Russian and Ukrainian artists were LGBTQ+, such as the composer Peter Tchaikovsky, the novelist Nikolai Gogol (1809–1852), the feminist editor Anna Yevreinova (1844–1919), the Symbolist poet Polyxena Soloviova (1867–1924), the actress Alla Nazimova (1879–1945), the bohemian Jewish poet Sofia Parnok (1885–1933), the novelist Lidia Zinovieva-Annibal (1866–1907), the ballet impresario Sergei Diaghilev (1872–1929), and the filmmaker Sergei Eisenstein (1898–1948), among others.[111] The Polish ballet dancer Vaslav Nijinsky (c. 1890–1950) was also an erotic and gender non-conformist, and recently unearthed homoerotic love letters penned by Frederic Chopin (1810–1849) suggest the Polish composer enjoyed the company of other men, too.[112] Moreover, the Georgian Iosef Zhughashvili (1878–1953), who would become the despot Stalin, was bisexual with repressed homosexual tendencies.[113] For this reason, he resented the camp evident in Eisenstein's *Ivan the Terrible* (1944), a historical figure with whom he identified. Accordingly, the film's second part, despite finishing production in 1946, would only be released in 1958, over five years after Stalin's death.[114]

Then again, despite the patriarchal and homonegative social imaginaries promoted by Tsarism, Victorianism, and Bolshevism alike, Eros can never be totally denied, repressed, or contained.[115] In fact, during the carnival-esque ethos of the February 1917 Revolution, civilian and military protesters spontaneously embraced and kissed each other on the streets of St. Petersburg, and sex workers propositioned clients with newfound appeals to fraternity.[116] Pasternak's depiction of the final meeting between Strelnikov and the titular character of *Doctor Zhivago* (1957) is highly homoerotic, full of phallic imagery, a sense of reunion, and even a blending of Zhivago together with Strelnikov's wife, Larissa Antipova—an homage, perhaps, to Tolstoy's *The Cossacks* (1863; see Chapter 4 below).[117]

On the one hand, the authenticity of such queer relations across fundamental political differences imparts Pasternak and Tolstoy's common interest in male comrades who fight jointly for the Reclusian "Universal Republic."[118] On the other, the emblematic confrontations between Zhivago and Strelnikov replay the political and sexual tensions between the revolutionary-humanist figure of Jesus the Liberator and the bureaucratic Grand Inquisitor.[119] In *The Brothers Karamazov* (1880), Dostoevsky portrays the Grand Inquisitor interrogating Jesus upon his mythical return to Earth. This supreme cleric admits to his enthrallment to the lure of sovereignty and the putatively "powerful and intelligent spirit" of Satan, even as he deceives humanity through the active denial of its freedom, all the while claiming to rule in his teacher's name.[120]

Based on the intense bonds forged while fighting in the First Cavalry Army during the Russian Civil War, up to two thousand partisans communed together in the Red Lighthouse of the Volga River basin in the 1920s.[121] In *Red Cavalry* (1926), the Russian-Jewish journalist Isaac Babel's (1894–1940) fictionalized account of time embedded with this same army during the Polish-Soviet War (1919–1921), the author describes his protagonist's admiration for the "vigorous and dashing" Cossack Dyakov, chief of the Remount Service. Babel adds that, with the young shepherd and celebrated veteran known as "Sashka the Christ," his *alter ego* had "greeted the morning light and accompanied the setting sun quite often by now."[122] According to Lee Siegel, "Babel turns the he-man Cossacks into sexually repressed men who sublimate their [gay] desire[s] [...] into acts of atrocity."[123]

Despite formal decriminalization, the Communists arrested various sailors in 1921 for their supposed participation in pederastic sex parties in Petrograd.[124] Ivan Yermolaev, a camp sailor from the Red (or revolutionary) Fleet, was a hairdresser, syndicalist, poet, and "literary man" who took up "peaceful" civil engineering after release from imprisonment in 1924, secondary to his participation in the Kronstadt Commune of 1921.[125] The anarcha-feminist Emma Goldman, praised for her visionary "defense of homosexual love before the general public" in the US, had at least one lesbian relationship in life.[126] Now, we should view Tolstoy as an integral member of the long-lived International Homosexual Conspiracy, which advocates for same-sex union while agitating for a "new and better society."[127]

However, reflecting the intimate link between trauma and taboo that compels a dampening of one's erotic self-expression, out of fear of alienating one's family or society, Count Tolstoy was in reality a semi-closeted case.[128] Indeed, the "Tolstoy family secret" persisted until the Russian Freudian Vasily Rozanov (1856–1919) divulged the poet's queerness, based on conversations with the Ukrainian Itzhak Feinermann (1864–1925), one of the artist's confidants.[129] According to Tolstoy's close friend, Marya Alexandrovna Schmidt, "Lev Nikolaevich was very fond of [Feinermann]": "it used to be [that] he was lying on the grass, disheveled, his black shirt tucked into his pants, and Lev Nikolaevich was sitting nearby," admiring him.[130] At the same time, the count was not "openly and defiantly gay," as the historian Dan Healey characterizes his fellow noble from the next generation, Mikhail Alekseevich Kuzmin, as being. Kuzmin wrote *Wings* (1906), the "first modern coming-out story with a happy ending in any language." This courageous individual only escaped Stalin's executioners due to his succumbing to pneumonia in 1936.[131] The NKVD arrested and tortured his partner, Yuri Yurkun, for seven months in 1938, before summarily executing him.[132]

By contrast, having married Sofia Andreevna Behrs in 1862 and siring 13 children with her (eight of whom survived to adulthood), Lev Nikolaevich Tolstoy sublimated his homoerotic feelings through the heavy use of camp and the integration of emblematic male-bonding experiences as counter-symbols in his literary works. He also did so by forming homophilic bonds with other men, whether they would be his junior or senior partners.[133] In the words of Nina Nikitina, senior researcher at the Yasnaya Polyana estate, "Tolstoy's intimate space had blurred boundaries," and his hypersexual "psychophysics" had "androgynous" dimensions.[134] Freud might have said that he conveyed "psychical hermaphroditism."[135] In a March 2020 interview, Russian journalist Nikolai Uskov likewise recognized that Tolstoy had "constantly struggled with his homosexuality"—though not without adding the requisite nod to the Putin regime's extreme homonegativity.[136] (In a similar context, during a September 2013 television interview, President Putin quipped that Tchaikovsky's queerness was "not the reason we love him."[137])

Therefore, rather than strictly platonic or homosocial, non-genital attachments, Tolstoy evidently felt emotional and sexual attraction for other men. He "read love signs all the time and was in their power."[138]

Queer Tolstoyan Eroticism

In *Childhood* (1852), his first book, Tolstoy recalls how he was smitten by Sergius Ivanin, "whose striking good looks had captivated me from the first, and I felt an irresistible attraction towards him. Only to see him filled me with pleasure [...]. Awake or asleep, I was forever dreaming of him." Nevertheless, he tells no one about his first love then—not even Sergius. Ultimately, Levochka laments his failure to express his attraction to Serëzha, and so open the possibility for it to be reciprocated. In his anguish, Tolstoy juxtaposes free love to social conventions of hyper-masculinity, heteronormativity, and self-denial: "I deprived myself of the pure delight of a fresh, childish instinct for the absurd purpose of trying to resemble grown-up [straight] people."[139] Repeating similar patterns, in a February 1849 letter to his brother Sergei, the youth complains that, in St. Petersburg, "one cannot find a man with whom one could lead an aimless life [...]."[140] For his youthful friend Gautier, who had inherited his father's bookshop in Moscow, Tolstoy reports "be [ing] thrown into a fever when he entered the room." Likewise, for Dmitri Dyakov, whom he had met in Kazan as a young man, Lev Nikolaevich recalls one night desiring to "kiss him and cry." Nevertheless, he confesses, "[m]y love for Islavin ruined for me the whole 8 months of my life in St. Petersburg."[141] This was so, not only because of the unsatisfying nature of the bond in question, but also because others noticed and shunned him for his supposedly deviant attachment.[142]

Sexologists must "often rely on inference, given the lacunae left by discretion and erasure compelled by social stigma," discretion, taboo, and history's "blank spots." Despite the (hetero)sexualization of life in the post-Soviet context, this dynamic holds true, especially within contexts as intensely homophobic as hegemonic Russian culture, which has lent its support to the enduring criminalization of, and incitement against, the LGBTQ+ community, at least since Soviet times.[143] That being said, the evidence from Tolstoy's private diaries and letters is confessional and conclusive, emerging chronologically during Erik Erikson's fifth stage of psychosocial development, when the developing adolescent or young adult struggles with identity vs. role confusion. The tantalizing nature of Tolstoy's literary relationships with Islavin and Ivanin—the latter character, having been based on his childhood attachment to General Alexander I. Musin-Pushkin (1827–1903), with whom the future artist liked to "play soldier"—is evidently reproduced in the epic *War and Peace*. This can be seen particularly in Prince Andrei's brief erotic approximation with Captain Tushin, as in Count Rostov's masochistic desire to serve the Tsar.[144]

In this vein, in the autobiographical short story "Father Sergius," written in the 1890s and only published posthumously, the artist declares that his *alter ego* Kasatsky, a promising military officer, is "seized by the same rapture" upon seeing the "tall erect figure" of the Tsar that "he experienced later on when he met the woman he loved."[145] Undoubtedly, in his art, Lev Nikolaevich often daydreams of being subordinated to a dominant Other, reflecting signs of a desired "passive homosexual phantasy." While conveying the author's desire for union with a strong man, this recurrent theme could also be read as an ascetic warning about what his follower, the Russo-Soviet philosopher Simon L. Frank (1877–1950), would term a "mass hypnosis resulting from a submission to power."[146] It simultaneously conveys the concept of Eros as creator *and* destroyer.[147]

Perhaps reflecting the imprint of intimacy with his mother, the influence from his aunts, and his resulting immersion in "[f]eminine imagery" in early life, the young Lev embraced an ethics of care and non-violence, and he rejected Oedipal ideas of gender polarity and normative sexuality. As a consequence, Tolstoy's gay attachments were not fleeting but enduring, manifesting the "longing for brotherhood which characterized him from childhood to old age."[148] Though the writer admits as a young adult that he "experiences this feeling" more rarely and less passionately than before, it nonetheless persisted then, and long thereafter, echoing childhood experiences.[149]

For instance, with his siblings as a young boy, Levochka played an "Ant-Brother" game that involved hiding from the world and cuddling together in the dark.[150] According to Nikitina, this was "Tolstoy's first, timid, and poetic erotic experience."[151] Five years after recording his love for Dyakov in his diary, he expresses jealousy and regret, "think[ing] of *the happiness that might have been mine* and which has fallen to the share of that excellent fellow [Princess] A. Obolensk[aya]."[152] Whereas female characters in his early literary works are "all emblematic residents who embody and reveal the way to divine love," in his later, short fiction, "these female figures are replaced by male peasants who serve the same function [...]."[153]

According to his biographer Andrei Zorin, Count Tolstoy's youthful heterosexual liaisons mostly involved female sex workers, "servants, peasants, [and Roma] and Cossacks girls," such that his encounter with Sofia Andreevna Behrs represented "the first time in his life" that "he felt a strong erotic attraction to a woman of his own social standing."[154] However, Countess Tolstaya will indirectly explore her suspicions about her husband's bisexuality in her short story "Songs Without Words," written in the early 1890s as a critical response to Tolstoy's "Kreutzer Sonata" (1889), which normalizes and even idealizes femicide. At the conclusion of "Songs Without Words," Sofia Andreevna's ego-persona (or *alter ego*) suffers in a mental ward, as her object of affection, an emotionally unavailable artist with autistic characteristics, plans to travel abroad with his junior male partner.[155] In fact, in his encounters with the composer Sergei Ivanovich Taneev (1856–1915), a student of Tchaikovsky and confidant to the countess, Lev Nikolaevich confronted a double of sorts: a queer artist interested in music and Esperanto, the international language that had been invented by the Pole L. L. Zamenhof (1859–1917) in the hopes of encouraging world peace.

Ironically, just as Sofia Andreevna attached to Taneev amid the grief of their son Ivan's death in 1895, so Tolstoy grew close with his enthusiastic follower, Vladimir Grigorievich Chertkov (1854–1936), a wealthy proprietor and former military officer whom he met in 1883. Vladimir Grigorievich was childhood friends with Tsar Alexander III (r. 1881–1894), who would exchange visits to the Chertkov family mansion in Petersburg for invitations to the Romanov palace in Crimea—on land expropriated from the indigenous Tatars. Rumor even had it that Chertkov was Alexander II's son, born out of wedlock.[156] Tolstoy and Chertkov would collaborate closely until his death. Concretely, this partnership resulted in the founding in 1885 of "The Intermediary" (Посредник) publishing house, established on non-profit grounds with the allowance given Chertkov by his mother, Elizaveta Ivanovna, toward the end of distributing affordable, straightforward, and quality readings for literate peasants and workers.[157] Within four years of its founding, the tremendously successful Intermediary had sold 12 million volumes.[158]

Indeed, the significance of this relationship comes through in Feinermann's 1912 film, *The Departure of a Grand Old Man.* As well, Tolstoy's personal physician Dushan Makovitsky (1866–1921) and daughter Alexandra (1884–1979) respectively observed how "overjoyed" or "buoyant" the man would become at receiving either word or visit from Chertkov, and the writer explicitly told his junior would-be partner in an 1884 letter how much he loved him and would like to live with him. Picking up on this love-bond, Countess Tolstaya would openly accuse Chertkov and her husband of having a gay affair.[159] After his death, Sofia Andreevna came to realize that her partner had "preferred Chertkov at the end of his life." She reports visiting his grave to plead for forgiveness for having been "unable to make him happier at the end of his life" by accepting Chertkov as his true beloved.[160]

As with studies on Malcolm X's erotic life, the argument of *Queer Tolstoy* is not meant to deny the artist's heterosexual attachments, experiences, or fantasies. These might include his reported loss of virginity with a female sex worker at a brothel to which his elder brothers Nikolai and Sergei had brought him at age 14, his platonic attachment to Zinaida Molostvova in Kazan, the hyper-sexual phases of his marriage with Sofia Andreevna, and the emblematic significance of Natasha's dance in *War and Peace*, through which the countess revitalizes herself after a loss of love and self-love.[161] Rather, the novelty of our approach is to uncover overt and sublimated bisexual queerness in Tolstoy's life-experiences and literature, and to link the artist's erotic dissidence with his anarchist politics and anti-militarist ideal.

Arguably, Tolstoy's sexual debut at a brothel, though with a heterosexual object-choice, permitted a "safe" release of male homoeroticism, given that it was his brothers who put him up to it.[162] Moreover, Tolstoy dreamt repeatedly in his final year of life about a young, androgynous Tatar woman who had been his lover during his service in the Crimean War.[163] Through his literary art, which his brother Nikolai had inspired him to create, referring to a mythical "green stick" that would liberate humanity, Tolstoy served as an encyclopedic "injustice collector." He denounced the abuses of the powerful and sought to promote human unity across erotic and class lines, in an attempt to preserve self-esteem in the face of trauma, loss, and isolation.[164] By sublimating his libido, Tolstoy could dedicate himself to research, and by engaging in creative writing, he gave voice to his dreams and worries.[165] Thomas Newlin remarks on the link in Tolstoy's psychogeography between the phallic-utopian "green stick" which would encode human happiness, and his own self-concept as an artist and social critic.[166] In this sense, our "tempest-tossed soul" employed "preaching, anger, [and] indignation" not only to destabilize despotism, but also as a means of psychotherapy.[167]

A Brief History of Tolstoy's Homoerotic Life

Bruce Perry, author of *Malcolm: The Life of a Man who Changed Black America* (1991), finds that Malcolm X had "suggested ties with five homosexual counterparts" prior to his imprisonment and subsequent conversion to Islam.[168] In like fashion, we count at least 19 significant same-sex relationships over the course of Tolstoy's life. In parallel to the aforementioned figures of St. Moses and Don Quixote, the Russian artist's habitual desire to break radically away from his family, marriage, and upbringing, whether seen reflected in his journey as a young man to the Caucasus, or in his final flight from home in 1910, likely signaled deep sexual frustration.[169]

As a young boy, Lev Nikolaevich was impressed by the beauty and character of his renegade relative Fëdor Ivanovich Tolstoy (1782–1846), an officer within the elite Preobrazhensky Guards who had sailed around the globe on the warship *Nadezhda* ("Hope"). Perhaps unconsciously, the young Lev, "still enmeshed in feudal property relations," was excited by hearing Fëdor Ivanovich's stories and vicariously experiencing same-sex intimacy and intrigue on the high seas.[170] Lev Nikolaevich would base the character Fëdr Dolokhov in *War and Peace* on this "extraordinary, lawless, and attractive man," and fantasize about having a gay relationship enshrining comrade-love with him on at least one occasion: namely, in his depictions of the spontaneous infatuation of his adolescent *alter ego*, Petya Rostov. On the symbolic front, Petya joins Dolokhov on a daring mission to rescue their compatriots from imprisonment and execution by the retreating French, thus evincing an autonomous interest in homosexuality and liberation.[171]

The relationship between Lev and his childhood serf-companion Vanusha, who was effectively fettered to his master as the family moved from Moscow to Kazan in 1841, may have had homoerotic dimensions as well.[172] Now dubbed the "Third Capital of Russia," after Moscow and St. Petersburg, Kazan evinces "perhaps the clearest illustration of Russia's identity as a transcontinental, multiethnic country straddling both Europe and Asia."[173] As if channeling Eros, during his visit to Kazan in 1862 en route to Siberia to serve with the Amur Cossack Army, the future anarcho-communist Peter Kropotkin (1842–1921) remarked on the "pretty" Tatar boys and "pleasant faces" of men he encountered in the city.[174] In this light, during his stay there in his adolescence, Tolstoy presumably encountered the customary same-sex relations practiced among Muslims and Christians alike in Central Asia and the Caucasus at this time.[175] In a diary entry written in Tiflis (now Tbilisi, Georgia) in 1851, the disinhibited youth confesses to his frequent emotional and sexual attachments to other men, and lists nine comrades by name, most of them fellow university students, while mentioning "many others."[176]

Furthermore, Count Tolstoy viewed the robust serf Ufan as a muse for his kenotic, Populist dream of becoming a peasant, and even adopted the bonded agricultural worker's name as a verb expressing this ideal: to "ufanize."[177] His university friend Dmitri Dyakov, for whom he felt deep ecstasy, was one of the few friends who continued to visit Tolstoy after his wedding.[178] In Chechnya, the youth befriended the Russian-loyalist local Sado Miserbiyev, who became his *kunak*, or blood-brother. Sado may have inspired Lukashka's Dionysian character in *The Cossacks*, and served as model for the tragic minor character Sado in *Hadji Murat*.[179] Tolstoy wrote his own version of "A Prisoner of the Caucasus" (1872), based on a near-miss he experienced while riding ahead of Russian infantry alongside Sado (see Chapter 4 below).[180]

Besides these, the poet and officer Afanasy Fet (1820–1892) bought an estate close to Yasnaya Polyana in the 1850s to live near the artist. A reactionary *krepostnik* landlord who opposed the emancipation of the serfs, Fet expressed jealousy over Tolstoy's marriage to Sofia Andreevna. Despite their political disagreements, the pair would continue exchanging thinly veiled love letters for decades after 1862, the year of Tolstoy's wedding—thus proving Freud's point that, despite conscious heterosexual object-choice, "the homosexual tendencies are not [...] done away with or brought to a stop."[181] Likewise, the conservative historian Nikolai N. Strakhov, who never married, became "an ardent convert to Tolstoy's way of thinking and an eager assistant in all his enterprises."[182] With Peter I. Tchaikovsky, a fellow estranged artist, Tolstoy shared a platonic approximation. Both suffered similarly turbulent straight marriages, although Tchaikovsky's was more short-lived than Tolstoy's.[183] In reality, the post-revolutionary Bolshevik State viewed both men's art suspiciously: in 1923, Nadezhda Krupskaya (1869–1939), Lenin's partner, circulated an order to withdraw "counterrevolutionary and art-destructive literature" from municipal libraries. This forbidden list included all of Tolstoy, save for his novels.[184] Plus, Tchaikovsky's music was marginalized, for its melancholic tones were supposedly incompatible with global revolution.[185]

For Vasily Alexeev, a former militant organizer from the Chaikovsky Circle, the disowned son of a noble, and a principled revolutionary, Tolstoy developed a profound affection. Having hired Alexeev as a tutor for his children in 1877, the poet came to greatly admire his younger counterpart, with whom he shared intense political and personal goals. They even corresponded openly about their loving tenderness.[186] In similar fashion, en route to visit the Bakunins at their Priamukhino estate near Tver in the fall of 1881, Tolstoy impulsively deviated his journey to meet the acquaintance of the non-conformist peasant Vasily Siutayev upon first learning of him. Countess Tolstaya looks back on this encounter, noting the strong anti-depressant effect it had on her husband, inspiring him by example, and giving him the courage to proceed with his desired transition to ascetic renunciation.[187] Psychosexually, we presume that Tolstoy's improved mood upon his return from visiting with Siutayev was related to the blending of same-sex love and cooperative labor among Russian *muzhiki*, or male peasants.[188]

Equally importantly, the plant-based Russian mathematician V. K. Heins, otherwise known as William Frey, had left the Tsarist Empire to found a communal-agricultural colony in the US, volunteered at Chaikovsky's exilic farm in Kansas, and then returned to Russia in 1885. Frey and Tolstoy spent "five unforgettable days" together in October 1885, and under their visitor's influence, Lev and his daughters Masha and Tanya, Chertkov, and many Tolstoyans became vegetarians.[189] That same year, Lev Nikolaevich welcomed the 19-year old Orthodox Jew I. B. Feinermann, whose figure, passion, and manner of speech he found pleasing, to Yasnaya Polyana as a volunteer. Feinermann became one of the "dark ones"—peasant Tolstoyans, Jews, and freethinkers—whose presence on the manor vexed the countess.[190]

Feinermann converted to Christianity so as to be able to teach at Yasnaya Polyana, but even after his baptism, he was still barred from the job. Regardless, he chose to stay on the estate and work with the *muzhiki*. After a time, he returned to his hometown of Kremenchug in Ukraine to preach Tolstoyanism to the People.[191] Later, he went on to pen several controversial articles about his relationship with the artist, and he wrote *The Departure of a Grand Old Man* (1912) as a short film about Tolstoy's last days under the pseudonym Teneromo. *Departure* portrays Countess Tolstaya unsympathetically as a self-absorbed proprietor, and her marriage with Tolstoy as tempestuous and nonsensical, while it depicts the elder's bond with Chertkov and the *muzhiki* as sympathetic, authentic, and homoerotic.[192] For these and other reasons, including scenes laying bare the married couple's suicidal impulses, *Departure* provoked "an unprecedented public scandal," and Tolstoy's children called it "an outrageous desecration of the memory of their father."[193]

In a perhaps less emotionally charged way, Lev Nikolaevich took "joy" in his correspondence with John Kenworthy, a former businessman who co-founded the Croydon Brotherhood Church in Essex, England, in 1894.[194] This Church hosted activities, such as youth meetings and exercise classes; published their own writings, together with Tolstoy's; and promoted cooperative production. At Purleigh, which exists to this day, the first English Tolstoyan commune was established the same year.[195] What is more, according to literary critic Peter M. Bitsilli (1879–1953), Tolstoy and Anton Chekhov were Russia's "artists of life." Having met in 1895, they shared an intimate spiritual bond and a commitment to bringing about the Kingdom of God.[196] Demonstrating introjection of Tolstoyan utopianism and the "rationalist utopia of the Enlightenment," Chekhov's play *The Cherry Orchard* (1904) portrays a three-age interpretation of history.[197] In this drama, the feudal lord's private cherry orchard is devastated by capitalists in the name of profit, but then returns on a higher level as a "new garden [...] where all will find a new happiness in new surroundings."[198]

Along similar lines, the writer Maxim Gorky (1868–1936) felt "boundless admiration and fascination" for his elder, but he loathed the artist's followers, especially Chertkov. For his part, Tolstoy found "both Gorky and Chekhov pleasant, especially the former," and considered the journalist a "real man of the people," one blessed with "a great talent." Even so, Gorky and Tolstoy differed on the roles they saw for Western philosophy and the intelligentsia on the one hand, and the peasantry and Slavophilism on the other, in terms of Russia's past, present, and future. Gorky sought to overcome Russia's supposedly "Asiatic" inheritance through the modernization of the economy and State. As a result, he would side with the Marxist Bolsheviks over the *Narodnik* Socialist-Revolutionaries in the Russian Revolution. Later, despite sympathizing with the Kronstadt sailors in 1921, he would disgracefully welcome Stalin's imposition of forcible collectivization. As well, in response to Chekhov's 1922 sympathetic volume on Tolstoy's final home-leaving, Gorky wrote a "vigorous defense" of Sofia Andreevna.[199] This is not to mention his extremely homophobic 1934 article, "Proletarian Humanism," which we will discuss below in Chapter 6.

Next, Lev Nikolaevich met the painter Nikolai N. Gay (1831–1894) during his travels in Rome in 1861. Seeking to reunite with and "embrace" Tolstoy, whose "word [had] set [him] aflame," the depressed Gay, who was married with a wife, abandoned his farm in Ukraine for Moscow in 1882.[200] Under his fantasied partner's influence, whom he described as the "only one [...] for me," Gay adopted a plant-based diet and began to perform manual labor. Count Tolstoy would send Gay unambiguous sexual innuendo in letters written in 1887 and 1889, especially phallic imagery.[201] In turn in a manner traditionally expected of a romantic partner, Gay would complain, before passing away in 1894, that his counterpart "is thinking for the whole human race, but no consideration is paid to his spiritual needs at all."[202]

In January 1910, Valentin Fedorovich Bulgakov (1886–1966) arrived at Yasnaya Polyana to serve as Tolstoy's secretary during the latter's final months. Bulgakov describes his elder's "almost fulsome" greeting, and the pleasure Tolstoy took in attending to the weary traveler by "putting a blanket around my knees" and "fetching tea for me." Thus, Bulgakov attests to Tolstoy's aptitude for nursing, anticipating Carpenter's discovery from history and anthropology that those of "intermediate" or non-normative sexuality and/or gender have often functioned as priests, shamans, or healers.[203] Thanks to his elder's warm welcome, Bulgakov thinks, "This [is] a man I could easily love." Sofia Andreevna herself felt that Bulgakov was attracted to Tolstoy, while in turn, Chertkov's secretary, P. A. Sergeenko (1854–1930), believed that Tolstoy admired his assistant. Notably, Tolstoy did not use to invite his previous youthful secretary, Nikolai Gusev (1882–1967), to accompany him on trips to the *zaseka*, as he would Bulgakov, who conceded that his elder was "so curious" about him.[204]

Finally, during Tolstoy's last year of life, the artist corresponded with Mohandas K. Gandhi (1869–1948), with whom he shared many spiritual and political affinities: namely, an emphasis on "human brotherhood, race equality, resistance to tyranny and hatred of war."[205] Arguably living out the homoerotic "apprentice complex" and reflecting the relatively strong role played by identification in love between men, Gandhi celebrated the centenary of the prose writer's birth in 1928 by describing him in a speech as one of the three most influential people in his life.[206] However, reflecting the dangers of gay hyper-masculinity, Tolstoy and Gandhi converged in their sexist views on the woman question. Plus, Lev Nikolaevich's ambivalence over Great-Russian chauvinism has its parallel in the legitimization that Gandhi arguably provided to the starkly hierarchical ideology of Brahmanism, despite his humanization of the Hindu caste system's most oppressed, the *Avarna* ("untouchables"), as *Harijan* ("God's children").[207] Far more radically than the Mahatma, Dr. B. R. Ambedkar (1881–1956) espoused an anti-authoritarian interpretation of Buddhism focused on the outright annihilation of caste.[208] Ambedkar himself was reportedly moved to tears while reading Aylmer Maude's *Life of Tolstoy* (1908/1930), a major source for this text.[209]

Therefore, out of the 19 same-sex bonds here surveyed—a sum which likely indicates only the "tip of the iceberg" of this return of the repressed—we count two relationships with homosocial features, 12 homophilic relationships, and five homosexual bonds that provided satisfaction and meaning in Tolstoy's life.[210] Beyond these, the writer himself confesses to having loved at least eight other men at Kazan University, making for a minimum total of 27 same-sex relationships.

Undoubtedly, the boundaries separating homosociality, homophilia, and homosexuality are fluid, as Eros manifests itself in many different ways. This could be through love for a partner, love for a friend or relative, love for one's country or collective, love for humanity, or even a sublimated love for philosophy, art, religion, or cause.[211] When it comes to Tolstoy's queer desires, we cannot say to what extent his libido was sated. In reality, his passions for male company and for sexual and emotional intimacy with his fellow men are constant enough.

Notes

1 Maude 1987b: 428.
2 Berdyaev 1966: 86; Berdyaev 2009: 11–12.
3 Medzhibovskaya 2008: 35.
4 Ken; Byrd 120.
5 Orwin 1993: 212; Honneth; Gustafson 1986: 456; Зверев и Туниманов 38; Grodetskaya 100.
6 Shestov.
7 Maude 1987b: 410; Evtuhov et al. 237–8.
8 Gustafson 1986: 440; Rancour-Laferriere 1995: 39; Malia 327; Berdyaev 2009: 9; Hall 169.
9 Berdyaev 1966: 87.
10 Bulgakov 39; Smith D 148; Hall 164–6; Rubin.
11 Hamburg 12.
12 Quoted in Medzhibovskaya 2010: 29.
13 Maude 1987b: 121; 1987a: 370.
14 Bartlett 2011: 345–6, 409.
15 Luxemburg 1–2.
16 Maude 1987b: 415.
17 Johansson 1990j; Dynes 1990b; Yousef; Berdyaev 1966.
18 Mole 2; Healey 4–15.
19 Figes and Kolonitskii 30; Venturi 142; Figes 2002: xxvii; Berdyaev 1966: 38.
20 Feuerbach 70, 79.
21 Hall 218.
22 Maude 1987a: 256; Mandelker.
23 DeYoung.
24 Freud 1953; Maude 1987b: 304.
25 Gustafson 1986: 432.
26 Rancour-Laferriere 1995: 3.
27 Nealon 4; Chitty 22–6, 32.
28 Tavis 107–8; Gustafson 1986: 190, 397; Capra 173.
29 Gustafson 1986: 11–21, 96.
30 Maude 1987a: 14–17, 197.
31 Bartlett 2011: 58–9.
32 Chodorow 1999: 44. After all, Isaac Newton suffered childhood abandonment, but went on to make stunning contributions to mathematics and physics (Williams).
33 Hall 167–72; Pietikainen 1–2; Freud 2013: 34; Berdyaev 1966: 14; Triandis.
34 Triandis.
35 Evtuhov et al.
36 Matthew 4: 8–11; Berdyaev 2009: 139.

37 Healey 101; Smolski et al.
38 Rancour-Laferriere 1995: 25–6; Karlinsky.
39 Orwin 2002b: 2, 30; Pietikainen 6, 22; Bartlett 2011: 340; Honneth 60.
40 Gustafson 1986: 318–23; Hrdy.
41 Jakim 272; Berdyaev 2009: 18.
42 Berdyaev 2009: 147–8.
43 Tolstoy 1985: 241.
44 Gustafson 1986: 274.
45 *Ibid* 429; Medzhibovskaya 2004; Benjamin 177.
46 Love 2007; Chouliaraki; Reitz.
47 Gustafson 1986: xi; Maude 1987a: 419.
48 Orwin 2002a: 49–50, 53; Stites 1990: 9.
49 Vergara 22; Smolski et al.
50 Lundskow; Bartlett 2011: 386; Honneth 51.
51 Rancour-Laferriere 1995: 45–6.
52 Stites 1990: 138; Mazurin 67; Maximov 195.
53 Venturi; Lundskow; Bulgakov.
54 Békés et al.
55 Rancour-Laferriere 1995: 95; Figes 2002: 88–98.
56 Shafer 63–79.
57 Shestov.
58 Maude 1987b: 183, 240–1.
59 Christoyannopoulos 2011: 203–4.
60 Rancour-Laferriere 1998: 2, 32.
61 Cortina 405; Freud 2016: 91.
62 Shelley; Baldwin.
63 Freud 1953: 420; Maude 1987a: 49.
64 Gustafson 1986: 3.
65 Maude 1987a: 234–5.
66 *Ibid* 363.
67 Bartlett 2011: 154–63.
68 Maude 1987b: 178.
69 Freud 2016: 75.
70 Grodetskaya 97.
71 Gustafson 1986: 349.
72 Bullock 105–6, 120.
73 Healey; Mole 5.
74 Karlinsky 1136.
75 Rubin 148; Leeder.
76 Maude 1987a: 276–7.
77 Tolstoy 1985: 32 (emphasis added).
78 Rancour-Laferriere 1985: 353. Likewise, the Black LGBTQ+ campaigner Ted Brown (b. 1950), a member of the Gay Liberation Front who organized the UK's first Pride march in London in 1972, acknowledges his mother for "imbuing him with the spirit of revolutionary love and rejection of bigotry" (Okundaye).
79 Rancour-Laferriere 1995: 3, 28: Donaldson 1990b; Medzhibovskaya 2005: 43; Stites 1989.
80 Шевелев (emphasis added).
81 Forrest 70.
82 Bulgakov 29; Ramnath; Figes and Kolonitskii 73.
83 Dynes 1990i: 398; Fiedler 5–9.
84 Fiedler 7–8.
85 Nealon 9; Berdyaev 2009: 55–7.
86 Zakaria.
87 Chitty 34–6, 57, 71, 148–9.
88 Shively 1990a.

89 Herzen 44n13, 62.
90 Burgen.
91 Chitty 76–7. According to journalist Tim Reid, before the Taliban took over Kandahar in 1994, the city had been considered the "homosexual capital of South Asia" (Reid). Now, the Taliban have taken over the city yet again.
92 Nealon 10.
93 McGrattan; O'Dowd.
94 Shafer 145–50.
95 Ahmed; Koshiw.
96 Pasternak 401, 546.
97 Figes and Kolonitskii 74–5; Mendelsohn.
98 Cohn 284–9; Freud 1953.
99 Freud 1964: 57; Lanzieri and Hildebrant 282.
100 Chitty 73–5.
101 Tolstoy 1985: 31–2.
102 Lieven 2000: 218.
103 Massad 11.
104 Shantz and Williams 161; Bartlett 2011: 102; Phelps.
105 Gettone 1404; Clay 215; Zatat.
106 Pushkin 458.
107 Evtuhov et al. 28–9; Gilman-Opalsky 67.
108 Karlinsky.
109 Healey 21–2, 78–81, 112–15, 187, 202–3; Mole 2.
110 Healey 35, 93, 108.
111 Karlinsky; Johansson 1990q; Healey; Mole 10.
112 Oltermann and Walker.
113 Feldman.
114 Rancour-Laferriere 1988.
115 Healey 112–14.
116 Figes and Kolonitskii 42–59.
117 Pasternak 541–9.
118 Clark 2021.
119 Berdyaev 1966; Pelikan.
120 Berdyaev 2009; Dostoevsky 1990: 246–60.
121 Freud 2016: 61; Stites 1989: 211.
122 Babel 30, 80.
123 Siegel.
124 Healey 38–46.
125 Леонтьев.
126 Kennedy 91; Wexler; Falk.
127 Roberts 80–2.
128 Williams et al.
129 Никитина 95.
130 Толстой 1928–1964, vol. 85, 253n5.
131 Healey 17, 47, 101; Johansson 1990g.
132 Healey 190.
133 Gerth and Mills; Hamburg 128.
134 Никитина 79, 88, 95.
135 Freud 2016: 63.
136 Книжный чел.
137 Bullock 103.
138 Никитина 85.
139 Tolstoy 2006b.
140 Maude 1987a: 51. In this sense, Tolstoy feels himself "as a woman in search of a man" (Freud 2016: 64).

141 Tolstoy 1985: 32.
142 Никитина 96–7.
143 Bullock 104–5; Phelps 679; Healey 1; Khazov; Khazov-Cassia; Shakhidzhanian and Reiter; Kondakov.
144 Громова-Опульская 400.
145 Tolstoy 2009a.
146 Freud 1961b: 39; Benjamin; Malatesta; Medzhibovskaya 2004: 22.
147 Pietikainen 83.
148 Johansson 1990d; Gustafson 1986: 13; Maude 1987b: 140; Rancour-Laferriere 1988; Benjamin; Никитина 97.
149 Tolstoy 1985: 32.
150 Maude 1987a: 18.
151 Никитина 81.
152 Maude 1987a: 155 (emphasis added).
153 Gustafson 1986: 202.
154 Zorin 20, 59.
155 Tolstaya 2014a. To this point, two 2015 studies corroborate Countess Tolstaya's hypothesis about the link between creativity/prodigy and autism (University of East Anglia; Ruthsatz et al.).
156 Bartlett 2011: 306–66; Evtuhov et al. 399.
157 Zorin 126–9; Bartlett 2011: 315.
158 Figes 2002: 260.
159 Parini 123–4, 131–6, 140; Bartlett 2011: 360–2; Tolstaia 574.
160 Tolstaia 668–70.
161 Maude 1987a: 34–66; Bartlett 2011: 73, 99; Figes 2002; Phelps; Rancour-Laferriere 1988.
162 Rancour-Laferriere 1985: 344.
163 Parini 72–3, 279–80.
164 Johansson 1990e.
165 Freud 1961b: 30; Freud 1953.
166 Newlin 368–74.
167 Shestov.
168 Phelps 665.
169 Bartlett 2011: 300–1.
170 Chitty 134.
171 Bartlett 2011: 49–51; Tolstoy 2010: 205, 1127–38; Figes and Kolonitskii 1; Museu Marítim de Barcelona.
172 Maude 1987a: 33.
173 Chausovsky.
174 Kropotkin 2022: 14.
175 Healey 97–8.
176 Tolstoy 1985: 32, 488n41. Kropotkin makes an analogous confession in 1863 in the town of Chita in the Far East: namely, that "I am not created for women, and women are not created for me" (Kropotkin 2022: 60).
177 Maude 1987a: 199.
178 *Ibid* 41, 317; Zorin 78.
179 Bartlett 2011: 102; Maude 1987a: 70–2.
180 Tolstoy 2005: 287.
181 Maude 1987a: 140, 284–317, 373–4; Freud 2013: 87.
182 Zorin 87.
183 Johansson 1990q; Maude 1987a: 363–5.
184 Maximov 221–2; Bartlett 2011: 431–47.
185 Bullock 107.
186 Bartlett 2011: 258–64; Maude 1987a: 381; 1987b: 13–14, 85–7.
187 Maude 1987b: 83–5.
188 Healey 27, 49.

189 Maude 1987b: 167–9; Bartlett 2011: x, 350.
190 Maude 1987b: 174–5; Tolstoy 1985: 218–19; Figes and Kolonitskii 35.
191 Матонин 69; Толстой 1928–1964, vol. 85, 253n5.
192 Teneromo.
193 Матонин 70.
194 Bartlett 2011: 362.
195 Osgood.
196 Шевелев; Harris 90.
197 Sternhell 258.
198 Kropotkin 1991: 345–6.
199 McLean 2002: 27–8; Tolstoy 1985: 346, 360, 448; Figes 1996: 767; Kropotkin 1991: 120.
200 Maude 1987b: 116; Tolstoy 2010: 257.
201 Bartlett 2011: 142, 297–308.
202 Maude 1987b: 205, 243–9, 267–75, 339.
203 Parini 46–8, 90; Carpenter 1919: 14.
204 Parini 68, 83–4.
205 Balasubramanian 67. This is not to overlook either Gandhi's anti-Black racism, or Tolstoy's ambivalence toward Asians or Jews (Desai and Vahed). For more about Tolstoy's approximation with, and critique of, Orientalism, see Chapter 4.
206 Rancour-Laferriere 1985: 345–52; Balasubramanian 66–8.
207 Shaw.
208 Ramnath.
209 Yusufji.
210 Rancour-Laferriere 1985: 348. Though limited by their preliminary and speculative nature, these categories are as follows: homosocial: Vanusha, Kenworthy; homophilic: Fëdor Ivanovich Tolstoy, Ufan, Sado Miserbiyev, Frey, Fet, Strakhov, Tchaikovsky, Siutayev, Gorky, Chekhov, Bulgakov, Gandhi; homosexual: Dyakov, Alexeev, Feinermann, Gay, Chertkov.
211 Berdyaev 2009: 55–6; Gilman-Opalsky 144; Chitty 169; Freud 1961a: 184.

3

THE LIFE AND DEATH OF A "HOLY FOOL"

Besides being a religious anarcho-Populist and a political and sexual dissident, Count Tolstoy idealized the Asiatic-Russian figure of the "holy fool" (юродивый) in his art, reflecting his wish to become a "revolutionary saint" himself.[1] He had met many monks, nuns, *Stranniki* (religious wanderers), beggars, and other "God's folk" at Yasnaya Polayana through his Aunt Aline, who invited such pilgrims to visit and stay on the estate—hence, lending it certain communal characteristics.[2] These fools are akin to the "masterless men" of early-modern England, many of whom had been displaced by the enclosure of the commons that facilitated the rise of capitalism.[3] They resemble preachers or itinerant friars, more than cloistered monks or nuns, who remain sequestered from the social world. As such, Christian holy fools commingle with the People as followers of Jesus of Nazareth and prefigure the Kingdom of God by renouncing family life and possessions, and by committing themselves to fearless truth-telling and social critique.[4] The *yurodivy* practices a "specifically provocative or exhibitionist" form of depressive moral masochism, through ridicule of the dominant order and its master symbols.[5] Abraham Maslow's parallel concept of the self-actualizer presupposes self-moving individuals who resist dominant social relations.[6]

Tolstoy sympathized with his fellow gentry insurgent *Don Quixote* (1605/1615), who "lives for his brothers, [and] for opposing the forces hostile to humanity," in Turgenev's view.[7] Disenchanted with early modernity, Miguel de Cervantes' good-natured gentleman loses himself in books of chivalry, momentously decides to become a medieval knight-errant, and "travel[s] about the world with his armour and his arms and his horse in search of adventures, [...] redressing all kinds of grievances."[8] In this sense, Quixote shows how the study of philosophy, when combined with intellectual pride, can lead to madness.[9] This literary anti-hero is the epitome of the holy fool: an artistic, "creative deviant" who "is not adjusted to his [*sic*] own time and throws out a challenge to it," enjoining an enhancement of

DOI: 10.4324/9781003328964-3

spiritual consciousness.[10] Typically, the holy fool is a "[n]on-movement anarchist," a trickster akin to the *heyoka*, or sacred clown, of the Lakota and Dakota, who undermines the political order and calls on listeners to shift allegiances.[11]

Three contemporary examples might be the Russian elder Elena Andreevna Osipova, who since 2002 has protested Vladimir Putin's authoritarianism and wars in public using art; the fearless Russian anarcha-feminists of Pussy Riot (2011–present); and the young Syrian rapper Amir al-Mu'arri (1999–present), who has likewise critiqued the Assad regime's authoritarianism in his music.[12] Some historical examples of courageous self-actualizers, revolutionary saints, and holy fools might include Teresa of Ávila (1515–1582), Nawal el-Saadawi (1931–2021), Martin Luther King, Jr. (1929–1968), Albert Einstein (1879–1955), Ursula K. Le Guin (1929–2018), and Desmond Tutu (1931–2021).[13]

Fools stand for personal self-determination and "the triumph over the determination of the social group [...]." They embody "activity, opposition, victory over the dragging burden of the world," "the triumph of freedom," and the "refusal to acquiesce in slavery, and repudiation of the enslaving majesty of the world." They are judges of the world. Like Quixote, the fool "direct[s one's] rage at that which is truly deserving: inequality, oppression, and injustice." In this way, the fool's "inner borderline protects [the self] from falling prey to the abuses of the past." The *yurodivy* reminds us that the self-realization of personality involves suffering, antithesis, and loss, and that the supreme value is "active resistance to the power of the world, which desires to tear personality to pieces." These fools thus parody the successful employment of hierarchical power, instrumental reason, and the lure and slavery of sovereignty, all the while warning us that the Kingdom of Caesar cannot tolerate new or free ways of thinking or living.[14] Psychosexually, the "creative and courageous" *yurodivy* sublimates one's polymorphous-perverse desires into an avowal of subversiveness. The protagonist of Andrei Tarkovsky's film *Stalker* (1979) is a prototypical sacred clown, who considers the entire world a prison, and finds meaning in leaving his wife and daughter behind to guide male visitors on spiritual journeys to a mysterious "Zone," the apparent site of an industrial accident.[15]

Alluding in 1862 to classical Greece, early Christianity, Jean-Jacques Rousseau (1712–1778), pre-Petrine Russia, and the Old Believers, Tolstoy announced that "*[o]ur ideal is behind, not ahead of us*."[16] Consequently, his optimistic attitude toward the past is Romantic, in line with classical authors, and linked to the anti-modern utopianism of the Slavophiles, who looked back nostalgically to the pre-Tsarist past. As such, Tolstoy's spirit is reminiscent of the Christian hero, who looks backward for inspiration rather than forward, as the intelligent-humanistic hero does.[17]

Pushkin's heroine Tatyana Larina, who partially inspired Tolstoy's *Anna Karenina* (1875–1877), channels the iconoclasm of the holy fool in *Evgeny Onegin* (1825–1832). This occurs when she regretfully tells her would-be lover, the titular character, that she would happily trade "[a]ll this glitter and noise and revelry" for a "shelf with books, an unkempt garden"—the place where she first met Onegin.[18]

Surrounded by luxury and artifice, Tolstoy similarly searched for simplicity and authenticity throughout much of his life. Peering back into antiquity, Lev Nikolaevich identified especially closely with Socrates (c. 470–399 BCE) for his "opposition to unaccountable power," and his penetrating, discerning method.[19] As a token of his appreciation of this philosophical "ancestor of Voltaire," in 1885, Tolstoy collaborated with the revolutionary educator Alexandra M. Kalmykova (1849–1926) on a biography of this classical Greek thinker.[20] Moreover, the paradoxically Dionysian *and* sex-negative aspects of Socrates's life resonated for him. For example, in the *Symposium*, Aristodemos is taken aback at the sight of Socrates wearing evening shoes, as the philosopher typically would travel barefoot. Alluding to the young Agathon, Socrates explains that he has made an exception, so that he could be presentable for "a pretty man!" Even so, imparting the sexual renunciation of the holy fool, young Alcibiades complains that Socrates oddly avoided consummating his presumed newfound erotic bond with him, a "blooming beauty," because the elder cared not for whether a junior male partner be handsome, rich, or famous![21] Such flirtatiousness and anxious-avoidant attachment patterns characterized the count's approach to the libido, as well.

Reflecting his *dikost*—which can be variously translated as "wildness," eccentricity, shyness, daring, queerness, iconoclasm, or neurodivergence—Tolstoy felt drawn to the asceticism of Diogenes the Cynic (c. 404–323 BCE), who rejected marriage, family, law, and custom.[22] As a *dikii* man, the count was a horizontal individualist who was focused on building personal autonomy through the defiance of various collectives he found oppressive.[23] In light of the contrarianism with which Lev Nikolaevich often approached his fellow Russian *intelligents*, it is probable that Turgenev alludes to Tolstoy's very own *dikost* in his poem "The Fool," when he comments, "'Spiteful! malignant!' his friends began to say of [him]. 'But what a brain!'"[24]

Above all, the prose writer identified with Jesus the Nazarene. The Galilean whom Tolstoy met in the Gospels is a "lone crusader swimming against the current of public opinion, a 'humble sectarian' with whom he could identify."[25] Like the writer, Jesus was, according to the Gospel, still unmarried in his early 30s, and had mostly associated himself with other men before launching his ministry, which in turn was largely homosocial. In reality, Jesus and Tolstoy were both visionary, prophetic humanists who would change the world. They valorized humility and patience as virtues of the social ethos.[26]

Attesting to his iconoclasm, Count Tolstoy once exclaimed that his stays with nomadic Muslim Bashkirs on the Eurasian steppe near Samara had been far more pleasurable than his time spent listening to speeches in the Houses of Parliament in London.[27] Like his historical role-models, then, Tolstoy acted transgressively "against corrupt norms on behalf of Christian morality," in the estimation of his friend Nikolai Grot.[28] Similarly, the philosopher Simon Frank hailed Lev Nikolaevich as a "great religious and ethical thinker," whose example has much to teach us about the "categorical lack of compromise."[29]

Tolstoy's journey inward toward embracing holy foolishness followed from a logical conclusion: that it is impossible to live as a true Christian in a conventional, sadomasochistic society. In this sense, the conscience informed by authentic Christianity cannot readily accept history's oppressiveness.[30] Specifically, for the count, there was a fundamental contradiction between his economic privilege as a landlord, and his desire to become a free man like Jesus the Nazarene, who was self-governing but not enslaving.[31] As well, the example of his relative Pushkin was decisive, for Russia's national poet was "one of the first noblemen to shun [State] service and take up writing as a 'trade,'" a move for which he was subjected to great opprobrium.[32] For an aristocrat to become an artist was to reject one's class, and to pursue social justice ran counter to the societal expectations of the artist.[33] Our subject, for his part, did both.

In psychoanalytical terms, the phenomenon of holy foolishness is closely related to what might be termed "moral masochism," or an openness to sacrifice that is actually satisfying to oneself. Paradoxically, the phenomenon of moral masochism responds to feelings of guilt that demand "some compensatory behavior," which in turn functions as an anti-depressant.[34] Some examples of penitent behavior in Tolstoy's biography would include transitioning to a plant-based diet ("gastronomic asceticism"); replacing hunting with "mushrooming"; giving up smoking and the imbibing of alcohol; and attempting to repress the libido—insofar as this is possible—according to the Daoist doctrine of *wu-wei*, or non-action.[35]

Developmental and Psychosocial Dimensions of Tolstoy's Anarchism

In "Creative Writers and Day-Dreaming" (1908), Freud suggests that literary artists revisit their early experiences with play through their ongoing creativity, such that we should "look for the first traces of imaginative activity as early as in childhood."[36] In this sense, Tolstoy's anarchism may date back to his infancy, and to what he implausibly refers to as his first memory, and the "strongest impression of [his] life": of being bound, like Jesus, in swaddling clothes.[37]

> I lie bound and wish to stretch out my arms, but cannot. I scream and cry, and my screams are disagreeable to myself but I cannot stop. Some one—I do not remember who—bends over me. This all happens in semi-darkness. I only know there are two people there. My cries affect them: they are agitated by my screams but do not untie me as I want them to, and I scream still louder. To them it seems necessary that I should be bound, but I know it is unnecessary and I wish to prove this to them and again burst into cries [...]. I feel the injustice and cruelty—not of people, for they pity me, but—of fate, and I pity myself [...]. I desire freedom, it would harm no one, but I who need strength am weak, while they are strong.[38]

This spectral "some one" whom Tolstoy cannot name is assuredly his mother, the "prototypical 'master'" of the newborn infant, who is the "prototypical 'slave.'"[39] If we compare this retelling of how Tolstoy overcame infantile amnesia with Leonardo da Vinci's recalling of an episode during which he spontaneously sucked the tail of a kite that had flown into his cradle, we see expressions of polymorphously perverse sexuality from the beginning of life in both cases. If da Vinci's story conveys passive homosexuality and avian biophilia, Tolstoy's account emphasizes his lifelong struggles with sadomasochistic attachment.[40] Levochka's instinctual need to express himself through the free movement of the limbs, and to prove this need to his caretakers, leads him retrospectively to depict himself as crying and rebelling against his restraints, foreshadowing subsequent defiance and rebellion. He intimates that he has rejected the expected introjection of obedience to the laws of civilization from the very beginning: he rebels both on his own behalf, and that of humanity.[41] Consequently, we can say that the neonatal Lev, in the self-concept of his older self, hints at his affinities with the revolutionary character structure proposed by the psychoanalyst Erich Fromm (1900–1980), which affirms love for life and productive social critique, as opposed to the submissiveness expected of conformists.[42]

Moreover, the resistance of this pre-individuated being to the type of "second womb" represented by swaddling clothes may emblematically signify Lev Nikolaevich's anarchist rebellion against Russia's authoritarian political culture. According to the Russo-Soviet writer Vasili S. Grossman (1905–1964), the psychosocial legacy of fatalism and passivity amounts to the primary obstacle for breaking the cycle that has underpinned the desolation and suffering that marks Russian history.[43] Through his recollective allegory, which can be interpreted as a struggle not only against coerced forms of socialization but also death, the "ultimate enslavement," Count Tolstoy proudly proclaims the ostensible dignity of Russian aristocratic self-assertion—without immediately acknowledging how this would-be heroism is dependent on the enslavement of the serfs.[44] At the same time, his apocryphal origin story implicitly critiques not just the suffering to which he is subjected, but also the abuse to which he will subject his future dependents, such as peasants and female partners. This illustrates not only the use of displacement as a defense mechanism, but also the internal dynamism of the sadomasochistic relationship—that is, that a "sadist is always at the same time a masochist."[45]

Developmentally speaking, the childhood trauma involved in Tolstoy's orphancy surely contributed to the future artist's shyness and sensitivity.[46] According to the German idealist G. W. F. Hegel (1770–1831), the turning inward of the mind (*Er-innerung*) in search of divine reason can be a natural response of the organism to alienating external phenomena (*Ent-fremdung*). In like manner, Kantian physics postulate internal rather than external forms of causation.[47] For his part, Sigmund Freud, the father of psychoanalysis, saw "erot[ic] masochism" in the self-contained response to destructive, stressful, and tempting external stimuli.[48] In turn, his radical colleague Otto Gross held the psychoutopian view that inner revolution is a "prerequisite for the political revolution."[49] Likewise, Ali Shariati stresses the "divine spark" within that "refuses to submit to irrational and oppressive authority," that "seeks a better and more reconciled peaceful future," and that "refuses to be extinguished under the jackboot of tyranny [...]."[50] All of these concepts resonated for Tolstoy, as well.

Within the mother-child dyad, among partners, or on the individual level, the inner realm can function as a safe "transitional space" for psychological exploration and experimentation.[51] The artist's characteristic focus on this inner realm manifests Orthodox Christian, proto-nationalist influences, reflecting the apophatic creed about the world's wickedness, and the imprint of his ascetic brother Dmitri, also known as Mitenka, who was "serious, thoughtful, pure, and resolute." Rather than look up to Mitenka, though, who represented *dikost* and the free man, the young Lev was more compelled by the influence of Sergei and conformist convention more broadly.[52]

Despite the very real risks involved in resisting inherited authoritarianism, Tolstoy in his older age believed ardently that the possibility of redemption lies within all of us, individually and collectively. Like Gross, though, he thought that this struggle begins internally, as the title of *The Kingdom of God Is Within You* (1893) suggests. In an 1878 essay entitled "The Fundamental Concepts of Psychology," his friend Strakhov centers the inner realm which they both held in high esteem. He does so by reinterpreting René Descartes' hypothesis about the link between thought and existence—"I think; therefore, I am"—as incorporating the "whole totality of psychic, subjective phenomena," or the soul.[53] For Count Tolstoy, the "inner law" amounts to "reason, conscience, love, the good, God."[54] Likewise, the Tolstoyan labor lawyer Clarence S. Darrow (1857–1938) proposed that, "[t]o change the individual[,] you must change the heart."[55]

In keeping with the artist's essential anarchism, Lev Nikolaevich's emphasis on the inner realm proclaims a radical distrust of pyramidally organized social institutions. Tolstoy's biographer Aylmer Maude writes that the repentant landlord "had an inveterate distrust of officialism" and "saw an antithesis between the attempt to organize society [hierarchically] and the attempt to reform oneself and to live a good life."[56] In the same way that Tolstoy's fiction heralds a conscious psychosexual struggle with moral and political despotism—undertaken at the personal and collective levels in a revolutionary effort to elucidate one's ego-identity, change the world, and so retain physical and psychical health—it also evinces a repetitive idealization of the frustration of one's emotional needs, in accordance with Christian monastic traditions and psychological masochism.[57] As we shall see, this is a recurring problem for Tolstoy, considering that withdrawal from intersubjectivity promotes psychic disintegration and the breakdown of mutual recognition and understanding.[58]

According to Maude, who was more politically moderate than his mentor, Lev Nikolaevich came to adopt anarchism due to a constellation of class and psychical factors: his aristocratic privilege, his physical isolation in the Tula countryside, his characteristic male narcissism, and his "detachment from the real business of life."[59] Historians Peter Struve and Richard Stites would appear to agree, for they center the intelligentsia's "absolute dissociation" from Tsarist society, sense of superfluousness, and loneliness in the development of its revolutionary maximalism.[60] Along similar lines, according to Abdullah Öcalan (b. 1947), founder of the Kurdistan Workers' Party (PKK), anarchism approximates "a sect which protects itself from the evils of the system."[61] Herzen's biographer Martin Malia clarifies that, under Tsarism, the "denial of the state was naturally the first problem of politics," such that Russian radicals adopted anarchism as the logical antithesis to autocracy.[62] Furthermore, the Christian anarchist Berdyaev, the philosopher Sergei Bulgakov, and the British historian Isaiah Berlin explain that the despotic ban on all political activity in Imperial Russia impelled both the momentous birth of the intelligentsia, and the development of "the most radical socialist and anarchist ideas" within it. Such explanations foregrounding the symbolic sphere and the social imaginary echo the findings of French historians Roger Chartier and Jacques Revel, who stress the centrality of mental representations in historical change.[63]

Precisely as a result of Nicholas I's severe reaction after the 1848 European Revolutions, in keeping with the Tsar's self-concept as heir of Peter I, Russian dissidents became convinced that no negotiation or approximation with authority was possible. For this reason, they often followed their hero, the utopian socialist Charles Fourier (1772–1837), in envisioning the ideal future as stateless.[64] In a similar way, the biographer Richard F. Gustafson frames Tolstoy's separation from the rest of humanity as owing primarily to the man's privilege—leading to his energetic compensatory attempts to overcome such separation through art, pedagogy, eroticism, and politics.[65] Psychosocially, the poet's lifelong negotiation of estrangement vs. residence is a restatement of the separation-abandonment conflict which grips outsiders and/or masochists more prominently than others. In Tolstoy's case, the centrality of this conflict suggests the persistence of unresolved infantile trauma over maternal loss, loneliness, and connection developing into a prolonged mid-life conflict and then crisis regarding Erikson's sixth psychosocial stage: that is, intimacy vs. isolation.[66]

While certainly given to masochistic self-sabotage, Lev Nikolaevich would also make a life of rejecting imposed circumstances, in an affirmation of an anti-masochistic spirit. Examples abound of such instinctual rebelliousness, whether we consider his agonizing over being locked up in the closet by his French tutor, Prospère Saint-Thomas; howling as a young boy in protest against his mother's cousin, a Volkonsky hussar, who was restraining him; arguing with his superior officers during the siege of Sevastopol; or philosophically avowing autonomy, Christian anarchism, and non-cooperation with the State.[67] By all means reproducing the repressive legacy of the swaddling clothes, Tsarist censors marred Tolstoy's very first published writings, *Childhood* (1852) and "The Raid" (1853).[68]

With the abuse of power in mind, Tolstoy summarized the dilemma seemingly faced by all of us who are subjected to hierarchy in an 1881 letter to Vasili Alexeev: that is, "either [to] let one's hands drop and suffer passively, yielding to despair, or [to] make peace with evil, befogging oneself with cards and chatter and bustle [...]."[69] However, in his best art, Lev Nikolaevich presents a third option: namely, to reject passivity by exhorting dignified individual and collective struggles for self-determination, life, reason, and love against the "overwhelming force" of moral, erotic, and political forms of despotism in history and the present.[70] These were struggles he had participated in his whole life, without surrender.[71]

Christian Anarchism as Self-Assertion in the Face of Death and Loss

According to Berlin (1909–1997), Tolstoy's adult life can be divided into two distinct phases: "first comes the author of immortal masterpieces, later the prophet of personal and social regeneration; first the aristocratic writer, the difficult, somewhat unapproachable, troubled novelist of genius; then the sage—dogmatic, perverse, exaggerated, but wielding a vast influence, particularly in his own country—a world institution of unique importance."[72] Still, as useful as it might be, to adopt this two-phase model of Tolstoy's life and career would be to overlook his early period, when he wrote the "Sevastopol Sketches" (1855) and *The Cossacks* (1863), even before *War and Peace* (1869). All of these texts from the first half of the artist's life suggest the need for social reconstruction, in a progressively emblematic or allegorical manner.[73] The Slavist Lisa Knapp therefore proposes a three-phase model for understanding Tolstoy's biography—one that integrates the writer's often-ignored early works.[74] These three phases, then, would include his early (1852–1863), middle (1869–1877), and late (1878–1910) periods.

In our view, the bridge connecting the second and third stages of Tolstoy's life and career is the artist's commitment to Christian anarchism. This ideological system can surely be gleaned in his early writings, and it evidently blossoms in the novelist's late, openly prophetic period, when the writer sought to prove to the world the truth of his ideas by modeling what he considered righteous thought and conduct.[75] Questioning the divisions that Berlin and Knapp uphold between Lev Nikolaevich's first/middle and second/third periods, respectively, we thus concur with Gustafson that "the later [works] clarify the earlier [ones]," and that "*Tolstoy is not two, but one.*"[76]

The eludication by this "Christian warrior for the good" of his anarchist vision for society can be described as consistent with the scholar Donna Tussing Orwin's (b. 1947) identification of the artist's "lifelong effort to secure dignity for the human individual." It also speaks to his quests for faith, and his journey to come to terms with reality, his own existence, and his purpose.[77] The didacticism of Tolstoy's late writings, composed following his conversion to the belief that humanity must consciously "unite Nature and Morality," contrasts with the psychological realism of his earlier works, written during a time when the prose poet believed nature and human existence themselves to be moral, and as such, to need only description.[78]

Anticipating the novelist's prophetic period, Lev Nikolaevich was fascinated in childhood with his older brother Nikolai's fantasy about possessing the key to a Golden Age where "there would be no more disease, no trouble."[79] In this world, "everyone would love each other," and "everyone would become *ant-brothers*."[80] Nikolai told the five-year old Levochka and his two elder brothers that the key to this secret was written on a green stick that was buried at the edge of the *zaseka* old-growth forest located a mile from Yasnaya Polyana. Three decades later, it was in the apiary located in this effective sanctuary that Tolstoy would first think about *War and Peace*, and it was to this same *zaseka* that the artist had considered fleeing and settling for the purposes of writing. It was there, in his laboratory of life, that he was buried.[81]

Whether the "ant-brothers" (муравейные братья) envisioned and anticipated jointly by Nikolai and Lev referred more to the species of social insects; the Muravëv brothers (Муравьёв братья), famous Freemasons and Decembrists; or the Moravian Brethren, founded with the support of Count Nikolaus Ludwig von Zinzendorf (1700–1760)—who, like Tolstoy, renounced his property in favor of fellowship and service to others—the truth of the matter is that the artist believed in a universalist vision of this "ant-brother" ideal. In consonance with the popular Russian utopia about the mythical *Belovode* kingdom, freed of war and oppression, Lev Nikolaevich ecstatically foresaw "all people huddled together loving one another," with "all [of humanity] under the wide dome of heaven."[82] Likewise, the princess-intellectual who founded the Krinitsa *Kommuna* on the Black Sea in the 1870s sought "an enormous commune covering all the earth and to bring contentment to all."[83] More recently, the former Ukrainian parliamentarian Alex Riabchyn remarked that, in the face of the ruthless Russian attack that began in February 2022, the Ukrainian people are coming together like "a huge amount of ants."[84]

In this vein, Count Tolstoy would often infuse anarcho-Populist, utopian, and Christian-anarchist views into his art using symbolic imagery and naturalistic language centering "swarm life," which represents the collective nature of thoughts, emotions, history, and movements.[85] The artist's recurrent use of motifs relating to bees is also connected with the "past unconscious" significance of the Solovetsky Monastery, which is considered the original entry-point whereby bees were introduced to Rus' in the fifteenth century. Located on an island on the White Sea 160 kilometers south of the Arctic Circle, Solovetsky was the death-place of Tolstoy's ancestor, Peter Andreevich Tolstoy, as a former minister-turned-enemy of the State, together with his son Ivan, who met the same fate as his father.[86]

As suggested above, Tolstoy's advocacy of Christian love and interpersonal tenderness may have constituted coping mechanisms for dealing with the loss of his mother as a toddler.[87] While the premature death of Marya Nikolaevna Volkonskaya before his second birthday will leave Lev Nikolaevich with lifelong depressive anxiety (тоска, or "toska") and speculatively contribute to his aggressiveness toward women, it is significant that he was breastfed not by his mother, even while she lived, but rather by a peasant named Avdotia Ziabreva.[88] As such, he quite literally was nursed by the *Narod*—as he would later be saved from drowning in the Volga River by peasant women. Indeed, some of his last words in life reportedly were, "What about the peasants?"[89] In parallel, Alexander Pushkin learned folk tales and traditions from the peasant nurse who raised him, and he integrated these into his poetry. Herzen and many other gentry socialists raised in Imperial Russia emblematically described the residence they felt as children when allying with the serfs of their household against their parents.[90]

In a dialectical sense, the Yasnaya Polyana manor, being an "almost self-sufficient kingdom," provided a sheltered environment for Tolstoy's childhood, although the serfs were effectively "colonial subjects in their own land."[91] While inspired by the gardener Akim, whom they considered a "holy fool" of sorts, Lev and his brothers reveled in the time they spent in the estate's woods, ponds, and gardens, and with the cattle-herder Matryona and her peasant family, connecting thus in an idyllic sense with a "second family" comprised of fellow humans, animals, and ecosystems. The young Lev was also affected by the plight of Mitka Kopylov, the family coachman, who was seen forced to abandon life in Moscow to return to work in the fields of Yasnaya Polyana to support his family, following his brother's conscription by the State. Moreover, the future writer took umbrage in his youth at the normalization of corporal punishment against serfs on the manor. Witnessing persistent feudal violence being meted out against female and elder serfs upon his return to Yasnaya Polyana after his first visit to Western Europe in 1857 weighed heavily on the count.[92]

Implicitly in his early literary works and openly in his late period, Count Tolstoy advocated universal brotherhood, internationalism, the abolition of private property, and the injunction not to resist evil by violence in response to oppression, exploitation, or abuse (non-resistance).[93] Remarkably, however, he was an opponent of gender equality. In effect, Lev Nikolaevich transitioned to publicly and explicitly proclaiming his sexist, Christian-anarchist political ideal following a prolonged existential crisis that began in the 1870s, through which he confronted his own mortality. Tolstoy saw in the inexorability of human finitude a fundamental challenge to the very idea of the meaning of life, and he intimately explores these concerns in his "Confession" (1879) and novella, "The Death of Ivan Ilych" (1886). The latter story was based on the untimely death of his brother Nikolai Nikolaevich, age 37, due to tuberculosis.[94]

The author's concern with corporal suffering, agony, and mortality, both among human and non-human animals, permeates his literary output, spanning the "Sevastopol Sketches" through his major novels, to his short stories, plays, and essays. Lending support to Freud's views on Eros and Thanatos, Tolstoy's twin obsessions with sexuality and finitude arguably underpin much of his creativeness. As well, this fixation on mortality confirms William James' recognition that the fear of death, as the "worm at the core" of human aspirations to happiness, is universal and ever-present among human beings, casting a shroud of terror and an ultimate sense of powerlessness among us all.[95] Operating in accord with the basic instinct toward self-preservation, such death-anxiety manifests both productively—for instance, as sympathy toward children and the will to relatedness—and destructively, as through authoritarianism and suicidality.[96]

Not only this, but we humans seek "heroic transcendence" of the knowledge that we all will one day "lose the battle against death" by sublimating such anxiety, together with the libido, into shared cultural views and institutions like art, religion, language, politics, and science that afford us meaning, purpose, and self-esteem in this life. Our participation in, and contributions to, culture opens the possibility for either symbolic or literal immortality after death.[97] Therefore, for Tolstoy to compose *War and Peace* and other works as a means of creative transcendence of death can be taken as an affirmation of his humanity, linking his artistic output to the memory of "Paleolithic warlessness."[98]

Through his study of the way he believed peasants to confront death—that is, by means of "faith"—and with the intensification of the Populist movement against Tsarism and landlordism raging, Tolstoy "converted" to Christianity in the late 1870s by recommitting himself to the message of the Gospels, especially through his "*love for the peasant masses*."[99] In this way, Lev Nikolaevich proposes the observation of the teachings of Jesus the Nazarene as an authentic response to the reality of death. As his psychobiographer Daniel Rancour-Laferriere notes, the artist hence emphasizes solidarity with the *Narod* as a paradoxically masochistic, generous, and exhibitionist method of easing his depressive anxiety and death-anxiety.[100]

By idealizing the peasantry while denouncing the State, militarism, capitalism, and landlordism and espousing Christian anarchism as a reconstructive social alternative, Tolstoy affirms his basic need for "self-esteem as *the* condition for his life," signaling his distinct vision for society as a "codified hero system" that would encourage humanistic respect and mutual recognition. He furthermore identifies with the *Narod*, both to announce his intention to carry out revolutionary class suicide, and to seek solace in "collectivistic cultures [that] are less open to this type of [death] anxiety."[101]

Count Lev Tolstoy: A Rousseauvist Pedagogist

Inspired by Berthold Auerbach's novel *A New Life* (1851), which features a renegade aristocrat who opts to become a rural school-teacher, Tolstoy created an educational program for peasant children at Yasnaya Polyana beginning in the 1860s. Based on Jean-Jacques Rousseau's writings, the count's curriculum sought to advance knowledge, freedom, agency, and the flattening of hierarchies; a more natural and mutualistic than compulsory and sadomasochistic relationship between students and teachers; and the integration of a healthy measure of *dikost* and play.[102] According to one of his former students, Tolstoy "allowed the children to sit where they wanted, get up when they wanted and answer questions all together."[103] Such a free-spirited atmosphere exhibited the novelist's commitment to the Eastern Christian concept of participation as a central element of faith, and his sense that moral education and literacy are key to social change.[104] In contrast to what Paolo Freire (1921–1997) would later term the "banking concept" of education, Kropotkin explains that Tolstoy insisted that teachers must adapt their lessons to the needs and aptitudes of each individual child.[105]

In a sense, Tolstoy's pedagogical theory approximated that of his fellow *Narodnik* Peter Lavrov, who foresaw popular education as preparing social revolution, despite Lev Nikolaevich's disagreement with Lavrov's privileging of the opinions of the intelligentsia over those of the peasants.[106] When he was appointed by the liberal governor of Tula as Arbiter of the Peace following Tsar Alexander II's emancipation of the serfs, Lev Nikolaevich followed Populist principles by typically siding with the peasants over his fellow landlords in disputes, philanthropically redistributing part of the lands owned by his family, and opening over 20 peasant schools, based on radical pedagogical principles.[107] For these reasons, Tolstoy's fellow proprietors came to despise him, such that his tenure as Arbiter remained brief.[108] Both to study foreign pedagogical methods, and to visit his dying brother Nikolai, who was receiving treatment in Germany for tuberculosis, Tolstoy went abroad for a second (and last) time in 1860, traveling to Berlin, Paris, Marseille, London, and Brussels. In 1908, as an 80-year-old man, he would once again hold classes for village children.[109]

Equally importantly, Tolstoy's progressive ideals resonate in the tireless labor the prose poet poured into the production of the child-centered *ABC* (Азбука, 1872/1875), a volume he esteemed even more highly than *War and Peace* as his most important life-project. This textbook sold a million copies by the time of his passing.[110] Likewise, one of his last projects in life, which was sadly uncompleted, was to compile an encyclopedia for working people.[111] In this sense, there is considerable reason for skepticism about Berlin's attempts to equate Tolstoy with the French reactionary Joseph de Maistre (1753–1821): namely, his egalitarian interpretation of Christianity; his philosophical and religious opposition to war, class inequality, and statism; his emphasis on the importance of autonomy and self-determination; his good-faith commitment to the education of peasant children in a society wherein less than six percent of the rural population was estimated as being literate in the 1850s; his work with the non-profit educational Intermediary Press (Посредник), and his editing and revising of the *ABC*; his composing *What Then Must We Do?* (1886), a volume which emphasizes just how "unendurably wrong" are caste systems and class society; and his journalistic and practical relief efforts during the famines of 1873 and 1891–2.[112] As the literary critic Nikolai Mikhailovsky (1842–1904) observed in 1882, remarking on the political convergence of Tolstoy and the anarchist Pierre-Joseph Proudhon (1809–1865), despite the vastness of differences in their classes and life-experiences:

> If he [Tolstoy] still arrived at [anarchism] in spite of all that, then however he may have contradicted himself, you must recognize that he is an honourable and powerful thinker in whom we may feel confidence.[113]

Despite the numerous problems with Proudhon's theory—from advocacy of private property to the promotion of sexism, sex-negativity, and anti-Semitism—Mikhailovsky does have a point. At the same time, in a manner revealing of the count's contradictions and fragmented sense of identity, Tolstoy left his schooling project behind to write *Anna Karenina*, which he in turn set aside to compose the long essay, "On Popular Education" (1874).

The Christian-Anarchist Threat to Church and State

In keeping with the writer's anarcho-Populist political and erotic sympathies, in the epilogue to *War and Peace*, Lev Nikolaevich condemns the historical subjection of the People to the arbitrary will of despots who are legitimized by religion. His argument is reminiscent of Proudhon's atheism, and it presages Mikhail Bakunin's analysis in "God and the State."[114] Moreover, in this *magnum opus*, known as the

"Russian *Iliad*," Lev Nikolaevich develops his anarcho-Populist theory of "*the masses versus the heroes*," as revealed to him through his research on the war of 1812, during which the Napoleonic invaders were repelled by the *Narod* rather than its leadership.[115]

Such as it is, Tolstoy's Christian anarchism is in keeping with Enlightenment rationalism: it considers Jesus of Nazareth to have been a great moral teacher with an essential ethical message to teach humanity, rather than any sort of king or demi-god. As a consequence, Tolstoyan Christianity contests the legitimizing ideology of most, if not all, churches, which the poet likens to "sentinels keeping guard over a captive."[116] Such rationalist critique opposes the bureaucratic *rationalization* of the life-world, which the sociologist Max Weber defined as the wielding of formal law to operationalize capitalism and the State.[117] By recovering the ethical teachings he discovers in the Gospel of Matthew, Lev Nikolaevich repudiates Paul of Tarsus's infamous distortion of the meaning of the Nazarene's life.[118] Removed of "all gnosticism and mysticism," Tolstoy's vision of Christianity thus represents a "spiritual teaching about the universal spirit which leads [humanity] to a higher life—a life of equality and of friendly relations with all." He sees in the concept of God the "universal desire for welfare which is the source of all life."[119]

Above all, Kropotkin is right to observe that Lev Nikolaevich's writings constitute a "*passionate resistance against the different forms of evil*" that surrounded him.[120] In this sense, the historian Jaroslav Pelikan may be right to identify Tolstoy's account as the "most widely celebrated" rediscovery of Jesus as Liberator: "the one who challenged every social system and called it to account before the judgment of God."[121] This conception of Jesus as revolutionary prophet and Liberator of humanity clashes fundamentally with Paul's injunction that Christians respect the constituted authorities.[122] Such distortions of Jesus's insurgent message arguably mirror the conscious attempts made by Paul, whose mind "was of an administrative, organizing type," to transform the ethical anarchist system of the Galilean into an institutionalized dogma emphasizing the rabbi's supposed divinity.[123]

Like Jesus, many saints, and countless of his compatriots and followers, Count Tolstoy suffered for his unique reinterpretation of Christianity and attendant, relentless criticism of the State and Church, which is made especially openly in *Resurrection* (1899). Practically speaking, the artist exhorted equality and a rejection of State and private property to a peasant community on the Eurasian steppe in 1883, and with his family set up over two-hundred plant-based field kitchens to support peasants affected by the 1891–1892 famine that struck the Russian Empire—just as the State discouraged ordinary Russians from rendering aid. Retaliation for these autonomous actions was swift: the Tsarist secret police opened a file on Tolstoy and raided Yasnaya Polyana in 1862; the Holy Synod excommunicated him in 1901, at the behest of Metropolitan Antony of St. Petersburg, who feared a mass defection of the clergy to Tolstoyanism; and the State censored and even burned his writings, banned a lecture he had planned to give to the Russian Literature Society in 1883, and placed him under direct surveillance during the last quarter-century of his life.[124]

Forthwith, the sage began to receive death threats, including a public one raised by the Bishop of Kronstadt. In general, the Tsarist State sought to retaliate more firmly against Tolstoy's supporters than against the count himself.[125] But exceptions to this rule exist. In 1891, Lev Nikolaevich narrowly escaped imprisonment, and likely death, in the Suzdal monastery, secondary to the publication of an explicitly anti-statist essay of his in an English periodical. It was only thanks to the timely intervention of his high-ranking second cousin Alexandra Tolstaya ("Alexandrine") that his life was spared.[126] On the other hand, due to the artist's courage, example, and sacrifice during the 1891–2 famine, his popularity crested among peasants and the intelligentsia alike, with Chekhov hailing Lev Nikolaevich as a "giant and a Jupiter."[127] Ironically, Tolstoy's excommunication backfired, provoking the mass-illegal printings of the author's religious writings in the provinces of the Tsarist Empire, and elevating *Resurrection* to the highest-selling novel of the era.[128]

In so transforming himself into enemy of State and Church, Tolstoy closely followed in the steps of his relative Sergei Grigorievich Volkonsky, a Decembrist radical who was similarly monitored on a continuous basis upon his return to European Russia in 1856, after having been subjected to hard labor in Siberia for three decades. Like his distant cousin, who was saved by Alexandrine's intercession, Volkonsky only narrowly avoided the common fate of his co-conspirators—namely, execution—due to the influence of his mother. A similar story could be told about Bakunin, whose prison term the new Tsar Alexander II commuted to permanent exile in Siberia in 1857 following a personal appeal for clemency from the prisoner, plus two formal pleas for transfer submitted by his mother as his advocate.[129] Rather than support Jung's emphasis on the father-figure, then, the fates of these three Russian radicals suggests the significance of the *mother and allomother* in the destiny of the individual.[130]

Amid the "dozens of unrealized plots" Tolstoy had been composing in his final years, numerous stories with strong anarchist themes that are tied to his childhood marvel at the wonder of creation stand out prominently. Such constellations are conveyed in his 1886 short story "Ivan the Fool," which depicts a kingdom lacking armed forces, money, or intelligentsia. This realm is visited by the devil, but his project of raising an army fails "because the people refuse to pledge allegiance."[131] Plus, in correspondence with the hieromonk (or Orthodox priest-monk) John of Penza in 1907, Tolstoy openly calls for the destruction of both Church and State. His last fictional work was an untitled manuscript featuring a former hieromonk who breaks with the Church and becomes a revolutionary agitator and fighter, but who is ultimately captured and killed by the State. (As we will see in the next chapter, this plot closely follows that of *Hadji Murat* [1912].) It was this story, featuring a priest "who was converted by a free thinking man," about which the dying Tolstoy wrote his final, feverish notes in life.[132] As with the resolution of "Master and Man" (1895), when the bourgeois Brekhunov sacrifices himself by embracing the peasant Nikita to keep him warm during a winter storm, this manuscript communicates the idealization of the spiritual homosexual, who is abstinent and given to martyrdom.[133]

Employing homoerotic subtext and autobiographical disclosure in this "swan song," Lev Nikolaevich elucidates the convergence of the messianic values of the Russian intelligentsia with militant-ascetic and monastic traditions: like the monk, the hero "shuns reality, flees the world, and lives apart from actual, historical, everyday life in a world of phantoms, dreams and pious faith."[134] Yet another unfinished work at life's end includes the "Posthumous Note of the Elder Fëdor Kuzmich," which presents the writer's take on Tsar Alexander I's supposed faking of his own death—being an abdication with anarchist implications.[135]

Tolstoyan Anarchism and the Russian Revolution

Perhaps ironically, over the decades, many Russian radicals remained deeply suspicious of Tolstoy, considering him more of "a count, an officer and a reactionary" than "one of themselves," his "boldest protests against the political system, his heterodoxies, [and] his destructive nihilism," or maximalism, notwithstanding.[136] This is no doubt in part due to Lev Nikolaevich's critique of the idea of revolutionary insurrection because of the counter-violence proposed by this theory, taken together with his assumption that insurrection can only result in the reproduction of minority rule and an even worse despotism than had previously existed.[137] In *The Kingdom of God Is Within You*, the essayist observes that all historical revolutions "are merely the seizure of power by evil men and their domination over the good," while in "Thou Shalt Not Kill" (1900), the author closes ranks and implicitly criticizes Gaetano Bresci (1869–1901), an Italian-American associate of the anarcho-communist writer and activist Errico Malatesta (1853–1932), for having assassinated King Umberto I. He does so, even while recognizing that the crimes for which any State ruler is responsible are incomparably worse than "the murders committed by Anarchists."[138]

Whereas such statements likely reflect the thinker's apt critique of Jacobinism and its mimicry currents within contemporary Russian radicalism, they also presage Freud's formulation of the primal horde, whereby a stylized group of sons rise up to kill their autocratic father, only to reinstate his rule through the establishment of law, due to their guilty feelings and identificatory love for him.[139] In other words, political revolution seeks to emancipate humanity, but almost invariably ends up re-enslaving it through the establishment of new master symbols, reconstituted ruling classes, and the employment of terror. While there is no doubt, for instance, that the Orthodox Church facilitated serfdom and Tsarist despotism for centuries, these crimes may not necessarily "justify the hangman,"

> and the protests against the slavish subjection of the Church in the old kingdom of Caesar certainly cannot lead to the demand for slavish subjection to a new kingdom of Caesar, although this may call itself communist.[140]

Although such points are compelling and consistent with Lev Nikolaevich's overall affinities for anti-authoritarianism and libertarianism, Tolstoy's argument against revolution here is admittedly contrived. He perceives false continuities between "the men of Versailles" and the Parisian Communards on the one hand, and between Empress Catherine II and the insurgent peasant leader Yemelyan Pugachëv, who claimed to be Catherine's late husband, Tsar Peter III, on the other. Then again, these questionable equivalencies illuminate the intersection of Lev Nikolaevich's pacifism, ethical critique, and maximalist anti-statism. The artist believes that "[t]o seize power and retain it, it is necessary to love power. But love of power goes not with goodness but with the opposite qualities—pride, cunning, and cruelty."[141] Yet, in reality, the Paris Commune's program was decentralist, not statist, and numerous observers have lamented the Central Committee of the Commune's timid decision *not* to march on Versailles and expropriate the Bank of France.[142] In this light, for Tolstoy to dismiss the Commune is consistent with his established contrarianism and self-defeating tendencies, relative to his interest in anarchism.

However, following the abortive 1905 Russian Revolution, the thinker would revise his position somewhat, holding out the possibility that there might be a social revolution which actually could create "something quite new, such as the abolition of *all* Government," beyond simply reproducing oppression indefinitely into the future.[143] Even before the uprising, in July 1904, the thinker privately proclaimed: "One must first of all throw a certain amount off a heavily laden wagon in order to be able to overturn it. The time has come not to throw things off gradually any more, but to overturn the wagon."[144]

Tolstoy's critiques contributed profoundly to undermining the Romanov dynasty and preparing the February 1917 Revolution, which succeeded in overthrowing Tsarism, after his death.[145] In his final years, Lev Nikolaevich continued to advocate conscientious objection to military conscription and non-cooperation with Tsarism, feudalism, and capitalism, calling on his followers to refuse participation in structures of exploitation and oppression.[146] Ultimately, the sage's influence would inform the Mexican Revolution of 1910, and it was undoubtedly central to the Russian Revolution. The insurgent General Emiliano Zapata himself acknowledged Tolstoy's *Kingdom of God* as an inspiration to revolutionary movements in both Mexico and Russia.[147] In a mesmerizing way, Lev Nikolaevich's example would inspire peasants and intellectuals to establish agrarian communes after the democratic February 1917 Revolution deposed Tsarist despotism. Even in the fictional *Star Trek* universe, an allegory for cosmic communism, a twenty-fourth century Federation starship is named after Tolstoy.[148]

Estrangement, Flight, and Death

In his zeal to observe his principles, and reflecting his impulsivity and disregard for convention as a so-called "mad genius," Lev Nikolaevich, whom Kropotkin called "the most touchingly loved man in the world," paradoxically isolated himself from his friends, children, and wife at life's end.[149] Alongside sexual, psychological, and ideological conflicts in their marriage, Countess Sofia Tolstaya's opposition to her husband's emergent transition from being a "great artist" to "play[ing] at being

Robinson Crusoe" was a decisive factor in her husband's home-leaving from Yasnaya Polyana at the end of October 1910.[150] As her brother Stepan Andreevich explained, the countess "involuntarily [had] developed a dread and abhorrence" of Tolstoy's political doctrine, because it competed with her for his affection, called into question her status as wife and copyist of a world-renowned writer, and threatened her financial future, together with that of the eight surviving children she had borne the troubled artist.[151] Seeking solace from the distressing present, then, she sought to return to the more blissful past, during the early years of their marriage, when she and her husband had loved each other passionately and collaborated intimately—before the appearance, that is, of Chertkov.[152] Given her powerlessness over the course of her husband's end of life, though, she focused on how the distribution of property would affect the family's interests.

Given the circumstances, not only did Countess Tolstaya find her partner's idealization of class suicide, world-renunciation, and non-exclusive, universal love eccentric, but she also resented his attachment to his followers and well-wishers—the "dark ones"—for distracting him from his family and writing.[153] Tolstaya would often chastise her husband for paradoxically neglecting his own children through his performances as an ostensible "holy fool," as well as his championing of the rights of others. In fact, the countess viewed her husband's as a "sham Christianity, founded on hatred for those closest to you."[154] His daughter Masha, who had copied her father's writings by hand, taught peasants, served as a rural nurse, and then died of pneumonia in her father's arms at the age of 35, felt similarly aggrieved by this contradiction.[155]

In spite of the love between Lev Nikolaevich and Sofia Andreevna, and their common commitment to the causes of anti-militarism and humanism, it was apparent by the end of Tolstoy's life that his views were more radical than hers on the land question and the religious question.[156] In 1891, Tolstoy relented by transferring the rights to his works published before 1881 to his wife, and renouncing the copyright to all new writings, while giving up his estates and property in land not by returning these to the *Narod*, but rather by dividing them up among Sofia Andreevna and their children.[157]

However, these terms still did not satisfy him. The writer's final will, prepared by Vladimir Chertkov three months before the artist left home for the last time, and signed in secrecy, stipulated that *all* his literary works should be transferred to his daughter Alexandra, Chertkov's closest ally in the family. However, the question of the will opened an unsolvable rift within its signatory himself, who agonized about how it would effectively divest his wife from being his literary heir. At the same time, he did not choose to either tell her about it *or* destroy it. Tormented by this dilemma, "t[orn] to pieces" by Chertkov's bullying, and longing to consummate his renunciatory-homoerotic ideal either in the Optina Pustin monastery or with his communist followers in the Caucasus, Lev Nikolaevich ultimately chose to sacrifice his marriage and commitment to heterosexual life—both of which had caused him such torment for so long—to observe his solidarity with the malnourished peasantry and embrace his identity as a "militant monk."[158]

The well-known result of Tolstoy's flight from Yasnaya Polyana in late October 1910 was his death of pneumonia ten days later near the Astapovo train station.[159] Truly, the pathos of this moment brings to mind the literary-historical deaths of Anna Karenina *and* Jesus the Nazarene, being "voyage[s] into madness, terror, absurdity, and self-dispossession."[160] In Feinermann's cinematic depiction, *The Departure of a Grand Old Man* (1912), the final straw was Tolstoy's learning of the physical abuse of a peasant mother and child perpetrated by the Circassian guard Akhet, whom Sofia Andreevna had hired to enforce her dominion over the land.[161] According to his own diaries, though, the elder decided to abandon home over indignation at his wife's rustling through his papers and surveillance of his person, supposedly for reasons of health.[162] Leaving Yasnaya Polyana in the middle of the night on his 82nd birthday, rather like the Hadji Murat he so admired, the elder had not planned to reconcile with the Orthodox Church. Instead, he sought finally to bring his existence into relative accord with his ascetic ideals, by living simply, praying, meditating, and continuing to write.

Toward these ends, he reunited at the Shamordino Convent with his sister Marya Nikolaevna, who had become a nun in 1889 over grief at the loss of her son Nikolai.[163] Opting to see his sister first before boarding a train southbound to the Caucasus, from where he might try to leave the Empire, the imperious sage contradicted the recommendations of his physician Dushan Makovitsky, who had proposed that they travel south straightaway.[164] Inescapably, from a medical point of view, Tolstoy's flight was high-risk, for he had been suffering from seizures in the run-up to his departure.[165] Caught in a rainstorm while awaiting a railway transfer before visiting with Marya one last time, the sage contracted pneumonia and died within days in Ryazan province at the home of the Astapovo station-master, who was himself a follower of the writer's, in the presence of Chertkov, his physicians, and his children Sasha, Tanya, and Sergei. After all, the antibiotics used to treat bacterial infections would not be discovered until nearly two decades after his death.

Just as the infantile Lev had unsuccessfully resisted the feeling of being bound by swaddling clothes, so could his elder self not realize his wishes: specifically, to end his life in poverty and tranquility, much less live to see a free society.[166] In reality, Tolstoy's status as Stranger persisted—with brief respites—from cradle to grave.[167] The man expired "in agony, oppressed by the burden of […] his sense of perpetual moral error": "the most tragic of the great writers, a desperate old man," who wandered to his death in the countryside, observing the *Strannik* ideal, like a Russian King Lear.[168]

That being said, during his life review with his sister Masha, as imagined by Feinermann, Tolstoy takes pride in his work to promote peasant education, his boot-making apprenticeship under a *muzhik*, and agricultural labor—but not marriage or family life.[169] In Astapovo, the moribund Lev Nikolaevich began transcribing a French motto in his final diary entry: *Fais ce dois, adv…* ("Do what's right, come what may"). Such lucid Kantianism synergized with the man's characteristic Rousseauvism to produce Tolstoy's loud pronouncement, the day before passing away, that "there are many other people besides Lev Tolstoy in this world, and you only attend to Lev!"[170]

The artist rendered homage to Enlightenment *philosophe* Voltaire (1694–1778), the "apostle of humanity," in refusing to reconcile with the abbot sent by the Holy Synod—although his caretakers did not appear to give him a choice either way. He remained true to his own concern with intoxicated states of consciousness by resisting morphine analgesia, and sought both peace and escape through consummation of his own finitude.[171] Ultimately, Tolstoy's end of life conveyed the artist's ideal of revolutionary suicide, or "what those who were revolted, like him, [...] ought to do."[172]

According to the Tolstoyan scholar L. D. Gromova-Opul'skaia (b. 1925), the artist's death and departure represented a protest against both Church and State, as well as the teacher's own family, who did not "sufficiently value [him] as a creative force."[173] Then again, shocked by her husband's flight, Sofia Andreevna attempted to drown herself in the pond near their home. Rescued by Sasha and Bulgakov, she survived, and hired a private train to transport herself, three of her children, a nurse, a psychiatrist, and some servants from Tula to Astapovo. Barred by Chertkov and company from seeing her husband, who was not informed of her presence until the very end, the countess was tragically permitted to visit him only once he had lost consciousness for the last time.[174] Despite the lines of Gromova-Opul'skaia and Chertkov, Tolstoy in his final letter to his wife writes, "I love and pity you with all my heart, but I can't do otherwise than as I am doing."[175] In keeping with these dual feelings of fear and sympathy, there is no doubt that the countess was on Tolstoy's mind in his final days.[176]

Tolstoy's Funeral and Burial

After Lev Nikolaevich Tolstoy passed away in the Astapovo station-master's home on November 7, 1910, the State quickly mobilized to transfer his body by special locomotive to the sole place that would accept his body. Owing to his excommunication by the Holy Synod and consequent denial—like Voltaire—of either a Christian funeral or burial, Tolstoy could only be interred at Yasnaya Polyana.[177] During this moving pilgrimage signifying an entrance into existential time, or what the anarcha-feminist writer Ursula Le Guin calls the "joining of temporal and eternal," thousands paid their last respects to the artist, having traveled to the Zaseka station near Yasnaya Polyana by day and night, even in the freezing cold, to be physically present.[178] Multitudes rendered homage to the prose writer at each station through which the train bearing Tolstoy's corpse passed.[179] Upon the carriage's arrival to the last station, Tolstoy's sons transferred his coffin to the peasants, who would bury him the following day in his final resting place of the *zaseka*, near his brother Nikolai's fabled "green stick."

In Moscow, news of the prose poet's death led to widespread wildcat strikes, the closure of theaters, student demonstrations, marches, processions, and public calls for the abolition of the death penalty, as of the corporal punishment meted out against political prisoners in Siberia.[180] Whereas the Holy Synod banned all memorial services for Tolstoy, Tsar Nicholas II, the Duma, and the Council of State hypocritically mourned his death.[181] Nicholas reportedly feared an uprising, such that he ordered the reinforcement of the police and militias, and the imposition of strict censorship.[182]

Remarkably, all of Lev Nikolaevich's kith and kin were present at his funeral: along with his immediate family, his extended family of the *Narod* and common people, including peasants, factory workers, and intellectuals, as well as aristocrats, of all ages. Villagers from Yasnaya Polyana maintained a vigil throughout the night, anticipating the nocturnal bonfires of the February Days of 1917, which would keep the anti-Tsarist street-fighting crowds warm. A local peasant remarked that the night after Tolstoy's passing was reminiscent of Easter, when Orthodox Christians typically stay up all night to celebrate the symbolic idea of resurrection. As during the future Revolution, "[o]ne had the sense of a miracle close by, next to you, around you."[183]

Five thousand mourners paid their last respects before the artist's burial took place the following afternoon. These included two local *muzhiki*, who brandished a banner emblazoned with the following eulogy: "Lev Nikolaevich! The Memory of Your Goodness Will not Die Amongst the Orphaned Peasants of Yasnaya Polyana!"[184] Tolstoy's internment was accompanied by the common singing of "Eternal Memory," but, in accordance with Sofia Andreevna's instructions, no speeches were made, much less was a religious service held. There were no priests or icons present. Hence, even in death, Lev Nikolaevich "pointed the way to a new world."[185]

Notes

1 Figes and Kolonitskii 74–5.
2 In an expression of Christian piety, Aline would customarily redistribute her money, maintain a simple diet, and disregard her physical appearance (Bartlett 2011: 41–2).
3 Anderson 10–11.
4 Berdyaev 1966: 58; Bartlett 2011: 332–3; Figes 2002: 371–6.
5 Rancour-Laferriere 1995: 21–8; Clark 2019: 301; Gerth and Mills 276.
6 Foster R.
7 Kropotkin 1991: 110–11.
8 Cervantes 25–7.
9 Kusters.
10 Cervantes 507; Becker 220; Atterbury; Berdyaev 2009; Efird.
11 Shantz and Williams 165; Gerth and Mills 298–301; Nelson.
12 Петлянова.
13 Al Yafai; Dare; Aldris.
14 Shantz and Williams 107; Berdyaev 2009: 24–8, 49–52, 67, 139–53; 1 Corinthians 6; Dodds.
15 Artukoglu and Szejko. Compare the guide's lamentation to *Izvestia* no. 10 (March 12, 1921), written by Kronstadt rebels days before the Bolsheviks drowned their Commune in blood: "Russia in its entirety has been transformed into an immense prison" (Voline 512).
16 Poole 106, emphasis in original; Medzhibovskaya 2004.
17 Berdyaev 2009; Berlin 1999; Pietikainen 11; Stites 1989; Bulgakov 34.
18 Sloane 1991: 20.
19 Byrd 124.
20 Sternhell 123; Knapp 1991: 25n2.
21 Plato 2015: 73, 121; Plato 360 BCE; Gilman-Opalsky 81.
22 Bartlett 2011: 48, 77–8; Stites 1989; Hall 143.
23 Triandis.
24 Turgenev 1878a.

25 Bartlett 2011: 285–6.
26 Horner; Lundskow; Bulgakov 38; Clark 2013.
27 Bartlett 2011: 238.
28 Medzhibovskaya 2004: 20.
29 Medzhibovkaya 2005: 49.
30 Bartlett 2011: 342; Berdyaev 1966: 131.
31 Berdyaev 2009: 61–71.
32 Figes 2002: 79.
33 Bartlett 2011: 118.
34 Rancour-Laferriere 1995: 30, 43; 1998: 20–1.
35 Tolstoy 1985: 221; Denner 2011: 97.
36 Freud 1953: 420, 427.
37 Zorin 7–8; Maude 1987a: 11.
38 Maude 1987: 10–11.
39 Rancour-Laferriere 1995: 96.
40 Freud 2016: 81–2; Freud 1961b: 32–9; de Lauretis.
41 Benjamin 5; Freud 2013: 107–8.
42 Rancour-Laferriere 1995: 49–50, 96; Chodorow 1999; Lundskow; Fromm 1969: 163–5.
43 Rancour-Laferriere 1995: xi, 116–19.
44 *Ibid* 53.
45 Maude 1987a: 199; Chancer 2020; Freud 2016: 72.
46 Zorin 12–13.
47 Reitz 60, 122–3; McLaughlin 159.
48 Freud 1995: 278.
49 Pietikainen 90.
50 Byrd and Miri 2.
51 Benjamin.
52 Evtuhov et al. 362; Maude 1987a: 44–55; Berdyaev 2009.
53 Orwin 1993: 208.
54 Gustafson 1986: 272.
55 Darrow and Lewis 2003: 85.
56 Maude 1987b: 111.
57 Spiegel 230; Békés et al.
58 Benjamin 19–21.
59 Maude 1987a: 59–60.
60 Struve 118; Stites 1989.
61 CNT.
62 Malia 363.
63 Berdyaev 1966: 20, 65; Bulgakov 27–8; Berlin 1978: 18–19; Figes and Kolonitskii 6; Gerth and Mills.
64 Kobrin; Jameson 241.
65 Gustafson 1986: 16.
66 Kokobobo; Békés et al.; Chodorow 1999: 260.
67 Bartlett 2011: 48, 59; Zorin 32; Gustafson 1986: 33.
68 Maude 1987a: 88.
69 Maude 1987b: 86.
70 Gustafson 1986: 392, 453.
71 Zorin 182.
72 Berlin 1978: 27–8; Orwin 2002d: xii.
73 Gustafson 1986: xiii.
74 Knapp 2002: 161–2.
75 Orwin 2002c: 235; Figes 2002: 342.
76 Gustafson 1986: xiv, 7 (emphasis added).
77 Orwin 2002d: 235; Orwin 1993: 217; Gustafson 1986: 5.
78 Orwin 1993: 211; 2002: 57–8.

79 Maude 1987a: 18.
80 Newlin 367 (emphasis added).
81 Maude 1987b: 177; Zorin 205; Newlin 367.
82 Bartlett 2011: 53–4; Maude 1987a: 19; Gustafson 1986: 9.
83 Wesson 345; Stites 1989: 206.
84 Harding.
85 Newlin.
86 Bartlett 2011: 17–18. Similarly, the Bolshevik State would banish followers of Tolstoy and rebellious Kronstadt sailors to the Solovetsky islands, and kill bishops and priests there, after the October 1917 Revolution (Berdyaev 1966: 167).
87 Newlin; Gustafson 1986.
88 Rancour-Laferriere 1998: 49.
89 Bartlett 2011: 78; Figes 2002: 353.
90 Figes 2002: 83, 119–30; Herzen.
91 Evtuhov et al. 378.
92 Bartlett 2011: 40–63, 136.
93 Tolstoy 1960.
94 Tolstoy 1987: 231n4.
95 Becker 13–20, 87.
96 *Ibid*; Chancer 1992; Solomon et al.; Benjamin.
97 Becker 209; Solomon et al. x–9.
98 Solomon et al. 68–84, 221; Hrdy 20.
99 Christoyannopoulos 2006; Kropotkin 1991, 142–4 (emphasis in original); Orwin 2002a: 50.
100 Tolstoy 2004: 256; Rancour-Laferriere 1998: 31–2.
101 Becker 7; Tillich 42; Maude 1987b: 220.
102 Tolstoy 1987: 8, 231n5; Maude 1987a: 241–77.
103 Bartlett 2011: 48, 144–6, 198.
104 Gustafson 1986; Maude 1987a: 267–8.
105 Kropotkin 1991: 127.
106 Berdyaev 1966: 43–70.
107 Figes 2002: 238–9; Bartlett 2011: 144–5.
108 Orwin 2002a: 51; Zorin 48–9; Maude 1987a: 236.
109 Maude 1987a: 207–23; 1987b: 450.
110 Bartlett 2011: 197–218.
111 Polosina 60.
112 Kropotkin 1991, 151; Tolstoy 1987: 8; Bartlett 2011: 9, 140, 211–13; Maude 1987a: 342–3; 1987b: 89–199; Gustafson 1986; Sizova.
113 Maude 1987b: 118.
114 Tolstoy 2010: 1279.
115 Orwin 2002a: 50; Kropotkin 1991: 138 (emphasis in original).
116 Tolstoy 1942: 76.
117 Habermas 1981: 158.
118 Tolstoy 1886: 75; Aslan. After all, Paul was an apologist for slavery (Griffin).
119 Kropotkin 1991: 149–152.
120 *Ibid* 154 (emphasis in original).
121 Pelikan 209.
122 Romans 13: 1–7.
123 Maude 1987b: 39; Aslan.
124 Zorin 138; Bartlett 2011: 147, 290–387; Christoyannopoulos 2011: 203–4; Maude 1987b: 303; Figes 2002: 353–4; Pelikan 212; Orwin 2002a: 56; Johansson 1990s. To this day, in fact, Tolstoy remains excommunicated in Russia (Zolotov).
125 Figes 2002: 343–4; Bartlett 2011: 365–411.
126 Maude 1987b: 314–17.
127 Zorin 140.

128 Figes 2002: 343–4.
129 *Ibid* 90, 143; Leier 152; Goodwin 54.
130 Heuer; Hrdy.
131 Bartlett 2011: 333; Jahn 120.
132 Becker 50; Medzhibovskaya 2010: 17–20.
133 Tolstoy 2005: 271–9; Bullock 105.
134 Grant and Wade-Benzoni 613; Frank 150–1.
135 Medzhibovskaya 2010: 21.
136 Berlin 1978: 54.
137 Tolstoy 1960: 54–5, 234; Berdyaev 1966: 72.
138 Tolstoy 1960: 291; 1900; Bartlett 2011: 346).
139 Benjamin 143–4.
140 Berdyaev 1966: 175, 190–5.
141 Tolstoy 1960: 287–8.
142 Shafer.
143 Maude 1987b: 447 (emphasis in original).
144 Tolstoy 1985: 378.
145 Tolstoy 1987: 9; Berdyaev 1966: 174.
146 Kropotkin 1991: 157.
147 Zapata.
148 Roddenberry et al.
149 Johansson 1990a; Maude 1987b: 71; Fink et al.
150 Maude 1987b: 152.
151 Zorin 122–6, 197. In a January 1895 diary entry, Sofia Andreevna remarks, "I cannot help complaining that the things he preaches for people's happiness complicate life so much that it becomes harder and harder for me" (Maude 1987b: 540).
152 Parini 68.
153 Hamburg 123; LeBlanc 1993: 26.
154 LeBlanc 1993: 26.
155 Orwin 1993: 144; Bartlett 2011: 189–234, 311, 367–405; Maude 1987b: 237, 449.
156 Parini 137; Tolstaia 577–8, 646.
157 Zorin 142; Bartlett 2011: 5, 331.
158 Maude 1987b: 174, 235–76, 434–506; LeBlanc 1993: 27; Johansson 1990j; Johansson 1990p; Medzhibovskaya 2004: 26; Kropotkin 1991: 161; Книжный чел. In parallel, the gay Ukrainian writer Nikolai Gogol visited Optina Pustin on numerous occasions toward the end of his life (Rancour-Laferriere 1995: 27–8; Karlinsky).
159 Bartlett 2011: x, 4.
160 Eagleton 23.
161 Teneromo; Parini 141–2.
162 Tolstoy 1985: 469–70.
163 Bartlett 2011: x, 280.
164 Maude 1987b: 508; Zorin 202.
165 Parini 35, 217–18.
166 Zorin 7–8.
167 Gustafson 1986: 15.
168 Berlin 1978: 81.
169 Teneromo.
170 Zorin 205–10.
171 *Ibid*; Shafer 166; Maude 1987b: 510–13.
172 Kropotkin 1991: 163; Newton.
173 Gromova-Opul'skaia 2000: 80–2.
174 Tolstaia 648; Zorin 206–7; Parini 270–5.
175 Parini 243.
176 Maude 1987b: 512; Tolstoy 1985: 471.
177 Bartlett 2011: 413.

178 Le Guin 263.
179 Berdyaev 2009; Maude 1987b: 518.
180 Bartlett 2011: 413–15; Parini 283; Maude 1987b: 516.
181 Maude 1987b: 516.
182 Parini 282–3.
183 Figes and Kolonitskii 34, 42.
184 Bartlett 2011: 414.
185 *Ibid*; Parini 284.

4

HUMANISM, MILITARISM, AND IMPERIALISM IN *THE COSSACKS* AND *HADJI MURAT*

In this chapter, we will examine the humanistic, queer, and anti-imperialist themes that are present in two Tolstoyan novels about the Caucasus: namely, *The Cossacks* (1863) and *Hadji Murat* (1912).

As Tolstoy's first major success, the autobiographical work *The Cossacks* recounts the author's experiences fighting in the Russian military in Transcaucasia from 1851–1854, during the Russo-Caucasus War (1817–1864). The 24-year-old aristocrat and cadet Dmitri Andreich Olenin, the writer's double, whose name means "of the stag" or "deer" (олень), decides to abandon life in Moscow to be reassigned to the Eastern Caucasus following the failure of a heterosexual relationship.[1] Olenin has—much like Tolstoy at his age—never graduated from university, "chosen any career or ever [...] done anything much at all." Thus, he is an anti-hero, and the "typical Tolstoyan Stranger": "dull," "unhealthy," and a veritable "nightmare," in the estimation of Ivan Turgenev.[2]

On the other hand, the posthumously published *Hadji Murat* celebrates the robust titular character, based on his real-life counterpart (1818–1852), who was a Sufi Muslim Avar chieftain and *naib*, or lieutenant, to the anti-colonial Imam Shamil (1797–1871). As Avars, a "nomadic proto-Turkish people" who had migrated in the sixth century CE from Central Asia to the Eastern Caucasus, Murat and Shamil led the resistance during the Russo-Caucasus War, in which Tolstoy also fought—that is, on the other side.[3] The Dagestani insurgency against Russian imperialism was carried out by so-called *murids*, or Sufi militants, whose leaders (*murshids*) united the Chechens and Avars in a *jihad*. This resistance thrived for decades, in part due to the Russians' lack of familiarity with local geography.[4] Conveying Tolstoyan sympathy for these anti-imperialist struggles, as well as the cause of collective liberation, *Hadji Murat* expands on *The Cossacks*' condemnation of power politics and implicit avowal of self-determination for oppressed peoples. Plus, it appears to have a homoerotic origin story.

DOI: 10.4324/9781003328964-4

In his diary, Tolstoy explains that he was spurred to write the story after encountering a broken crimson "Tatar" thistle in the plowed fields. He remarks on the great "energy and life force" with which the injured flower had resisted his picking of it, and marvels at how this phallic substitute had stuck out and "defended its life to the end, alone in the midst of the whole field."[5] Here, Tolstoy is expressing admiration for his titular character, while also evidently describing himself, too, as a courageous but unaligned and out of place rebel.[6] While the artist's passionate attraction to Murat provides evidence for the close ties Freud perceived between self-love and gayness, in favor of the idea that "like attracts like," it also recalls his youthful bond with the Chechen Sado Miserbiyev, favoring the thesis that the "exotic becomes erotic."[7]

The Cossacks

The setting of the opening chapter of *The Cossacks* establishes the tale within the continuum of Russian tales about journeys to ostensibly "undiscovered lands." This tradition spans the aristocratic rebel Alexander Radishchev's (1749–1802) revolutionary denunciation of serfdom in the *Journey from Moscow to St. Petersburg* (1790); Ilya Repin's (1844–1930) momentous travels down the Volga River in the summer of 1870, during which he met the haulers who would serve as the subjects of the stark *Volga Barge Haulers* (1873) painting (see Figure 4.1); and the summer of 1874, when thousands of student radicals "went to the People" with an ill-fated revolutionary project.[8] In this way, the beginning of *The Cossacks* is almost reminiscent of the outset of Ernesto "Che" Guevara's *Motorcycle Diaries* (1951–1952), as the future revolutionary's bourgeois relatives and friends see him off before his life-changing journeys.[9] Curiously, Peter Kropotkin's *Siberian Diaries* (1862–1867) open in a similar way to Tolstoy's novella, as the cadet soon feels relieved upon abandoning St. Petersburg—much as Olenin does, after leaving Moscow.[10]

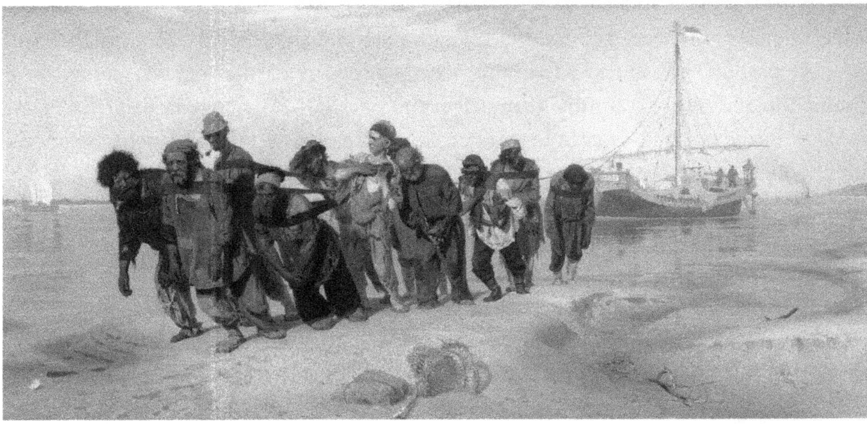

FIGURE 4.1 Ilya Repin, *Volga Barge Haulers* (1873)

The Cossacks of the Don, Volga, and Dnieper River basins, whose name is derived from the Turkic word *quzzaq* ("horseman," "guard," or "freeman"), represent communities of former serfs who had fled central Russia during the epoch of Moscow's State formation in the fifteenth through seventeenth centuries (see Map 1 above).[11] In southern Russia, Ukraine, and the Caucasus, on the frontiers of the Tsarist Empire, Cossacks founded self-governed "exilic spaces" instituting an "anti-bureaucratic," though colonial and patriarchal, socio-political and economic system.[12] Renowned as folk heroes who fought against Mongol and Ottoman slavers of Ukrainians, steppe-dwelling Cossacks created forms of "semi-anarchy on the fringes of organized society" that resembled piracy both through their democratic forms of self-rule and their defiant rejection of Russian and Turkic forms of bonded labor.[13]

Indeed, the Grebensk Cossacks whom Tolstoy joined were descended from Old Believers, otherwise known as sectarians, who had repudiated the centralizing ecclesiastical reforms imposed by the "Great Sovereign" Patriarch Nikon in the seventeenth century. This schism would split Orthodox Christianity in two. It was common among such Dissenters to view Tsar Peter I as the Anti-Christ, and many Old Believers joined the insurrection against serfdom led by Pugachëv from 1773–1774.[14] In *War and Peace*, the hero Prince Andrei Bolkonsky meditates on the southbound murmurations of serf families, as they fled the landlords' manors to establish new lives among "warm rivers," thus echoing the defection of sailors to pirates, and foreshadowing the utopian communes founded after the February 1917 Revolution.[15]

As autobiography and allegory, Olenin's trek south from central Russia presents "a Rousseau[v]ean, wish-fulfilling fantasy of a return to an Edenic state of innocence and purity" among the "savage beauty" of mountains and forests; the ostensibly natural, simple ways and beauty of the Peoples of the Caucasus; and the prospect of bisexual experimentation.[16] After all, the protagonist's identification with wandering deer reflects the author's "vague, voluptuous hope of catching *someone* in the bushes."[17] Lev Nikolaevich's story provoked shock through the contrast it establishes between the artifice and meaninglessness of the Russian Empire, symbolized by the noble Olenin's privilege, and the beauty of nature and the freedom and simplicity of Cossack peasant life.[18] As Rosamund Bartlett observes, the novella serves as a "metaphor of Tolstoy's spiritual journey in the decade before his marriage."[19]

At the story's outset, Olenin leaves behind the hypocrisy of his Moscow relations, and the enslavement and class exploitation his previous life had required, such that "the nearer he drew to the Caucasus, the happier his mood became."[20] He renounces convention to pursue truth: through estrangement and exile, he paradoxically seeks residence.[21] The novella can therefore be said to reflect Tolstoy's own putative encounters with a "God of Love *and* Reason" in the Caucasus, as well as to manifest Lev Nikolaevich's affinities for the well-known Russian idealist N. V. Stankevich's affirmation of a "religion of love."[22] Beyond being spatially remote from Moscow and St. Petersburg, the "rural idyll" in *The Cossacks*—located in "Novomlinsk," Tolstoy's name for the Starogladovskaya village in present-day Chechnya—is also depicted as *temporally* distant from these metropolitan centers.[23]

Perhaps ironically, then, the Russian cadet Olenin "seeks to merge with a hospitable 'primitive' [*sic*] culture which strikes him as being more natural and authentic than the sophisticated culture of his homeland."[24] Just as the migration of Russian peasants south and the forging of exilic Cossack spaces depended on the displacement of indigenous peoples, so does Olenin seek to flock to Transcaucasia, in search of a different life.[25] At the outset of the story, he is less conscious of the colonial dynamics whereby the Kremlin lords over the Caucasus, Tatarstan, Siberia, and the Arctic, but will soon be rudely awakened in Chechnya.[26]

Considering the novella's Romantic and internationalist dimensions, and its portrayal of Transcaucasia, being "one of the most beautiful regions" in the world, it is unsurprising that *The Cossacks* should have inspired Ernest Hemingway's "The Snows of Kilimanjaro" (1936) and *For Whom the Bell Tolls* (1940).[27] As for Tolstoy's own influences, scholar Philip Rogers shows how *The Cossacks* shares much in common with Johann Wolfgang von Goethe's *Sorrows of the Young Werther* (1774), in that both art-works concern themselves with "the failed quest" which the "young man of superior intellect and sensitivity" must confront.[28]

Thematically, *The Cossacks* can be considered a borderland romance, or a borderland counter-romance.[29] Lev Nikolaevich portrays the Eastern Caucasus as a contact zone in the encounter between imperial power and indigenous life. The Cossacks, having abolished serfdom among themselves, appear internally democratic and anarchic compared with Tsarist feudalism. Still, the main contradiction of Cossack autonomy—as Tolstoy recognizes—is that it based itself on serving the Tsarist State's imperialist aims of violently dominating and exploiting the Chechen, Ingush, Nogai, Avar, Adyghe (or Circassian), and Tatar peoples living in the Don and Volga basins, Crimea, and the Caucasus mountains. Like Mongol overlords of yore, who intermingled with their Rus' subjects, the Grebensk Cossacks in Tolstoy's story have adopted Circassian dress, intermarried with the Chechens, and taken up local customs, including the *kunak* system of honorary kinship or comradeship (see Figure 4.2).[30]

In 1763, following up on its conquest of the Tatar khanates, the Russian Empire under Catherine II had begun expanding into the northern Caucasus region. Initially, this aggression primarily targeted the Kabardian tribes of eastern Circassia, and did not include the western tribes or the northeast Caucasus (see Map 1).[31] Yet, following the example of Paul I, who annexed Georgia in 1801, Tsars Alexander I, Nicholas I, and Alexander II aimed to vanquish the mountain peoples of Transcaucasia, most of whom had converted to Islam centuries prior, in a bid to link the Christians of Georgia to the Empire.[32] The subsequent Russo-Caucasus War would be marked by genocidal crimes against the Adyghe by Russian forces—including Cossack settlers—under the command of Generals Sergei A. Bulgakov (?–1824) and Alexei P. Yermolov (1777–1861), who annihilated approximately half of all Circassians.[33]

Despite this violent context, upon arrival to the Don River basin, Olenin remarks at the friendliness of "[a]ll the Cossacks," and how there is no need to consider social class when "jok[ing] and chat[ting]" with them. Even so, prior to arriving at his destination, the protagonist has imaginatively anticipated *both* achieving "glory" for the Russian military by slaying numerous "mountaineers," *and* himself defecting to become one of those mountaineers, thus "helping them to defend their independence against the Russians."[34] As such, we see the "common birthmarks" of Mikhail Lermontov's (1814–1841) poem "Izmail Bey" (1832) in Olenin's dichotomous thought-process, considering that the Romantic writer identified with the Adyghe Prince Izmail Bey, who is persecuted and ultimately assassinated by the allies of the same Russian military which both he and Tolstoy served.[35] Besides thinking about merging with the resistance to Russian imperialism, Olenin has fantasized about "the dream of a woman," initially imagining a "Circassian slave girl" whom he might formally educate and integrate into his former salon life in Moscow, before dismissing the idea as absurd upon reaching the host of the Terek River Grebensk Cossacks in Chechnya.[36]

In point of fact, the Adyghe muse conjuring Olenin may allude to the renowned poet Alexander Pushkin and Lermontov's own renderings of "The Prisoner of the Caucasus" (1822 and 1860, respectively), wherein a Russian officer is captured by an Adyghe militia but then assisted in his escape by a local woman who has fallen in love with him.[37] Below, we shall see that, as with the treatment of combat in the revolutionary "Sevastopol Sketches," Tolstoy's humanistic writings defamiliarize the stylized, mythological approach to the Caucasus previously established by Pushkin and Lermontov in the White-Russian imagination.[38]

Olenin's Revulsion at Colonial Violence, and Self-Discovery in the Stag's Lair

Within the Eastern Caucasus region, in the artist's reconstruction, Grebensk Cossack settlements are separated from those of the Muslim Chechens by the Terek River, and raids against the host from "*Abreks*" ("hostile" Chechens) are expected regularly. As frontier guards serving Tsarist imperialism, the male Grebensk Cossacks rotate duties at observation posts, using vertical power to surveil the indigenous population.[39] Lukashka, a striking young Cossack with whom Olenin will become *kunak* (or "comrade"), kills a Chechen "Abrek" trying to cross the Terek at night, much to the necrophilic pleasure of his Cossack comrades-in-arms.[40] Lukashka is expected to be awarded a medal for this act, and gains prestige as an eligible bachelor after having done so.[41]

For all this, Tolstoy realistically exposes and therefore implicitly critiques the objectification and dehumanization of the Other demanded by this process of in-group cohesion, which functions to serve Russian expansionism, without omitting the dynamic's homoerotic dimensions. Reflecting animalistic dehumanization and imperial ultraviolence, Lukashka's comrades refer to the murdered *djigit* (warrior, or brave) as a "fine fish" and a "nice brown one, too!" At the same time, admiring the body of the "Abrek," Lukashka tragically acknowledges, "He was a man, too!"[42]

When the deceased *djigit*'s brother crosses the Terek to accept his brother's corpse, the Chechen's morose contempt starkly contrasts with the "[l]aughter and joking" exhibited by the Cossacks. Being "alone among the Cossacks" in expressing compassion for the humanity of the Chechen and his brother, Olenin inquires about his Muslim neighbor's family through the interpreter, and comes to learn that, of the family's five brothers, the Russians had now killed three.[43] This experience leads him to a remarkably internationalist and Christian-anarchist realization:

> "What nonsense and muddle is this?" he thought. "A man kills another, and is happy, content, as though he'd performed the most magnificent deed. Is there really nothing to tell him that there is no cause for great joy in this? That happiness lies not in killing, but in sacrificing oneself?"[44]

While sympathetic toward the social freedom practiced by the Grebensk Cossacks of the Terek River, Tolstoy criticizes the settler-colonial dispossession they serve. Taken together with the author's loving portrayal of the Avar militant *Hadji Murat* (1912), as we will see below, Tolstoy's attitude toward Great-Russian imperialism appears more critical than ambivalent, as literary historian Anthony Anemone asserts.[45] In Freudian terms, Tolstoy resolved his war neuroses by affirming his peaceful ego and repudiating the imposed martial superego.[46] In this vein, Olenin's internal epiphany about Cossack violence opens a psychical door that will ultimately lead the protagonist to abandon his hosts. After all, the Cossacks had internalized the Mongol Empire's militarism, and they participated in all of the wars waged by Tsarist Russia between the eighteenth and twentieth centuries. During the Russian Civil War and on the Eastern Front in World War II, they fought for the Soviet State *and* its White and Nazi enemies.[47] Accordingly, the legacy of Cossack aggression has undoubtedly influenced the "Ruscism," or Russian fascism, that the post-Soviet Kremlin has unleashed in Chechnya, Syria, and Ukraine.[48]

Olenin's moment of clarity on the banks of the Terek River closely mirrors the youth's earlier experience in a stag's lair, when "conscience and consciousness come directly to [him] from nature," as Tolstoy's ego-persona "discovers the Earth."[49] During one afternoon of this "rural odyssey," while out hunting pheasants and so "mortify[ing] his flesh" with the retired Cossack "Uncle" Yeroshka—his mentor, father-figure, and possibly, elder male lover—Olenin and Yeroshka happen upon an elderly stag, frightening him away.[50] The next morning, Olenin returns just with his dog to the same place. After killing a number of pheasants, the protagonist suddenly undergoes an all-encompassing, oceanic feeling. The narrator remarks on the "outrageously lavish vegetation, this vast array of birds and beasts that filled the forest, this dark foliage, this hot, pungent air, these channels of muddy water that everywhere seeped from the Terek [...]."[51]

Basking in such embryonic and eco-sexual imagery, Olenin appears to be atoning for his violence against avian life. He encounters biophilia, or love of life, and nature as a *kalokagathon*: the unification of goodness, truth, and beauty.[52] The youth then enters the stag's lair, that "dark" and "damp place," where his initial experiences are suggestive of Nirvana, or embryonic life, when the "sums of excitation" are "ke[pt] as low as possible."[53] "He felt cool, comfortable; there was nothing in his mind, he had no desires."[54] In this remarkable scene, which discloses transitional, experimental space, "true prayer" and inner transformation help clarify

Olenin's identity and vocation.[55] Here, the implicit Kantian elements of the search for truth within oneself and in nature are truly palpable.[56] As he activates the "cool cognitive system" and reflects on death, Olenin experiences enhanced pro-social feelings.[57]

Applying a Frommian analysis, we discern that Tolstoy has intuitively chosen, as a young man, to embrace "freedom through ethical behavior" as an ideal, rather than affirm conformity, escapism, or sadistic oppression as answers to one's individuation-separation and death-anxiety.[58] He needed physical and psychological distance from the Cossack group to come to this conclusion. If only momentarily, the hero successfully discovers the importance of "*express[ing] his faculties in relation to the world rather than in his need to use the world as a means for [his] satisfaction.*"[59]

By identifying with his "beautiful" namesake the stag, in whose lair he is resting contemplatively, Olenin discovers both his individuality and his love for, and interconnectedness with, the rest of nature, at the same time as he confronts his common mortality with all other suffering beings. Through awareness of his finitude and the unity of all things, Olenin awakens like the young fictional pilgrim-prince Sudhana—who becomes a disciple of Guanyin, the Buddhist goddess of compassion—to "fin[d] kinship with all living beings."[60] Specifically, Tolstoy divines the will to relatedness and the legacy of his mother, Marya Volkonskaya, bringing to mind a more peaceful and loving context, relative to the bleakness of imperialist expansionism.[61] In this experience of metaphysical unity, reunion, and re-enchantment, Olenin recalls early life as a young infant, before the completion of the first stage of separation-individuation, which is typically experienced between the fourth and eighth months of life.[62] The hallowed dimensions of his time in the stag's lair, being linked to the memory of his late mother, follow logically in the psychoanalytic sense of exhibiting a desire for connection and symbiosis.

Contemplating his nature as a finite being, and thinking back to early life, in symbiosis with Princess Volkonskaya and his wet-nurse Avdotia Ziabreva, Olenin recalls Yeroshka's wise observation that "the grass will grow on your grave, and that's it," and so decides that he must be happy and "live in the best way."[63] Anticipating Pierre Bezukhov's outlook after his participation as an observer during the momentous battle of Borodino in *War and Peace*, the cadet concludes that the best way to live is through observing the Christian law of love.[64] In mindfully appreciating his own vulnerability and "oneness with the absolute," Olenin's compassionate commitment to (re)union with the Other is reinforced.[65]

"And is there any point in living for oneself," he thought, "when very soon one may die, and die without having done any good, and in such a way that no one will ever know?"[66]

Upon Olenin's exit from the stag's lair, the scene reveals itself as an allegory for the meaning of life in the face of death, as for the idealized "natural self outside of social regulation."[67] Psychologically, Olenin's new heroic self-concept emerges from a meditative encounter with the abyss of mortality.[68] It confirms the psychiatrist Stephanie Engel's view that the "call back to the memory of original narcissistic bliss pushes us toward a dream of the future."[69] The cadet is shown to be lost, and cannot find his companion dog; the night approaches, and the wind rages. The moon is hidden, as the sky is covered in clouds. Olenin fears capture or death at the hands of the Chechens. In Freudian terms, we thus see how the experience of the Nirvana principle in the cave "expresses the trend of the death instinct," or Thanatos.[70] Soon enough, though, he will find a tributary of the Terek and reunite with his dog, and thereafter return safely to the Nizhne-Protosk military post, as the sun reemerges, suggesting the return of Eros and, in Orwin's view, the "naturalness of human sociability."[71]

Inspired by his clarification of identity and vocation in the stag's lair, Olenin expresses his newfound social confidence by confronting Luka about his killing of the "Abrek": "What are you so pleased about? [...] What if it was your brother who'd been killed; would you be pleased?"[72] Whereas the Cossack responds by conceding that their brothers, too, die in war, this authentic interaction—building on Luka's own humanistic recognition of the *djigit*'s body—sparks a temporary homoerotic approximation between Olenin and Lukashka. Although Olenin is primarily infatuated in this tale with the Cossack Maryana, a "female noble savage" (in the Rousseauvean concept) who has her parallel in Maria in *For Whom the Bell Tolls*, he has an evident erotic attraction toward his *kunak* Lukashka as well, whom he considers "pleasant looking and talkative," and with whom he "involuntarily combine [s]" Maryana "in his [erotic] imagination."[73] Their bond recalls the custom of *matelotage*, or same-sex marriage among coequal male comrades, practiced by pirates on the Caribbean island of Tortuga (now Haiti) in the seventeenth and eighteenth centuries, as well as the "sacred marriage of males" featured in Melville's fiction.[74] Like Tolstoy himself, his *alter ego* also "oscillates [...] between heterosexual and homosexual feelings."[75]

Within the relatively autonomous social context of the Cossack host, which afforded women and men alike greater sexual and affective freedom than did social life in central Russia, Olenin feels more sexually liberated. Hence, in Maryanka (and presumably Lukashka, as well), he comes to "love nature, and the personification of all that is beautiful in nature."[76] As suggested above, Olenin's relationship with Yeroshka has homosocial and platonically erotic dimensions, in light of "Uncle's" slim figure, handsome looks, and embodiment of "spontaneous natural instinct" and a "bold and carefree life," all of which Olenin finds attractive.[77] In this vein, *Red Cavalry* (1926), Isaac Babel's journalistic account of being embedded with Cossacks during the Polish-Soviet War (1919–1921), presents plenty of evidence for homoerotic comrade-love among these warriors.[78] Consequently, the homophilic inter-generational relationship between Olenin and Yeroshka foreshadows the platonic bond between the young Prince Andrei Bolkonsky and the elder General Kutuzov in *War and Peace*.

Olenin's Estrangement from Russian Imperialism and Cossack Life

In contrast to the chaste Tolstoy, Hemingway in *For Whom the Bell Tolls* presents a passionate consummation of the erotic attraction between the Spaniard Maria and

Robert Jordan (Olenin's parallel), an idealistic US volunteer with the International Brigades. Their sexual fusion thus symbolizes the union between Spanish Republicans and their international supporters against the fascist menace represented by the combined forces of Francisco Franco, Benito Mussolini, and Adolf Hitler. In *The Cossacks*, however, Maryana is ultimately unavailable to Olenin, much like the Caucasus are to Russian imperial designs, as a result of collective indigenous resistance for over three-quarters of a century and beyond. The "natural woman" hence rejects the would-be master.[79] In Tolstoy's case, such failures of heterosexual union may have represented emblematic ways of communicating the writer's own gay feelings, thus lending weight to the Freudian concept of universal bisexuality, as anticipated by Melville's declaration in *Moby Dick* (1851): "Damn me, but all things are queer, come to think of 'em."[80]

Next, the cadet's gift of a horse to Lukashka, while well-intentioned and pleasurable for the self-abnegating Olenin, will estrange him from his Cossack counterpart and love interest. Upon receipt of the horse, Luka becomes suspicious of his *kunak*'s intentions. Ironically, then, through self-sacrifice, Olenin isolates himself from his peers and objects of affection.[81] Upon the arrival of one Prince Beletsky, "who liked wine and women," as an adjutant to the Terek region, the Cossacks immediately take a liking to him. They even grow to prefer Beletsky to Olenin, "who was a mystery to them," considering his eccentric, reclusive practices.[82] Implicitly, this psychosocial separation between the sensual Cossacks/Beletsky and the anti-militaristic, self-denying Olenin may constitute further hints about the queer sexuality of the latter, and therefore, of Tolstoy himself. Instead of pursuing women or wine, the youthful count unconventionally discovers in Chechnya that he "wished to merge into the Universal Being."[83] This past-unconscious desire for reunion, emanating from pre-individuated symbiosis with his mother and childhood union with his brothers, anticipates the Christian-anarchist philosophy he will convey using various techniques in this and many art-works to come.[84]

Indeed, though Olenin attempts to fit in by following Lermontov's example and adopting Circassian dress, he ultimately decides against "becoming" a Cossack and so endorsing their exilic response to the "alienation and discontents of modern social life." As much as he might prefer the idea of "be[ing] a simple Cossack, […] liv[ing] close to nature, […] do[ing] no harm to anyone, and even […] do[ing] good to others" to his previous ideas about serving the Tsarist State as a minister or commander as an adult, his idea of happiness centers self-denial, whereas the typical Cossack conception does not.[85] Above all, Tolstoy/Olenin recognize that they fundamentally cannot "make a home" in a society which demands that all of its males regularly shed blood—reflecting the author's judgment of the perceived violations of Christian love practiced in these communities.[86] Whereas Cossack autonomy is permitted as part of a loyalty bargain to the Tsarist State, Tolstoy/Olenin are disloyal to that same State.[87] Once Maryanka rejects the cadet's advances, after the latter is ostracized by Lukashka, Olenin's alienation becomes too great to bear.

Although the protagonist's initial naïveté about the Cossacks' role as "vanguard" of Russian expansionism is belied by the protagonist's subsequent experiences with the Chechens, we must distinguish between Olenin's early naïve inner monologue and Tolstoy's own perspective. While *The Cossacks* certainly qualifies as an example of the European and Orientalist adventure genre, following the lead of James Fenimore Cooper's *Pathfinder* (1841), it is plain that Tolstoy does not identify with either the means or ends of Russian expansionism in the region. Significantly, he experiences tender homoerotic love for the Chechen victims of Tsarist imperialism. In this sense, *The Cossacks* and *Hadji Murat* may constitute partial exceptions to the equations that the literary critics Edward Said and Anemone respectively make between Orientalist art, Romanticism, and imperialism.[88] In reality, *The Cossacks* presents compellingly direct and frank criticisms of Russian atrocities in Transcaucasia.

For instance, Yeroshka shares with Olenin what Tolstoy terms a poignant Tavlinsk song about a young Chechen shepherd returning to his *aul*, or village, one afternoon, only to find that the Russians had burnt it down entirely, killed all the men, and taken the women captive.[89] The source of this same story is in fact the first raid against the Chechens that Tolstoy participated in as a volunteer in 1852. The prose writer will return to portray it in *Hadji Murat* by relaying the heart-rending assault of the Russian military contingent on Sado's *aul*—illuminating imperialism at its most fundamental as a "murderous military operation."[90] Yeroshka's experience witnessing a broken cradle floating down the Terek River has countless parallels in Syria and Ukraine today, where the Russian military has committed countless war crimes and crimes against humanity, which are either sanitized or ignored by State media, and sometimes supported by the Russian public.[91]

In this sense, though *The Cossacks* is paradoxically written from the perspective of a White-Russian landowner embedded among Cossack frontier guards, we see that Tolstoy humanizes and even sympathizes with the indigenous and Muslim victims of Russian imperialism. To some extent, the feelings appear to have been mutual, for the Tolstoy Museum in Starogladovskaya was the only Chechen museum not to have had to close during the Second Chechen War (1999–2009).[92] Salavdi Zagibov, former director of the same Tolstoy Museum, praises Lev and his brother Nikolai for having "repeatedly saved Chechens" from Tsarist brutality. Countess Sofia A. Tolstaya likewise recalls that a Muslim from the Caucasus paid his respects to the artist's family in the weeks following Tolstoy's death, by bearing a wreath to Yasnaya Polyana.[93] Along similar lines, according to the writer's great-great-grandson:

> The Chechen people think that Tolstoy wrote most truthfully of the events that happened then and the character of the mountain peoples, their striving to be independent, for freedom, and their religious, ethnic and other particularities [...] Tolstoy, in spite of the fact that he was an aristocrat, a Russian count, was very democratic and open. He had friends among the Chechens.[94]

As a result of Olenin's failure to integrate socially with the Cossacks, and following the protagonist's discovery of the merely selective and therefore false love practiced by his hosts, an implicit value hierarchy is established which privileges the cadet at the top, and Yeroshka next, relative to the rest of the Grebensk Cossacks. This is classic compensatory behavior that is consistent with Tolstoy's well-known tendency to "collect injustice" as a means of coping with setback and loss.[95] Though the Cossacks' lives may be "unspoiled and natural," they are "not fully human," according to the writer—or, at least, not as human as Olenin—in that their "potential for reason [...] remains mostly undeveloped."[96] In Tolstoy's view, love and reason do not oppose but rather mutually support each other, such that love must be practiced in a cosmopolitan-internationalist way. For this reason, Tolstoy depicts Yeroshka as a more reasonable or "civilized" ex-Cossack. He is a "good gay" who has isolated himself from the Cossack host and its hegemonic values, and who reflects true humanity—as well as homoerotic longing—in his tearful farewell kisses to Olenin, when he twice reminds him of his love for him.[97]

(De)humanization of the Other

Ultimately, although Count Tolstoy may have intended to express solidarity with Chechens and Adyghes in *The Cossacks*, the reality is that his novella tends to represent the subaltern Other as *both* subject and object. In discovering that many Others are "semi-Asiatic" and "semi-European," the writer expresses his fascination with, and affinities for, the pluralist cultural inheritance shared by Russia, its neighbors, and colonial subjects.[98] At the same time, by affirming hierarchies of agency and ostensible civilization, the author stifles oppressed peoples in literary form, and so excludes them from full humanity. In self-defeating fashion, Tolstoy reifies and dehumanizes Cossack, Chechen, and Circassian alike, ironically serving the aims of Tsarist imperialism, and so undermining his vision of destabilizing Russian imperialism and militarism through internationalist, cross-class alliances, united fronts, and homoerotic bonds.[99]

As a "colonizer who refuses," Tolstoy is conflicted by his identity as a White-Russian, his desire to become a "free man" (*quzzaq*), and his semi-humanistic attitude toward the Chechens and other nations oppressed by the Empire.[100] Since he cannot join either the Cossack host or their indigenous rivals, he will suspend his life in Chechnya and return to Russia, where he will try to liberate the serfs bound to him, marry, and become a world-renowned writer, author of *War and Peace*. Later in life, as well, rather than visit German spas, the French Riviera, mineral springs in the Caucasus, or Yalta in Crimea, Tolstoy vacationed at least three times with the nomadic Bashkir peoples on the Eurasian steppe. He would even include his family in one of these holidays, for the purposes of cultural exchange. That being said, he also appropriated their lands as a Russian settler first when purchasing a large manor in Samara in 1871, and then again, when expanding the estate seven years later.[101]

Tolstoy's relationship with oppressed peoples is therefore complex. G. M. Hamburg details that the prose writer bought the Samara estate primarily to raise horses, and to oversee peasant cultivation of cereal crops.[102] Dynamically, though, alongside the city of Tula and the village of Begichevka, the Samara manor would serve as one of the hubs for famine relief organized by Tolstoy and his family in 1892–1893. Likewise, in an 1893 conversation with Russian-Armenian students about Turkish oppression of Armenians, the writer will challenge his interlocutors' chauvinism against Kurds. In the play *The Power of Darkness* (1886), he lauds the maternal care for a Kurdish war orphan practiced by the Russian ex-soldier Mitrich, to contrast with the infanticide which the female protagonists cruelly carry out.[103]

That being said, in a 1902 letter to Nicholas II, the writer declares that, although the Russian people may have progressed beyond any "need" for despotism, autocracy "may suit the needs of people cut off from the world somewhere in Central Africa [...]."[104] Tolstoy's sympathies with humanism notwithstanding, such a statement affirms white supremacy and presages fascist ideology about racial hierarchies.[105] These examples therefore help to illustrate the count's simultaneously humanizing *and dehumanizing* attitudes toward oppressed peoples. Like Pushkin, who unites the seeming polar-opposites of revolutionary poet and Tsarist apologist, Tolstoy thus perpetuates the Eurocentric division between "subject" (self) and "object" (Other) that Shariati and Achille Mbembe consider essential to imperial domination.[106] In this, he arguably anticipates the ambiguously "bad gay" T. E. Lawrence (1888–1935), a British Orientalist and military intelligence officer "whose sexual desire towards colonised people was built out of both admiration and exploitation."[107]

Through his Romantic insight into the artifice of high Russian society, and in his itinerant search for social alternatives, Olenin likely serves as a prototype for Pierre Bezukhov in *War and Peace*. Like Olenin, who must choose between "civilization" and "natural life," Bezukhov confronts the dilemma between upholding privilege and exploitation vs. renouncing these to accord with his (and Tolstoy's) stated principles of the leveling of social hierarchy, in keeping with a progressive yet at times chauvinist meta-narrative of emancipation, which flows from Lev and Pierre's common Kantianism.[108] Furthermore, as we shall see in Chapter 6, Olenin's homoerotic, cosmopolitan adventures in the Caucasus anticipate Prince Andrei Bolkonsky's proto-anarchist, psychosexual journey of self-discovery.

The critique of violence and love of nature are central to both works, reflecting the transference of maternal influence on Tolstoy's art—his "Oedipal" identification with the "archaic" mother over the "civilized" father.[109] The recurring motif of the Terek River returns in *War and Peace* as the Niemen River and the globe of life, connoting embryonic existence and symbolizing the *flow*, or continuous motion, of human history, which is collectively constructed by the *Narod*, rather than by the "great men" celebrated by despotic power (власть).

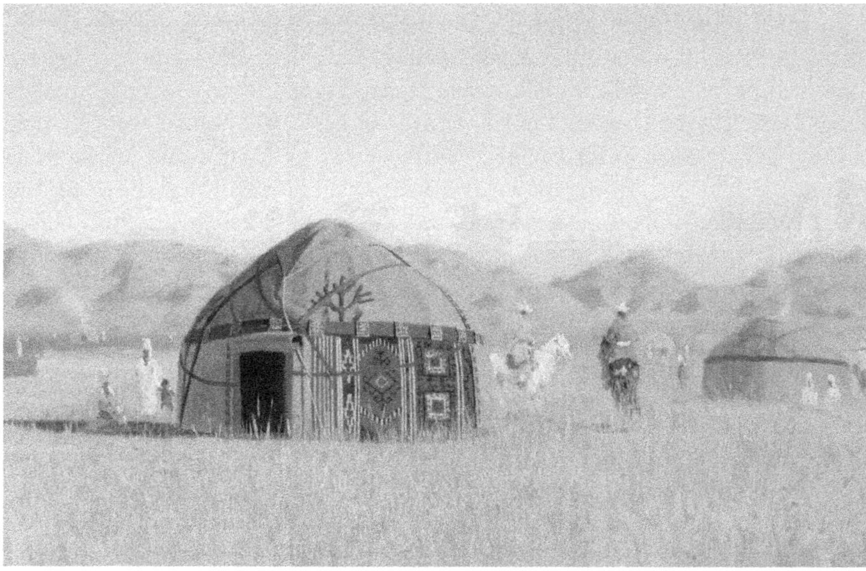

FIGURE 4.2 Vasili Vereshchagin, *Kyrgyz Tent on the Chu River* (1870)

Hadji Murat: A Political Novella that Preaches Anti-Militarism and Collective Liberation

Whereas *The Cossacks* expresses compassion and ambivalence about Russian chauvinism and the victims of Tsarist imperialism in the Caucasus, the posthumously published *Hadji Murat* (1912) unambiguously centers the titular character, a renowned Avar chieftain who reports to Imam Shamil. Murat has a reputation for courage against the Russian invaders, whom Tolstoy emblematically portrays as ruthless eagles.[110] According to John Foster, Jr., *Hadji Murat* is a "work of world literature conceived in a transnational spirit," evincing the author's "genuine will to examine another culture."[111] Hence, from the start of the novella, the writer's perspective is palpably Rousseauvist, Romantic, and critical of Russian imperialism.

Even so, it is not totally uncritical of the Avar resistance itself, in light of Shamil's authoritarianism, the petty tyranny evinced by his *murids* (Sufi militants), and the "deal with the devil" that Murat makes in allying himself with the Russians. Internally, the *jihad* will provide the rationale for its leaders to centralize power and eliminate rivals. Still, considering that Tolstoy appears to have identified with and even found Hadji Murat attractive, his championing in the novella of Murat—a partisan of the khanate which was defeated by Shamil's resurgent imamate—may betray the count's own conscious and unconscious biases in favor of "conservative agricultural sympathies."[112]

In Tolstoy's novella, which is set between November 1851 and May 1852, Murat defects to the Russian occupiers in the hopes that the imperial adjutant Prince Semën Mikhailovich Vorontsov, living in luxury in a Caucasian fortress, will negotiate the release of his family, whom Shamil has kidnapped, through a prisoner exchange. In a reverie, he further imagines that Vorontsov will provide him with an army with which to take revenge on Shamil, whose *murids* had killed his relatives—including his brother Osman—and allies in the khanate, which had aligned itself *with* the Russians against *jihad*. In this sense, his motives have to do more with family than with faith.[113] Murat even envisions recovering his prior privileged status by reviving the Avar khanate, installing himself as overlord of Avaria and Chechnya, and accepting rewards from the Tsar for having vanquished Shamil. Fearing death, desiring revenge and compensation, and resenting the imperial invader, he fantasizes about "not just being second, but first." With this in mind, Murat first surrenders himself, pledges himself to Nicholas I, and declares Prince Vorontsov his *sardar*, or military commander.[114]

Throughout this novella, numerous Russian officers view Hadji Murat with great suspicion. They are concerned that his ostensible defection may simply be a ruse to gather intelligence about their forces to plan future attacks against them. Defending his venture, Prince Voronstov disagrees, and the Tsar will back him up. Yet, in an illustration of the folly of power, the dissenting commanders turn out to be right. At the same time, within an environment of great artifice at the gubernatorial palace in Tiflis (now Tbilisi), Vorontsov's flatterers liken Hadji Murat to Napoleon's General Joachim Murat (1767–1815), the renowned cavalry commander, alluding to the Avar's protean status as victim, agent, *and* threat.[115]

Continuing this theme of satirizing the rich and powerful, Tolstoy describes the adjutant's father Mikhail Semënovich Vorontsov (1782–1856), a field-marshal from the Napoleonic Wars who was named the Tsar's vice-regent in the Caucasus in 1844, as someone incapable of "understand[ing] life without power and obedience."[116] More gravely, Tolstoy criticizes the violence of hierarchy, despotism, and capital punishment in his direct portrayal of Tsar Nicholas ordering the execution by flogging of a Polish student accused of assaulting his professor. The Tsar intends this harsh directive to serve to "*destroy this revolutionary spirit*" that the 1848 Revolutions had awakened in the People.[117]

Regarding the Russo-Caucasus War, Nicholas mandates a series of cruel orders to Vorontsov: namely, that he "*adhere firmly*" to the Tsar's "system of laying waste to habitations, destroying provisions in Chechnya, and harrying them with raids [...]."[118] In effect, Nicholas is demanding continued fidelity from his subordinates to the genocidal tactics that had been used for decades by that point to annihilate the Adyghe.[119] Apropos, Tolstoy does not fail to include a portrait of the next order of the day: the Tsar's "[a]pproving" of State retaliation against peasants of the Eastern Catholic faith in Ukraine and western Russia for having resisted conversion to Orthodoxy. They would be prosecuted for putative treason, a charge implying corporal punishment.[120]

Though evidently sympathizing with the causes of Chechen, Avar, and Circassian self-determination against Russian settler-colonialism, Tolstoy's tragic humanism also includes expressions of sorrow over the death of the Russian serf youth Petrukha Avdeev, who is mortally wounded by a Chechen, and of the sadness this causes his family. Lev Nikolaevich characterizes Avdeev as heartfelt in his homesickness, as in his cosmopolitan-internationalist friendliness toward the Chechens: "Really, they're just like Russians," he declares. "Nice lads." Nevertheless, Avdeev's youthful vitality yields absurdly to destruction, in keeping with Lev Nikolaevich's perspective that "soldiering [i]s like death."[121] In turn, the conscript's estrangement and end foreshadow the fate of the titular character.[122]

Indeed, the chapters in *Hadji Murat* reenacting the raid mandated by Tsar Nicholas, in which the author himself participated, represent one of Tolstoy's greatest denunciations of war. Following the Tsar's orders, a military contingent involving "four infantry battalions, two hundred Cossacks," and eight cannons invaded Chechnya in January 1852—such that the "beautiful, frightened" local animals flee before it.[123] Led by a cold officer who inures himself to human suffering, this detachment will burn down the very *aul* where Hadji Murat ironically had stayed as a guest while fleeing from Shamil just before presenting himself to the Russians. Sado, Murat's host, then returns from the mountains to the *aul* to find his *sakyla*, or earthen home, destroyed, the local spring wrecked, the mosque defaced, and his son murdered.[124]

Tolstoy characterizes the collective outrage and indignity felt by the Chechens who gather at the scene of this atrocity as "stronger than hatred." In reality, such rage constitutes a "refusal to recognize these Russian dogs as human beings," such that repelling them mercilessly with violence should be viewed as consistent with self-defense. At the same time, Tolstoy shows Shamil's *murids* as being overwhelmed by imperial forces, who lay waste to numerous *auls*, paradoxically with the intention of driving Chechens *away* from Shamil—in an illustration of the counter-insurgent strategies which have been applied by various repressive powers over the past half-century in Vietnam, Palestine, Afghanistan, Iraq, and Syria, as elsewhere.[125] In turn, we can appreciate the continuities between Tsarism and Lenino-Stalinist party dictatorship, considering that Stalin personally ordered the Bolshevik invasion of the independent, Menshevik-led Georgian Democratic Republic in 1921, and that Soviet leaders ignored Shamil (and presumably Murat too) in their curricula for historical education.[126]

At the climax of the story, Murat perceives the Russians' evident lack of interest in his proposal for an alliance, and so flees with a handful of his supporters to either "die or rescue his family." He and his comrades are soon tracked down, however, and surrounded both by Cossacks and militiamen allied to Shamil. Their odds notwithstanding, Murat and his comrades resist heroically until the very end, when they are overrun by the combined firepower of Cossacks and *murids*, who gloat over Murat's fresh corpse, and his now-captive colleagues, "like hunters over a slain animal."[127]

Beyond these victims themselves, and the sympathetic martyred serf-soldier Petrukha Avdeev, the only Russian character in this novella who views the corporal agony and political subjugation of Murat, the Avars, and the Chechens in a critical light is Marya Dmitrievna, a working-class partner of one of the Tsarist officers. She experiences an intensely mutual but not openly acknowledged sexual attraction with Hadji Murat toward the end of the novel—thus fostering a short-lived utopian and platonic romance, or a transient commune, which prefigures peaceful and cooperative international relations and unity in diversity.[128] She will condemn the Russians as "all butchers [...]. Real butchers" after encountering Murat's severed head.[129] As with John the Baptist, who was similarly decapitated by King Herod Antipas for his dissidence, the militant Chechen's mutilated corpse is sent to the Russian commanders as a master symbol or trophy sadistically affirming the established military hierarchy, the suppression of the Avar khanate, burgeoning Russian imperialism, and the coming defeat of Shamil, plus the great oppression that Tsarist occupation would entail. Like Petrukha Avdeev and Marya Dmitrievna, Tolstoy protests against all of this violence perpetrated by the Romanov dynasty, thus undermining the "grand Russian narrative" to which *War and Peace* had previously contributed.[130]

In sum, *Hadji Murat* critiques war and imperialism while implicitly summoning a simultaneous liberation of "progressive solidarities" and a cosmopolitan-internationalist alliance for non-cooperation among oppressed peoples, including the titular character himself, the humanistic conscript Petrukha Avdeev, and the thoughtful onlooker Marya Dmitrievna.[131] In depicting Dmitrievna as the voice of reason for rightly identifying imperialism with butchery, Tolstoy affirms values of care and compassion that are traditionally associated with femininity, thus betraying the masculine commitment to aggression—and, by extension, heterosexuality—expected of him. As a political novella, *Hadji Murat* encourages Dmitrievna and the audience simultaneously to construct an "International of good people," decolonize the Russian Empire, and resist the forces strangling humanity.

Notes

1 Tolstoy 2006a: 3–5.
2 *Ibid* 8; Gustafson 1986: 54; Maude 1987a: 295.
3 Tolstoy 2009: 121n4.
4 *Ibid* 120–1, 121n1; Evtuhov et al. 397–8; Bosworth 2001: 827.
5 Pevear ix.
6 Zorin 169; Foster J 195.
7 Freud 1961b: 54–5; Lanzieri and Hildebrant 282.
8 Evtuhov et al. 302–3; Figes 2002: 220–30.
9 Guevara.
10 Kropotkin 2022: 1.
11 Plokhy 75; Figes 2002: 386.
12 Grubačić and O'Hearn 54–8.
13 Evtuhov et al. 125; Plokhy 73–84.
14 Evtuhov et al. 184–5; Struve 115.
15 Tolstoy 2010: 772; Newlin 379; Chitty; Stites 1989.
16 Anemone 55; Maude 1987a: 64.
17 Никитина 79 (emphasis added).
18 Kropotkin 1991: 125.
19 Bartlett 2011: 159.
20 Tolstoy 2006a: 14.
21 Gustafson 1986: 55, 237.
22 Orwin 1993: 66–7 (emphasis in original).
23 Rogers 67n10; Первый канал.

24 Peterson 35.
25 Grubačić and O'Hearn; Newlin 379.
26 Michel.
27 Peterson; Shul'ts; Kropotkin 1991: 55.
28 Rogers 60.
29 Peterson 35; Kornblatt.
30 Peterson 38; Tolstoy 2006a: 18; Berlin 1978: 247; Pevear xii; Smolski et al.
31 Mola.
32 Maude 1987a: 62; Evtuhov et al. 396–8.
33 Evtuhov et al. 398; Mola.
34 Tolstoy 2006a: 12, 14–15.
35 Harris; Figes 2002: 387.
36 Tolstoy 2006a: 13.
37 Lönnqvist 2007: 75–6.
38 Bartlett 2011: 106–15.
39 Tolstoy 2006a: 17, 26, 31–4; Mbembe 2003.
40 Tolstoy 2006a: 38–42; Fromm 1973.
41 Tolstoy 2006a: 59, 86.
42 *Ibid* 43, 46; Fontesse et al.; Kaur.
43 Tolstoy 2006a: 97–9.
44 *Ibid* 99.
45 Anemone 53.
46 Schonfeld and Chang 10.
47 Bellamy 2001b.
48 Snyder.
49 Orwin 1993: 68; Clark 2019: 30.
50 Figes 2002: 107. Yeroshka's parallel in Hemingway's *For Whom the Bell Tolls* is Anselmo.
51 LeBlanc 1993: 6; Tolstoy 2006a: 92.
52 Orwin 1993: 68.
53 Freud 1995: 274.
54 Tolstoy 2006a: 92.
55 Benjamin: 127; Pietikainen 18; Gustafson 1986: 326–7.
56 Rogers 63. This is despite Freud's skepticism about Kant, whose categorical imperative the psychoanalyst viewed as an external introjection into the life of the individual (Freud 1995: 281–3). In contrast, Kropotkin would implicitly affirm Kant's view—common to Tolstoy as well—that "human personality constitutes [...] the ethical basis of morality and of law." That being said, Kant could not locate a basis for morality beyond the one he postulated as originating from the divine realm (Kropotkin 2012: 169–74).
57 Grant and Wade-Benzoni 606–9.
58 Friedman 97–8.
59 Fromm 1968: 69 (emphasis in original).
60 Tolstoy 2006a: 92–3; Capra; Gustafson 1986: 57.
61 Pietikainen; Eisler 19.
62 Wilson D 476; Benjamin 206.
63 Tolstoy 2006a: 68, 93. Consistent with this idea, following the death of his six-year-old son Ivan in 1895, Tolstoy would express in his diary his wish that his funeral and burial be simple and humble, lacking flowers, priests, or obituaries (Bartlett 2011: 358).
64 Orwin 2002c: 232; Tolstoy 2006a: 93–4. Tolstoy establishes a stark contrast between living for oneself and others. If one compares *The Cossacks* to "The Death of Ivan Ilych," one can see that the youthful Olenin grasps Tolstoy's account of true life with more time to spare, relative to the moribund Golovin (Figes 2002: 349).
65 Chouliaraki 202; Gustafson 1999: 124.
66 Tolstoy 2006a: 94.
67 Rogers 63.

68 Becker 11; Capra.
69 Engel 101.
70 Freud 1995: 274–5.
71 Orwin 1993: 92; Tolstoy 2006a: 94–5.
72 Tolstoy 2006a: 100.
73 Gustafson 1986: 54–8; Tolstoy 2006a: 100.
74 Chitty 101–3; Burgen; Fiedler.
75 Freud 2013: 63.
76 Tolstoy 2006a: 148; Bartlett 2011: 101.
77 Peterson 36; Tolstoy 2006a: 83, 91. The etymology of Yeroshka's name suggests he is "hallowed by God" in Tolstoy's estimation (Anemone 49).
78 Babel.
79 Peterson 36–7; Anemone 60.
80 Dynes 1990l; 1990m; 1990n; Melville 139.
81 Tolstoy 2006a: 103–5; Gustafson 1986: 59.
82 Tolstoy 2006a: 109–13.
83 Maude 1987a: 65.
84 Benjamin 153n.
85 Anemone 51; Tolstoy 2006a: 109–10, 122–3.
86 Orwin 1993: 85, 96; Rogers 61–2.
87 Grubačić and O'Hearn.
88 Tolstoy 2006a: 462n35; Anemone 53–8n17; Said.
89 Tolstoy 2006a: 130.
90 Tolstoy 1982; Bartlett 2011: 206; Evtuhov et al. 399.
91 Borshchevskaya.
92 Bartlett 2011: 7.
93 Kishkovsky; Bartlett 2011: 416–17.
94 Nazaryan.
95 Johansson 1990e.
96 Orwin 1993: 93.
97 Tolstoy 2006a: 181–2; Staples.
98 Figes 2002: 380–6.
99 Gandesha; Chouliaraki 88–91; Moore 79. These humanizing goals were ones Tolstoy shared with the realist war artist Vasili Vereshchagin (1804–1942), of Turkmen descent, whose paintings depicting the atrocities of the Russian conquest of Turkestan provoked great controversy among progressives and reactionaries alike (Figes 2002: 411–14).
100 Memmi.
101 Maude 1987a: 341, 351–5; 1987b: 13.
102 Hamburg 124.
103 Maude 1987b: 333–4; Tolstoy 2019: 59–60.
104 Maude 1987b: 423.
105 Stanley.
106 Poole; Bartlett 2011: 208–9, 234–66; Byrd and Miri 7; Mbembe 2016; Berdyaev 1966: 24.
107 Staples.
108 Peterson 36; Orwin 1993: 90; Dodson.
109 Benjamin 141–6.
110 Tolstoy 2009b: 3–6.
111 Foster J 185–7.
112 *Ibid* 189; Trotsky.
113 Tolstoy 2009b: 15, 49–57; Foster J 193.
114 Foster J 189–90; Tolstoy 2009b: 27–33, 45.
115 Tolstoy 2009b: 43, 46–54, 72.
116 *Ibid* 39, 121n8.
117 *Ibid* 71 (emphasis added).
118 *Ibid* 72 (emphasis added).

119 Mola.
120 Tolstoy 2009b: 72.
121 *Ibid* 12–14, 37–9.
122 Foster J 186.
123 Pevear xii–xiii; Tolstoy 2009b: 75.
124 Tolstoy 2009b:77–9.
125 *Ibid* 79, 85; Townshend 231–2.
126 Lee; Evtuhov et al. 772.
127 Tolstoy 2009b: 101, 116.
128 Foster J 197–9; Gilman-Opalsky.
129 Tolstoy 2009b: 109.
130 Foster J 179.
131 Ferguson A 197.

5

WAR AND PEACE

An Anarcho-Populist Verbal Icon

A synthesis between a wide-ranging epic novel and a Homeric *poema*, or prose poem, that depicts Imperial Russia's relationship to the Napoleonic Wars, Count Lev Nikolaevich Tolstoy's classic *War and Peace* (1869) was conceived during the author's experiences as a cadet in the Caucasus, and as an artillery officer in the Crimean War (1853–1856). In this latter role, Tolstoy participated in the siege of the Turkish fortress of Silistra (1854), and fought to resist the Anglo-Franco-Turkish siege of the Russian naval base of Sevastopol (1854–1855), from where he served as war correspondent. Indeed, based on his experiences in Crimea, he composed the anti-militarist "Sevastopol Sketches" (1855), which brought him "great fame."[1]

Although he would ultimately choose literature and the arts following the popular reception of *Childhood* (1852), Tolstoy had been considering a career as a military officer during the Crimean War, before he resigned in 1856 to focus instead on writing.[2] As Peter Kropotkin declares, "[h]e has therefore the right to speak of War: he knows it from within."[3] Uniquely, and consonant with his anarchist sympathies, Tolstoy seeks to portray war "from the bottom up, in its own time, replete with moments of local horror, suspense, and unexpected comic relief."[4]

The "incomparable realism" of *War and Peace*, sometimes considered the greatest novel of all time, celebrates life "as it is, not as it should be."[5] The *poema* reveals the full plenitude of its author's skills as a writer of artistic documentaries, one who "philosophize[s] through images," using a method his biographer Richard F. Gustafson terms *emblematic realism*, which is inseparable from the author's Eastern Christian worldview.[6] Ethical and normative questions permeate the plot of the work, which can be read as a "verbal icon," or theological form of symbolic communication, which reveals Tolstoy's "divine truth" indicting "our statist bourgeois civilisation," together with the hegemonic elements of masculine Occidental reason—particularly its "calculative and operationalist modes."[7] Ultimately, *War and Peace* is concerned with human unity; the defense of the

DOI: 10.4324/9781003328964-5

individual against history; and the heroic, spiritual-aristocratic life, defined as one given to self-sacrifice, magnanimity, and a readiness to descend to and integrate with the *Narod*, or People.[8]

In this chapter and the five that follow, we combine political history, social psychology, and psychobiography to read *War and Peace* as a humanistic protest against inter-imperialist intrigues, toxic masculinity, heterosexism, bureaucratic despotism, and class hierarchies. As we shall see, many of these themes and messages follow from Tolstoy's queer-anarchist proclivities.

Although the *poema* represents the outcome of exhaustive research revolving around the Russian Empire's intrigues and wars with Napoleon Bonaparte and his forces between 1805 and 1812, there is, as the queer novelist Virginia Woolf and Tolstoy's biographer Aylmer Maude, respectively, observe, "hardly any subject of human experience that is left out of *War and Peace*," which "treats of life's deepest experiences from the cradle to the grave."[9] The British-American novelist Henry James (1843–1916) viewed Tolstoy as "a reflector as vast as a natural lake," whereas the Irish writer James Joyce (1882–1941) likened the count to William Shakespeare, Henrik Ibsen, and Dante.[10] According to the Slavist Dan Ungurianu, the epic "rests on a very solid foundation" in terms of the historical record, and the historian Alan Forrest praises the "precision and vibrancy" rendered by the integration of memoirs written by soldiers in Bonaparte's *Grand Armée*, whose accounts Tolstoy had consulted in the creative process.[11] Still, beyond extended scenes of war—defined as "*actual*, *intentional*, and *widespread* armed conflict between political communities"—the "peaceful" or "domestic" narratives center the friendships and love-bonds of the novel's principal characters—namely, Count Pierre Bezukhov, Countess Natasha Rostova, Prince Andrei Bolkonsky, and Princess Marya Bolkonskaya—who "struggled not to lose hope" despite setbacks and in the face of death, symbolized by both the Napoleonic invasion and the inevitability of mortality.[12]

According to the literary critic Peter M. Bitsilli, rather than individuals per se, Tolstoy's heroes are "collective entities" simultaneously pervaded by and seeking to advance the causes and interests of themselves, their families, and the *Narod*. Seen in such light, the *poema*'s plot can be interpreted as a series of symbolic interactions linking characters with "larger entities," ideas, unconscious fantasies, and movements.[13] As a psychological novel, *War and Peace* features the confluent and "conflicting currents of [Tolstoy's] own mental life in several heroes" and heroines.[14] Applying the analysis of the German existentialist theologian Paul Tillich (1886–1965), these collective-gentry protagonists' various assertions, adventures, and tribulations may be interpreted as confirmation of the thesis that human life is "a continuous attempt to avoid despair," which is met by the postulated "courage of despair." Such courage is actualized through the affirmation of oneself by means of a "heroic affect" and an enthusiastic love for the universe.[15] In this light, the complex narrative of *War and Peace* can be viewed both as an intended "immortality vehicle" for its creator, and as an exposition of a "metaphysic of hope" that sustains author, characters, and audience alike.[16]

Tolstoy first enlisted voluntarily with Cossack military units in the Eastern Caucasus to service debts he had accumulated through gambling in 1851—an addiction which would compel him for over a decade.[17] Nonetheless, his diaries from Chechnya unambiguously evince his horrors over war and militarism, and may point to the origins of his religious pacifism.[18] As we have seen, *The Cossacks* (1863) and *Hadji Murat* (1912) express humanistic critiques of the violence of imperialism and settler-colonial dispossession.

Evidently, Tolstoy's distant cousin, Prince Sergei Grigorievich Volkonsky (1788–1865), a Major General and a Decembrist, served as the inspiration for Prince Andrei Bolkonsky's character. Speculatively, the basis of the poignant metaphysical reflections Bolkonsky experiences as he lies grievously wounded at the battle of Austerlitz (1805) in book one of *War and Peace* may lie in part in the epiphany the author reports having experienced during the siege of Sevastopol: namely, the idea of founding a new religion based on the actual teachings of Jesus the Nazarene, rather than church dogmas.[19] Freud might say that the stress of combat led Tolstoy to protect himself by "taking flight into a traumatic neurosis" by recalling childhood happiness, thus producing a utopian daydream linking "past, present, and future."[20]

A related element of this moving verbal image, as we shall see in the next chapter, is its implicit psychosexual dimensions: confronted with death, Andrei looks up into the atmosphere, experiences the boundlessness of life, and semi-consciously intuits his erotic non-conformism.[21] This scene, which emblematically links personal self-discovery and self-determination with self-actualization and radical re-enchantment, goes to the heart of Tolstoy's utopian purpose in *War and Peace*: at its best, this can be summarized briefly as advocacy for a free, political, and sexual union of honest, simple people against the imposed viciousness and repressiveness of private, bureaucratic power.[22]

Three decades after *War and Peace*, in *What Is Art?* (1868), a volume wherein he ironically disavows nearly all of his previous creations, Tolstoy expresses his enduring belief that the purpose of true art is to transmit feelings of Christian love far and wide.[23] On this account, then, in spite of the writer's late judgment, *War and Peace* constitutes true Tolstoyan art. In common with so many others of his art-works, the approach favored by Lev Nikolaevich in the *poema* is "spiritual, anti-materialist, [and] based on universal truths of love, non-violence and moral perfection."[24] Whereas the religious dimensions of Tolstoy's political philosophy deviated from the anti-theologism espoused by fellow Russian critics and revolutionaries like Vissarion Belinsky, Mikhail Bakunin, and Nikolai Chernyshevsky, the prose writer nevertheless psychologically sympathized with the Populist project of liberating the People.[25] This comes through resoundingly in *War and Peace*.

In *My Life* (1896), a slice-of-life examination of the noble son of an architect who adopts Tolstoyan principles, working to sustain himself on the railways and as a house-painter, Anton Chekhov summarizes his mentor's philosophy in this way: "what is wanted is that the strong should not enslave the weak, that the minority should not be a parasite on the majority, nor a vampire for ever sucking its vital sap [...]. [H]e believed the chief thing on earth was truth and justice."[26]

In a paradoxical sense, then, perhaps *both* the textologist Evelina Zaidenshnur's view of the novel's origins as "celebrating the courage of the Russian peasants and indirectly calling for their emancipation," *and* the conclusion of the Formalists Boris Eikhenbaum and Viktor Shklovsky, who saw the work as a "warning against the emancipation of the serfs and the violent revolution it might lead to," are right.[27] Although we must not ignore that Tolstoy's Formalist critics were writing their analyses within the totalitarian context of Stalinist Russia, we must equally not overlook the conservative aspects of Tolstoy's story, especially in terms of its portrayal of certain peasants, much less its view of the "woman question."

In reality, the *poema* appears to have been conceived through its creator's abandonment of his wife, Sofia Andreevna, during her first pregnancy in the spring and summer 1863, as the count took up study of the "swarm life" of bees in the apiary near Yasnaya Polyana.[28] In fact, in a January 1865 letter to his friend, the poet Afanasy Fet, Lev Nikolaevich confesses that he "love[s] her [Sofia Andreevna] less than [his] novel," *War and Peace*.[29] According to the findings of the late Slavist Kathryn Feuer (1926–1992), confirming those of Eikhenbaum and Shklovsky, Tolstoy had initially conceived of *War and Peace* as a polemic directed against Tsar Alexander II and the liberal intellectuals avowing reform of the land question and the emancipation of the serfs.[30] Whether or not Feuer and the Formalists are right, the final version, available to us now, prominently features an anarcho-Populist theory of history which centers everyday people in the very *construction of history*. Then again, the villainous depiction of the serfs at the Bolkonskys' Bogucharovo manor marries noble anxieties about agricultural revolt with the traditionalist depiction of Marya Bolkonskaya as a "damsel in distress."

That having been said, Count Tolstoy's account of the war of 1812 is much closer to that of the proud Decembrists, who saw it as a people's war, than to the obsequious reactionaries who interpreted Russia's triumph as the salvation and triumph of Tsarist autocracy. Whereas the State would celebrate the latter narrative by ordering the construction of numerous monstrous monuments in the Imperial style, *War and Peace* exists as a testament to national liberation, the individual and collective mind, and the centrality of complex "swarm life," or mass-movements, within human and natural history.[31] Consequently, at least in part, Lev Nikolaevich's impetus for composing *War and Peace* can be found in his desire to illuminate the stark contrast he perceived between "the 'real' texture of life, both of individuals and communities, [and] the 'unreal' picture presented by historians," following the writer's affinity for the socialist Alexander Herzen's expression about the "'pattern' on life's carpet."[32] The author's humanism is well-reflected in Kropotkin's comment: though the plot contains more than one hundred historical characters, each one is shown to have a distinctly unique personality.[33] Accordingly, Lev Nikolaevich's *poema* reflects the outcome of an encyclopedic style of research that weaves together metaphor and allegory at the individual and collective levels.[34] In this sense, the renowned art critic Eikhenbaum was right to view Tolstoy as a historical chronicler.[35] To this, we could add that the author's comprehensiveness may reflect his status as a traumatized veteran and a queer outsider.

Although it doubtlessly represents a "document of incomparable historical complexity," one way of thinking about the 15 narrative parts and two-part epilogue of *War and Peace* would be to divide it into three components: a "philosophical essay" about human history; a "family chronicle" about the aristocratic Bolkonskys and Rostovs (the Tolstoys); and a "historical novel about the Napoleonic wars," wherein the French Emperor confronts the Russian *Narod*, led by commander-in-chief General Mikhail Ilarionovich Kutuzov. Described by scholar Gary Morson as a "sort of Taoist sage on horseback," and by Gustafson as "the absolute Resident," Kutuzov—whose last name translates from Turkic to "madman"—may also represent one of the author's ego-personas, or *alter egos*, in the *poema*.[36] In line with the championing of Kutuzov and the *Narod, War and Peace* represents a stinging satire of class society, the landowning aristocracy from which Tolstoy hailed, academics such as the "scientific" German General Carl von Clausewitz (1780–1831), and even the oppositional intelligentsia, as represented by Tolstoy himself and his colleagues at *The Contemporary* in Petersburg.[37] Lev Nikolaevich could not get along with his many of his fellow *intelligents*, despite their common opposition to serfdom, owing largely to his narcissism and contrarianism.[38]

Like Miguel de Cervantes' *Don Quixote*, which the count read at the turn of the 1860s, Tolstoy's *War and Peace* "makes reality problematic" by challenging hegemonic political authority.[39] Overall, the *poema* embodies a critique of the war, militarism, and imperialism rationalized by von Clausewitz and other statist apologists, continuing from the themes explored in "The Sevastopol Sketches" (1855) and *The Cossacks* (1863). Ultimately, the intricate course of the work's plot represents the outcome of intensive Tolstoyan study of human history for answers to "the fundamental ethical problems which obsessed [the author] as they did every Russian thinker in the nineteenth century. *What is to be done? How should one live? Why are we here? What must we be and do?*"[40]

Preliminary Tolstoyan Critique of Russian Political History

One of the major themes in this *poema* is the "artificiality and mendacity" of social relations, particularly as observed among the ruling elite, which is conveyed in the text by use of the French language among upper-class Russians.[41] According to Chekhov's Tolstoyan protagonist in *My Life*, gentry life is fundamentally characterized by dishonesty and hypocrisy, and the landowners' estates are "nests of damnation [...] where children are tortured."[42] Tolstoy contrasts the "calm luxurious life" of the capital city of St. Petersburg—based fundamentally on class exploitation, having been erected atop wetlands through Peter I's mobilization of half a million serfs, and "concerned only about phantoms and reflections of real life"—with Smolensk, Borodino, and Moscow, where the *Narod* sacrifices itself to defend against Napoleon's invading forces.[43]

Like his fellow Slavophiles, Lev Nikolaevich bears witness to the vile underside of Imperial Russian history, as the People were tormented by Peter Romanov—a "revolutionary from above" who anticipated Lenin and Stalin. Implicitly, Lev

Nikolaevich inverts the objectification of humanity presupposed by the Kingdom of Caesar, asserting a Feuerbachian sense that "[g]reat kingdoms and mighty empires" are "nothing in comparison with human personality."[44] Tolstoy hence wields the theme of artifice to navigate between the vastly different worlds of the upper classes, with a pretentious and stultifying European cultural orientation, and the *Narod*, who are depicted as vitally serving as the repository of true Russian culture.

The allegorical juxtaposition between Petersburg's decadence on the one hand and the ostensible authenticity of "the big village" known as Moscow, and of the Empire's farmyards and fields on the other, by all means reflects Lev Nikolaevich's childhood in the countryside. It also conveys the artist's philosophical preference for the cultural-nationalist Slavophiles, who championed the putative superiority of pre-Petrine Russian society over the Westernizing impulses that influenced socialists like Herzen.[45] Along these lines, the Slavophile Nikolai Gogol (1809–1852) characteristically observed that Petersburg is "a perfect German," while Moscow "is a Russian nobleman."[46] As in *The Cossacks*, Tolstoy in *War and Peace* counterposes the "natural" (the *Narod*/peasantry, the Russian language, nature) from the "artificial" (Petersburg, the aristocracy, bureaucracies, militarism, France / French / the West).[47] The prose writer hence distinguishes between the social aristocracies of feudal-slave societies and the spiritual aristocracies comprised of holy fools who reject determination by family and inheritance, together with relations of master and slave.[48]

In biographical terms, Tolstoy's rural bias manifested in the writer's abandonment of St. Petersburg in 1856 after a short-lived bid there to connect with fellow artists and intellectuals, in favor of physical seclusion at Yasnaya Polyana, where Lev Nikolaevich disconnected from all political parties and factions.[49] In this withdrawal, Tolstoy followed the examples of his maternal grandfather, Nikolai Sergeivich Volkonsky (1753–1821), who had sought refuge from the oppressive world of statecraft at his Yasnaya Polyana estate, and of his brother Dmitri Nikolaevich (1827–1856), who retreated to the family estate at Shcherbachevka following demoralization in the Tsarist bureaucracy.[50] Despite that Tolstoy belonged to no formal political organization, he was nonetheless inspired by an activist passion to take advantage of Alexander II's call for landowners to "settle the issue [of serfdom] on their own estates" by drawing up a localized emancipation plan for the serfs at the family manor.[51]

Perhaps ironically, although Russia's defining national myths claim its culture to be a combination of Scandinavia and Byzantium (therefore incorporating Rome as well), Russian nationalists typically fail to mention the legacy of the Qipchak khanate, otherwise known as the "Golden Horde," which ruled Rus' for over two centuries. Despite such omission, late-Imperial archaeologists and anthropologists like D. N. Anuchin, N. I. Veselovsky, and Dmitri Zelenin suggested Asiatic origins for many animistic and folk beliefs of Russian steppe peasants. The critic Vladimir Stasov (1826–1906) similarly argued that Asian influences permeate Russian culture, including the *bylini*, Russia's national epics in song, and even Nikolai Rimsky-Korsakov's opera, *Sadko* (1898). Avant-garde Russian "Primitivist" painters such as Marc Chagall (1887–1985), Wassily Kandinsky (1866–1944), and Nicholas Roerich (1874–1947) reproduced and appropriated Russian peasant and

Asian tribal art-forms. Through his late study of anthropology, Karl Marx theorized "Indian forms of common property" as the ultimate origins of common-property regimes found among Slavs, Teutons, Celts, and Romans alike.[52]

Even if major Russian cultural, economic, and political institutions combine features from Scandinavia, Byzantium, the Roman Empire, and the Golden Horde, in the sense that Russian sadomasochistic political traditions meld "Byzantine" cringing with Viking ultraviolence, the specifically German influences on these same institutions should not be overlooked.[53] According to Bakunin, taking a sarcastic tone, the Russian Empire was formed through a blending of the "Tatar knout, Byzantine blessings, and German bureaucratic, military and police enlightenment."[54] As part of his Westernizing reforms, Peter I colonized the Orthodox Church by imposing a synodal regime copied from German Protestantism, and he installed Prussian officials into prominent posts. Such bureaucratization would be reinforced by the expansionist Tsarina Catherine II, herself a ruling-class Prussian from the principality of Anhalt-Zerbst.[55] For Berdyaev, Tsar Nicholas I typified "the Prussian officer type," and rumors that Tsarina Alexandra Fedorovna—born in Darmstadt, Germany, in 1872 as Princess Alix of Hesse and by Rhine—was conspiring with the German high command to thwart the Russians after the outbreak of World War I both demoralized the armed forces *and* animated a mass-movement of self-styled revolutionary Russian patriots, in turn contributing to the very collapse of the Romanov dynasty.[56]

Along these lines, Selenin, erstwhile friend to Prince Nekhlyudov, the protagonist in Tolstoy's novel *Resurrection* (1899), is a high-ranking *Ober-Procureur*, or State prosecutor, engaged by definition in the systematic oppression of the *Narod*. Consistent with his Slavophilic and syncretic worldview, Tolstoy satirically introduces into this work an elder general and baron "of German descent" who was decorated multiple times after committing atrocities against Chechens and Poles, in the interests of Tsarist expansionism.[57] Infamous are the German military's starvation siege and bombardment of Parisians during the Franco-Prussian War (1870–1871), and its collusion with the royalist Versaillais in the suppression of the Paris Commune through its release of prisoners of war as part of an international peace treaty.[58]

In parallel to the critique of Russian political culture, another major theme of *War and Peace* is the fallacy of the "great man" or "person"—whether ruler, intellectual, or general—who impels historical change by wielding the imperialistic will. According to Berdyaev and Morson, Tolstoy repudiates the "great man" as a "genius of objecti[fi]cation," and rejects the related concept of a direction to history.[59] For Peterson, Tolstoy's preoccupations are internalized and restated by Ernest Hemingway in *For Whom the Bell Tolls* (1940), a novel that presents a "shared representation of war as a populist, empirical phenomenon in which 'generals like Kutuzov and Golz are unimportant.'"[60] Moving backward in time, we see an antecedent for Tolstoy's humanizing approach in Gogol's recreation of the battle of *Borodino* in verse form (1837), as this poem features the point of view of peasant conscripts.[61] In a similar vein, Forrest writes knowingly that the count "is at his best in dealing with the human side of war, the pride and honor, the pain and sympathy felt by soldiers in battle."[62] In this sense, we can understand why Tolstoy's work might have been so popular with veterans from his day to that of ours, for it presents combat as an individual and collective human experience that the "tools of history [...] did not capture."[63]

Lev Nikolaevich's anarcho-Populist interpretation of history emphasizes the movement of nations and peoples rather than leaders, States, or empires in guiding its course. It emphasizes self-discovery, self-determination, and self-actualization in political, moral, and erotic terms. In contrast to the approach of the Tsarist-apologist statist historian Nikolai Karamzin (1766–1826), which was incidentally shared by Pushkin, Count Tolstoy affirms the democratic interpretation of Russian history advanced by the Decembrists and their followers in *War and Peace*.[64] As the historian Dominic Lieven observes, then, Tolstoy "indeed [was] an early exponent of 'history from below,'" one who concurred with the Decembrist Nikita Muravëv (1796–1843) in holding that "[h]istory belongs to the people."[65]

What is more, the artist's combination of anarcho-Populist sympathies with a "deep reverence for his ancestors" is reflected in his queer ego-personas Prince Bolkonsky and Pierre Bezukhov, both of whom experience same-sex attractions as they struggle passionately against Bonapartism and Tsarism. Using art therapy, then, Tolstoy disclosed his past and charted a course for his future, seeking to follow the political biography of his distant cousin, Prince Sergei Volkonsky.[66]

War and Peace: A Satire of Moral and Political Despotism

According to Orlando Figes, historian of Russia, Count Tolstoy's Populist vision in *War and Peace* communicates the ideals of the so-called "men of 1812." These landed aristocrats "discovered" the humanity of the peasantry through the latter's steadfast wartime resistance in the face of heavy losses before the *Grand Armée*. Through direct contact with the People—anticipating the revolutionary Populist youth of the 1870s, and echoing Siddhartha Gautama Buddha's life experiences outside the walls of his family's palace—these "men of 1812" confronted the radical evils of feudalism and serfdom, together with the dehumanizing social ideologies underpinning these institutions.[67] The conscience of several of these officers was lit upon their encounters with the forced-labor military settlements established for serf families by General Alexei Arakcheev (1769–1834), Minister of War, and especially in the wake of the serial massacres carried out by Arakcheev's forces against resistant peasants and mutineers alike.

Some officers eschewed their "French" upbringing, and the Russian Imperial military's mimicry of the stark hierarchies of the French royal army, by "Russifying" themselves and growing closer with their soldiers in the rank and file. Meanwhile, artists like Alexei Venetsianov (1780–1847) depicted the peasantry in their paintings in innovative ways, stressing the People's strength, individuality, and humanity. Prince Volkonsky, the so-called "peasant-prince" who was banished for three decades to penal-labor colonies in Siberian exile rather than be executed for his leadership in the Decembrist conspiracy, applied the lessons of 1812 and his travels abroad in Paris, Vienna, and London in a radically political way.[68]

If "art can be looked at as a record of belief," then Tolstoy's humanizing recognition of the labor and sacrifice of the *Narod*, and the poet's parallel exploration of the educated classes' journey of discovery of their own "Russianness," transmits the artist's Populist conception of the *Narod* as a single unit which—significantly enough—includes the gentry. According to scholar Robert S. Jansen, populist discourse can be found whenever there is a framing of a unified mass of distinct groups, whose competing interests are downplayed for the sake of unity.[69] In *War and Peace*, Tolstoy's vision oscillates between an idealized populist vision of the harmonious bonds of lord and slave that is consonant with the Slavophilic concept of *sobornost'* (соборность), and a profoundly communist call for the abolition of social classes—a conclusion to which Tolstoy consciously comes later in life.[70] Then again, as we shall see in the next chapter, Tolstoy's anarcho-Populist ideal prefigures classlessness and social freedom through the "socialism of consciousness" and the "Utopia of Eros" projected in his homoeroticization of soldiers and peasants, in keeping with a widespread sexual pluralism practiced among both groups—a custom which the State and Orthodox Church had sought in vain for centuries to suppress.[71]

To wit, the writer's Romantic idealization of medieval Muscovite society and of the peasant commune, his contempt for Napoleon and Bonapartism, *and* his paradoxical sympathy for Enlightenment ideals very much reflect the split identity of the nineteenth- and twentieth-century European Russian artist and intellectual.[72] In Tolstoy's case, while the equilibrium was dynamic over the course of life, and despite the count's rationalist critique of the clergy, plus his embodied, fateful struggle with the Orthodox Church, the balance was arguably tilted in favor of Slavophilism. This can be seen in the artist's visit to the Optina Pustin monastery for the first time, to meet with the elder Father Ambrosy, as he approached his spiritual crisis in 1877.[73]

War and Peace commences in July 1805, at a *soirée* among St. Petersburg's high society. This historical chronotope, or space-time, is suggestive of the pseudo-Enlightenment falsely advanced by Tsarina Catherine II (1762–1796), a hypocritical student of Voltaire who was guilty of numerous crimes. She entrenched serfdom in Russia to favor the nobility and State; exiled the *philosophe* Alexander Radishchev to Siberia, after having first ordered his execution, for his critical study of feudal slavery, the *Journey from St. Petersburg to Moscow* (1790), and the confiscation of all but 5 percent of the print run of this "literary bomb"; ignored women's education in the Empire; and first expanded the reaches of said Empire into the Caucasus, as part of an "offensive-defensive" strategy.[74]

Employing the motif of beginning *in medias res*, or in the middle of things, Lev Niklolaevich starts the *poema* with Anna Pavlovna Scherer, an associate of the Empress Marya Fëdorovna, hailing Russia's entry into the War of the Third Coalition (1803–1806) against Napoleon, as she welcomes Prince Vasili Kuragin to her evening party.[75] This is, therefore, an opening that features the symbolic violence of conventional society, which bases itself on war, conquest, and other historical injustices. On Tolstoy's account, respect for order is what makes possible the perpetuation of the vast inhumanities of "governed society": namely, "its wars, its penal colonies, its mass poverty, its abject slavery."[76]

Anna Pavlovna appears to have been modeled after Tolstoy's close friend and second cousin, Alexandra Tolstoya ("Alexandrine"), a lady-in-waiting to the Empress and a tutor to the Grand Duchess and her daughters. Having met after the writer's return from fighting in Sevastopol, Lev and Alexandrine visited again during the author's trip to Paris and Geneva in 1857. Like Herzen's travels in Italy and France during the 1848 Revolutions, this deprovincializing journey abroad greatly assisted in the development of the count's anarchism, especially after he witnessed a guillotining in Paris, and encountered militaristic forms of children's education in Marseille.[77] If, following Erich Fromm, the social theorist Christian Fuchs is right to observe that we humans use communication to "produce and reproduce sociality, social structures, groups, social systems, organizations, institutions, and society," and in turn to develop a social character, then it is evident that Tolstoy means to emphasize the non-productive, authoritarian orientation of the members of his own class at this gathering, obsessed as they are with observing decorum and securing a "control-property-power orientation."[78]

As an illustration of "honor without virtue, reason without wisdom, and pleasure without happiness," *War and Peace*'s opening scene serves two functional social goals.[79] Firstly, for Prince Vasili to arrange the introduction of soon-to-be Count Peter Kirillich Bezukhov ("Pierre") to his daughter Princess Hélène Kuragina, toward the end of exchanging her in marriage to Pierre in the interest of ensuring the perpetuation of his family's privilege; and secondly, for Anna Pavlovna to relay a favor requested from Princess Anna Mikhailovna Drubetskaya of Prince Vasili: namely, that he help reassign the princess's son Boris to the Imperial Guards before the impending campaign against Bonaparte.[80] These base interactions may represent homages on the poet's part to Gogol's *Inspector General* (1836/1842), a comedy which portrays petty bureaucrats in a small Russian town bribing a youth they wrongly presume to be the State inspector, so as to ingratiate themselves with him. In his stories, Gogol satirizes "nearly all manner of pompous, status-obsessed, careerist bureaucrats."[81]

In parallel, from the start of *War and Peace*, Tolstoy illuminates the centrality of performance, affect, nepotism, and authoritarianism in the life of the social aristocracy, who treat life as though it were a game, the point of which is the accumulation of land, symbolic capital, and power. Through such verbal images, the writer manifests his affinities with the "Producerist Populism" of the French revolutionary Abbe Sieyès and the anarchist Pierre-Joseph Proudhon, together with his related desires to "remov[e] [all] barriers to social communication," level inequality, and expand the realm of freedom.[82] Within these highly exclusive reaches of the gentry, according to the historians Catherine Evtuhov and David Goldfrank, "[r]ank, wealth, and court connections counted toward status more than pedigree or such titles as count(ess) or prince(ss), which were legion."[83] At the same time, the distinctions between princes and princesses on the one hand and counts and countesses on the other reflect the tensions between the ancestral landlord class privileged by the Golden Horde and the Europeanized nobility called into being by Peter I a century prior to the war of 1812, respectively.[84]

Applying Karl Wittfogel's admittedly chauvinist analysis of agromanagerial despotism, which the Sinologist termed invariably "Asiatic," the opening scene of *War and Peace* represents an exhibition of bureaucratic hedonism and hierarchical domination: "Here the state [is] the ultimate owner, in control of the 'means of production' […] and implicitly the people themselves." Here is exalted the authority of "powerful non-producers," the "olympianism of parasites," and the higher value attached by landed aristocrats to status than authenticity.[85] Princess Drubetskaya's class power is derived from State authority, and the aristocrats, living "like sultans," institute Ivan Goncharov's *Oblomovshchina*, the archetype of the idle, parasitic landlord—akin to the poet Rumi's "Huge Eater"—who "did nothing, but simply dozed, or went with his gun to shoot ducks on the millpond."[86]

As Tolstoy will assert in "Strider" (1885), a unique short story written from the perspective of a horse, such a scene bears "the unmistakable stamp of excess, ostentation and absence of intellectual interests."[87] His critique of aristocratic absurdity in turn echoes Chernyshevsky's straightforward formulation, voiced in the words of the mother of the female protagonist in *What Is to Be Done?* (1863): "Where there's idleness, there's vileness; where there's luxury, there's vileness."[88] Tolstoy's satire presages syndicalist discourses emphasizing "the fear of dependence and corruption, the association of luxury with egoism, and the debilitating consequences of the growth of the division of labor."[89] Like LGBTQ+ Syrians reflecting on the suicide of the queer Egyptian Sarah Hegazi in Canadian exile in June 2020, Tolstoy is rebelling against a "hypocritical […] society that claims morality while turning a blind eye to all the violence" it perpetuates.[90]

Tolstoy on Aristocratic Sexual Abuse

In keeping with the practices of patriarchal despotism, which reduce women's lives to the mere property of men—for them to "use and abuse," according to Roman precedents, "within the limits of the law," according to the misogynist Proudhon—Prince Vasili Kuragin is father to Anatole, a young Horse Guards officer. Anatole will notoriously attempt to seduce and abduct the young Countess Natasha Rostova after their meeting in the darkness of the opera house in Moscow, in what Tolstoy apparently considered to be "the crux" of the *poema*.[91] Together with the death of the elder General Prince Nikolai Andreevich Bolkonsky at his estate in the "Bald Hills" as Napoleon's army approaches, this near-miss, which provokes a sexist reaction that leads Natasha to attempt suicide, can be considered an allegory for Russia's fall to the French. The turn of events represents "ethical blindness, aesthetic stupefaction, and the profligacy of urban life," on Tolstoy's account, symbolizing Natasha's moral descent to Anatole's level, and the overwhelming of reason by eroticism.[92]

However, to be fair to Natasha Rostova *and* Tatiana Behrs (1846–1925)—Tolstoy's sister-in-law, on whom she is in part based—the character's openness to Kuragin's advances may reflect doubts over her relationship with Prince Andrei. These arise, in light of the one-year engagement period insisted upon by the elder Bolkonsky, dovetailing with her rude reception by his family at the Bald Hills manor. Facing such loss of love, Rostova becomes vulnerable to the loss of self, the intoxication of false love, and annihilation itself within the world of convention and operatic theater.[93] Seen this way, Natasha's tragedy recalls that of Shakespeare's Juliet; it is a depiction of a nearly completed "honor killing," whereby women's lives are sacrificed to (re)assert male authority. With this in mind, we must recognize how unethical it was for Lev Nikolaevich to debase his sister-in-law, Tanya, by using her unfortunate experience with the unscrupulous Anatole Shostak as the real-life inspiration for this sequence—without even having the decency to change the abuser's first name for his novel.[94]

The only time in the text that Natasha will speak French—the language in which Anna Pavlovna and Prince Vasili mostly converse at the novel's outset—is during her conversation with Hélène Kuragina, Anatole's sister, who essentially sets her up to fail. In this, she functions like Ghislaine Maxwell did for Jeffrey Epstein.[95] As a further illustration of aristocratic baseness, Lev Nikolaevich even hints that Hélène and Anatole have had an incestuous relationship. By the same token, later in the text, as Napoleon's *Grand Armée* approaches Moscow, French will cease to be used among the Russian aristocrats—with the exception of Hélène.[96] This French-language motif, then, ties the drivel expressed by Anna Pavlovna and Prince Vasili in the first chapter to the Machiavellianism of the Kuragins. If Anatole's attempt to abduct Natasha can be likened to Bonaparte's attempt to occupy Russia, a parallel that Sergei Prokofiev's operatic adaptations of *War and Peace* (1942–1953) accentuate, then Anatole's private chastisement by the "lumbering, bumbling, slightly ridiculous" Pierre Bezukhov—the work's principal anti-hero—can be likened to the *Narod*'s expulsion of the *Grand Armée*, as led by the "lumbering, bumbling, slightly ridiculous" General Kutuzov.[97]

Neither Tsarism nor Bonapartism!

Returning to the opening of *War and Peace*, Tolstoy appears to satirize Anna Pavlovna's fanatical devotion to Tsar Alexander I, whom she envisions "fulfill [ing] his vocation and crush[ing] the hydra of revolution" emanating from Europe. She naïvely prefers Alexander, who in her opinion "wants nothing for himself, but only desires the good of mankind," to Napoleon, a supposed "murderer and villain."[98] In this sense, Tolstoy appears to be illustrating and questioning the arbitrariness of preferring one emperor (or ruler) to another, as he implicitly will throughout the *poema*, reflecting his internationalism, humanism, and anarchism. He almost seems to be acknowledging that "[n]ative government [is] no more legitimate than any foreign one," thus proclaiming, like Shakespeare's Mercutio, a plague on both their houses. Whereas the primary goal of Bonaparte's imperialism was war, Alexander's own expansionism must not be overlooked.[99] Another parallel that can be traced between Bonaparte and Alexander is that both leaders seized power through coups in 1799 and 1801, respectively.

In Napoleon's case, the Corsican general who had risen through the ranks, supposedly in defense of the French Revolution, seized power through a military dictatorship. He ruled in a manner inspired by the Roman Empire, and utterly derailed the course of the Revolution.[100] For instance, the evidently Roman inspiration for the design of the helmets worn by Bonaparte's Imperial Guard Dragoons—a nineteenth-century version of the Praetorian Guard—constitutes a distinct visual bridge between the Roman and Napoleonic Empires. To this point, according to Alexis de Tocqueville (1805–1859), Bonaparte simply continued the tyrannical *ancien régime* on a "higher level."[101] "Modern dictators are revolutionary usurpers," explain the sociologists Hans Gerth and C. Wright Mills. In this sense, Tolstoy's depiction of Bonaparte as the consummate Stranger lends weight to Berdyaev's critique of Bonapartism as merely reproducing "the old [...] with a new mask on."[102]

For his part, Tsar Alexander I was installed by the gentry, who had assassinated his father Paul (Catherine II's son), in part as retaliation over his reassertion of mandatory State service for the nobility, and his decrees aimed at improving the condition of the serfs. In his youth, before being corrupted by the influence of Arakcheev, Tsar Alexander had relaxed censorship, empowered the Senate (a judicial and administrative body), and established a legislative State Council modeled after Napoleon's *Conseil d'Etat*.[103] Spearheaded by an "Unofficial Committee" that echoed the "Committee of Public Safety" in the French Revolution, Alexander's administration advanced reforms modeled on the bureaucratic and legal changes brought about by Bonaparte through his "Code Civil." In Russia, certainly, this Code was applied only selectively: Alexander and his ministers never mandated formal legal equality, religious toleration, or the abolition of hereditary nobility, much less equality for Jews.[104] That Tolstoy may have sought to illuminate some of the affinities between Napoleon and Alexander does not however mean that Lev Nikolaevich entirely equates the two causes they manage, in light of the sympathies for Russian chauvinism he at times conveys in *War and Peace*.

From the very outset of the *poema*, then, we can already tell that the subversive scope of Tolstoy's epic has far surpassed the artist's apparent original intent of composing a "delightful gentry romance" entitled *All's End That Ends Well*. Still, we are vexed: can it be that Tolstoy primarily sought to celebrate Russia's victory over the *Grand Armée* with his novel, as Evelina Zaidenshnur claims, and compensate for Russia's loss in the Crimean War?[105] Did he seek to reassert male dignity and so "remasculini[ze]" the Empire?[106]

Connotations of Character Names and Title

At the salon held at Anna Pavlovna's in the summer of 1805, Elizaveta Karlovna Bolkonskaya, Prince Andrei Nikolaevich Bolkonsky's wife—who is described as evidently pregnant, and as "a thoroughly attractive woman"—laments her partner's imminent departure in observation of his duties as a military officer in the War of the Third Coalition against Napoleon. In French, Lise implores, "Tell me: what is this dreadful war for?"[107] Besides the Bolkonskys, this chapter also introduces Pierre, who has been "educated abroad" in Switzerland, and who will become

Count Bezukhov upon his father's death early on in the plot. Therefore, at the outset of the *poema*, Pierre, who must discover who he is, and what life is, enters the scene to be at home, while Prince Andrei, who must learn what to do, is taking leave of an unsatisfying conventional marriage.[108]

Pierre's future wife, the strikingly alluring Princess Hélène Kuragina—so named, surely, for *The Iliad*'s Helen of Troy—first appears in the following chapter. Tolstoy focuses on Hélène's physical beauty by likening her bust to that of classical marble statues idealizing the female figure. In focusing especially on her imagined breasts—and emphasizing the connection between their form, Pierre's sexual arousal, and the anti-hero's emergent desire to marry the princess—the count demonstrates his Freudian view of Hélène (and presumably of his marital partner, Sofia Andreevna) as wife *and* mother, and discloses the mark of the loss of his own mother early in life. In this sense, Hélène is idealized as a "good breast-mother," according to the framing of the psychoanalyst Melanie Klein.[109]

Speculatively, we can say that Pierre is named for Pierre-Joseph Proudhon, whose visage he unmistakably resembles in the sequences depicting the French capture of Moscow in Sergei Bondarchuk's Academy Award winning cinematic adaptation of *War and Peace* (1966–1967). In this film, director Bondarchuk plays Pierre. His look also recalls that of the groundbreaking artist Alexei Venetsianov, whose realistic paintings of peasants inspired the *Narodnik* radicals. In a sense, as an orphan born into the upper aristocracy who ultimately chooses radicalism to ward off superfluity and resist oppression, Bezukhov blends elements from Proudhon, Herzen, and Tolstoy. Accordingly, in the prose poem, Pierre confronts the dualistic choice between serving the legacy of Tsar Peter Romanov vs. the anarcho-Populism of Herzen and his namesake Proudhon.

In fact, Lev Nikolaevich and Pierre-Joseph had met in Brussels in 1861 during Tolstoy's tour to study Western European educational methods, thanks to Herzen's letter of introduction. The title of *War and Peace* itself may have been either an homage to, or implicit critique of, Proudhon's 1861 text, *La guerre et la paix*. Another possibility is that the title reflects the influence of Herzen, who had published three articles using the same title in 1859.[110]

Still, compared with Proudhon, in terms of social class and biography, Pierre is undoubtedly Tolstoy's main *alter ego*, even if Lev Nikolaevich enthusiastically converged with the exiled French writer on matters ranging from politics to economics, gender, and sexuality. That being said, the count sets forth an anti-militarist, pacifist perspective in his *poema*, which clashes starkly with Proudhon's glorification of war, as well as with the vision of the fascist syndicalist Georges Sorel (1847–1922), who saluted the "revolutionary warriors" of the "great *Napoleonic battle[s]*."[111] Along these lines, if *War and Peace* is a critique of Proudhon's views on violence, it may equally be considered a critique of Proudhon's instrumentalist view of the industrial companies, "true armies of the Revolution," comprised of "soldier[s] in [their] battalion[s]," which the French anarchist foresaw replacing standing armies.[112]

At the *poema*'s opening salon, we will meet Prince Andrei, a "very handsome young" officer with a marked "strength of will" who had "read everything, knew everything, and had an opinion on everything."[113] He has "the mind of a master," and "believes in himself, distrusts emotion, and has a firm faith in the power of his reason to shape reality." Bolkonsky finds Anna Pavlovna's *soirée* thoroughly tiresome, and feels alienated from everyone but his wife and Pierre.[114] Like Bezukhov, Andrei is another double for the novelist, considering both Bolkonsky and Tolstoy's paradoxically aristocratic yet generally progressive standpoints, which to an extent stand for "class suicide." Their common disdain for the vanity of the upper classes from which they hail is beyond any doubt, such that Orwin knowingly perceives Andrei to be Tolstoy's "spokesman."[115] Prince Andrei's mission, according to Gustafson, is to follow Jesus the Galilean by leaving family and home behind, thus "rid[ding] himself of that past which is the source of his estrangement."[116] As we will propose in the following chapter, Andrei's political journey toward enlightenment dovetails with a journey toward psychosexual self-discovery and erotic self-determination that echoes Tolstoy's own.

Considering the multiple meanings of the Russian word **мир**, the title *War and Peace* (**Война и мир**) may also be translated as "War and World."[117] Inverting the sequence of the words—as is accepted practice in Russian—leaves us with "World and War," a formulation that is highly suggestive of *World War*. In turn, this bleak term may aptly describe the international political chaos of the Napoleonic Wars, linking it in breadth of death and destruction to the Mongol yoke, as detailed in such chronicles as the *Sermon on the Ruination of the Rus' Land* (c. 1238–1246) and the *Tale of the Destruction of Ryazan* (c. 1270s), as well as to the two world wars of the twentieth century, and even to Syria, Yemen, Ethiopia, and Ukraine in the twenty-first.[118]

According to Éric Alliez and Maurizio Lazzarato, war is the very ontological reality of capitalism.[119] Correlatively, in choosing this title, Count Tolstoy may have meant to comment on the centrality of warcraft to class society and State rule, in light of the axiomatic resort on the part of powerful States and ruling classes to imperialist violence, with the goal of securing pools of labor and "natural resources" against their rivals, whether these be other States or firms, as well as raising taxes, expanding the bureaucracy, and maximizing social control.[120] Considering the violence of Russian political history—from the Mongol Khanate to Tsarist conflicts with Persia and the Ottoman Empire; colonization of the Caucasus, Central Asia, and Eastern Europe; forcible collectivization, the Holodomor, and Stalin's Terror; the Soviet invasion and occupation of Afghanistan; and Putin's ongoing wars in Syria and Ukraine—together with the marked absence of pacifist and anti-militarist beliefs in Russian society, Tolstoy's title may mean to contrast utopian possibilities against stifling imperialist realities.[121]

In contrast, Evelina Zaidenshnur interprets Count Tolstoy's title as meaning "War and Community," in an allusion to the Russian *Narod*, and hence affirming Russian communitarian patriotism, while Alexander Gulin provides alternative equivalent inverted titles, including "Concord and Enmity" or "God and the Enemy of Humankind—the Devil."[122] Gustafson mentions further possibilities for *Peace*: "calm, harmony, union, all people together, the commune, [...] the universe."[123] Indeed, Война и мир may allude to the peasant utopia of the "universal commune."[124] Equally, the choice of title may be taken as an attempt on the author's part to focus the reader's attention on the existentially perplexing and high-risk "state in which we find ourselves," balancing between life and death.[125]

Introducing Protagonists and Concepts

Bezukhov, Pierre's last name, means "earless" in Russian (без ухов). This epithet itself may connect Pierre to the strong-willed and chivalric Don Quixote, to whom Ivan Turgenev likens the literary figure. Characteristically, neither Bezukhov nor Quixote listens to others.[126] Manifesting erotic dissidence, Bezukhov will serve also as a "Tolstoyan Sancho Panza" to Prince Andrei's Don Quixote.[127] Like Tolstoy, a wealthy landowning orphan, Pierre will inherit vast riches upon his father's death. As the *poema*'s anti-hero, Peter Kirillich is meant to combine the principles of ideal and real, sky and earth, "Imagination and Understanding."[128] Inspired by the German poet Johann Wolfgang von Goethe's theory of colors, which follows Kant's critiques of reason and judgment, Tolstoy has Natasha Rostova remark on the "dark blue and red" rays emanating from Bezukhov, symbolizing *Verstand* (scientific or intuitive understanding) and *Phantasie* (fantasy or imagination), respectively, according to Goethe's schema.[129] For Natasha, Petya, and Nikolai's surname, in earlier drafts of the *poema*, the count had tried Prostov ("simple"), before settling on a simplified version of the latter, Rostov, which also connotes the ancestral central Russian town, founded in the ninth century CE. Natasha's character is an amalgam of Tolstoy's wife Sofia *and* her sister Tanya, to whom the author was evidently attracted, as well.[130]

Echoing the self-critical poetry of the Populist Nikolai Nekrasov (1821–1878), who likewise hailed from privilege, Tolstoy exhibits his contempt for the gentry early on by portraying the crassness of the Kuragins. With Princess Katerina Semëvna, Pierre's cousin, they jointly scheme to secure the elder Count Bezukhov's inheritance for themselves.[131] To boot, Prince Boris Drubetskoy, Princess Anna Mikhailovna's son, is evidently more about "dinner parties and scandals than politics"—thus confirming Pushkin's comment on salons, at which "[n]o lasting truths or dissertations" are told.[132]

Bolkonsky and Tolstoy alike change over the course of their literary and historical lives. Initially, they are self-absorbed, selfish, and given to "a pleasant sense of repose among luxurious surroundings," but with time, they come to pursue progress as justice, echoing Proudhon, both internally and socially; heroism, defined as self-sacrifice; and self-perfection, following Kant's concept of the "human disposition toward moral perfection."[133] In parallel, Peter Kirillich Bezukhov undergoes a similar transformation to Andrei, from entering the novel as an aimless alcoholic brawler, to embracing Freemasonry and participation in the revolutionary Decembrist conspiracy by its end.

If Pierre embodies an equilibrium between *Verstand* and fantasy (blue and red, respectively), and General Kutuzov a predominance of *Verstand*, then Andrei exemplifies a predominance of *Vernunft* (yellow), or a speculative-metaphysical understanding, associated with knowledge, light, spirit, and sky. In this sense, Prince Andrei's speculation and dreaming belie the prose poet's public disavowal of metaphysics.[134] In parallel, David Sloane differentiates between Lev Nikolaevich's concepts of *reason* (разум) and *consciousness* (сознание), which may roughly correspond to *Verstand* and *Vernunft*, respectively.[135] In this way, Prince Andrei abides by his father, General Prince Nikolai Andreevich Bolkonsky, an "intelligent hero" exemplifying *Vernunft*/сознание who has been exiled to his estate by the "paradomania[c]" Paul I. Bondarchuk will represent the elder prince on the silver screen as highly reminiscent of Kant himself, in keeping with a known family portrait.[136]

Political Struggle at the *Soirée*, and Gay Bonding at the After-Party

During the opening *soirée*, the progressive youth face off with their reactionary elders. Once Anna Pavlovna communicates Princess Drubetskaya's private request for a favor from Prince Vasili, Pierre and Prince Andrei begin to argue with her and the exiled French viscount of Mortemart about politics. Those who would defend Tsarism in this case express outrage at the killing in March 1804 of the Duc d'Enghien, the heir to the Bourbon royal family, at the hands of Napoleon's gendarmes. At the same time, Pierre tells Anna Pavlovna that he finds unrealistic the "Abbé Morio's" (i.e., Kant's) proposals for "perpetual peace": namely, the idealist proposal, beyond mere peace treaties, for a "*pacific federation*" that would "end *all wars* for good." Even so, over the course of the *poema*, Pierre will trace the unity Kant saw in the ends of nature and freedom, and reject the "flattering [of] tyrants and abusing [of] humanity."[137] By portraying Pierre's initial reluctance to identify himself with the German idealist's theses, Tolstoy relays the anti-hero's initially counter-productive, unconscious identification with autocracy and attendant suspension of conscience—a psychological constellation that facilitates war and exploitation—regardless of his progressive impulses.[138]

In spite of such doubts about the future of cosmopolitanism, ones he will dynamically overcome as the plot advances, Pierre is a relatively more openly enthusiastic Jacobin and partisan of Napoleon than is Prince Andrei. That same evening, Bezukhov openly avows the importance of "the rights of man, emancipation from prejudices, and equality of citizenship."[139] At the salon in question—and perhaps unusually, for a Russian count-to-be—Pierre passionately declares that "[t]he [French] Revolution was a grand thing!" Anna Pavlovna will later disclose that Pierre would even pose as the martyred Jacobin leader Jean-Paul Marat (1743–1793) at one of her parties, in a profession of his revolutionary-republican sympathies.[140] In this way, Bezukhov doubles for Count Paul Stroganov (1774–1817), a Russian heir to a vast fortune who joined the Parisian *Club des Jacobins* in 1790, while anticipating the revolutionary republican leaders of the February 1917 Revolution.[141]

At the *soirée*, Peter Kirillich causes Scherer anxiety because, as a neurodivergent political dissident, he has difficulties with the "hidden curriculum" of conventional society, and is prone to disruptive outbursts against the taboos of polite society.[142]

Moreover, his philosophical commitment to the "producerist populist ideology" shared by Proudhon and the Jacobins—which divides the life-world into "virtuous producers" and "immoral parasites"—necessarily threatens Anna Pavlovna's social position, which after all represents an obstacle to the coming of "a harmonious and egalitarian community."[143] As if to mark the cycle of *samsara*, full of frustration and suffering (*dukkha*), this episode of ideological struggle will recur in the novel's conclusion, when Pierre and Nikolai Rostov argue for disobedience and obedience to the authorities, respectively. Ultimately, the threat of humanistic and proto-democratic communication overwhelming the normalization of feudal exploitation, as symbolized by the escalating political tensions at Anna Pavlovna's salon, is conspicuously derailed by Prince Ippolit Kuragin's nonsensical, contrived, and comical interruption.[144]

After the party, in Andrei's private quarters—the *andron*, or men's space, connotative of their androphilic bond—Pierre and Prince Andrei seek solace from convention by retreating into a homosocial and homophilic space to engage in humanistic communication, whereby people "listen to themselves and to each other" through mutual recognition.[145] That the "after-party" scene unfolds in the *andron* functions to convey both Andrei and Tolstoy's own homoerotic "emotional geography," considering how the White-Russian gentleman was often considered a "European" on the public stage and in grand reception rooms, and a "Russian" in the privacy of his study, parlor, or bedroom.[146]

Lying "from habit" on Andrei's sofa while reading a book by the bisexual strongman Julius Caesar, as if seductively symbolizing one-half of the same-sex couple who would typically recline together at Greek symposia, Bezukhov confides to his friend that he would not want to join the military effort against their common political hero, Napoleon.[147] (Such an acknowledgment of their common identification with Bonaparte, made in the context of Andrei's imminent departure to the military theater, is itself suggestively homoerotic.[148]) Implicitly recognizing the revolutionary nature of anarchy and the Kantian categorical imperative, Prince Andrei will reply by saying that "there would be no wars" if everyone were to fight based only on his or her convictions.

> "And that would be splendid," said Pierre.
> Prince Andrei smiled ironically.
> "Very likely it would be splendid, but it will never come about..."
> "Well, why are *you* going to the war?" asked Pierre.
> "What for? I don't know. I must [...]."[149]

Pierre's weighing whether to join the foreign service during this homophilic social intercourse may connote the gay sensuousness often practiced among diplomats of the "old school," hence linking queerness with anti-militarism.[150] More fundamentally, the exchange suggests that Tolstoy converges with Herman Melville, who emphasized the indistinct boundaries between platonic and homosexual male bonds, and that he agrees with his US counterpart's belief that male friendship is subversive.[151] With its Kantian-anarchist undertones, this dialogue implies the disloyalty of the LGBTQ+ and free-thinking communities to the State.[152] By all means, Pierre's dual repudiation of joining the Russian diplomatic corps and the Horse Guards symbolically mirrors Tolstoy's own self-assertion in calling the State and militarism to account: while he rejects these homosocial worlds along Rousseauvean lines for their ignorance and violence, he fantasizes about other worlds that would institute perpetual peace. Admittedly, his choice also reflects his privilege as a child of the aristocracy and a future landlord, living off the rent extracted from the forced labor of serfs.[153] The dialogue itself reflects the relative freedom afforded Russian nobles by Peter III, who "liberated" the nobility from the obligatory, lifetime sentence of State service that Peter I had imposed.[154]

Thus, at the outset of the *poema*, we see that Pierre's abstract philosophical musings, like Tolstoy's, are paradoxically made possible by exploitation. Later on in the novel, both counterparts of this "particular friendship" will contemplate opening the door to "revolutionary suicide" by renegotiating the terms of labor and land with the feudal slaves who are bound to them, while Pierre will survive his partner and become a Decembrist in his place.[155]

Hierarchy, Heroism, and Sexist Homoeroticism

By conceiving of justice as the renunciation of privilege, Count Tolstoy renders homage to his Decembrist relative, Prince Sergei Volkonsky, who hailed from one of Russia's wealthiest aristocratic families. Significantly, the Volkonskys claimed descent from Rurik (c. 830–70 CE), the Scandinavian Varangian prince who,

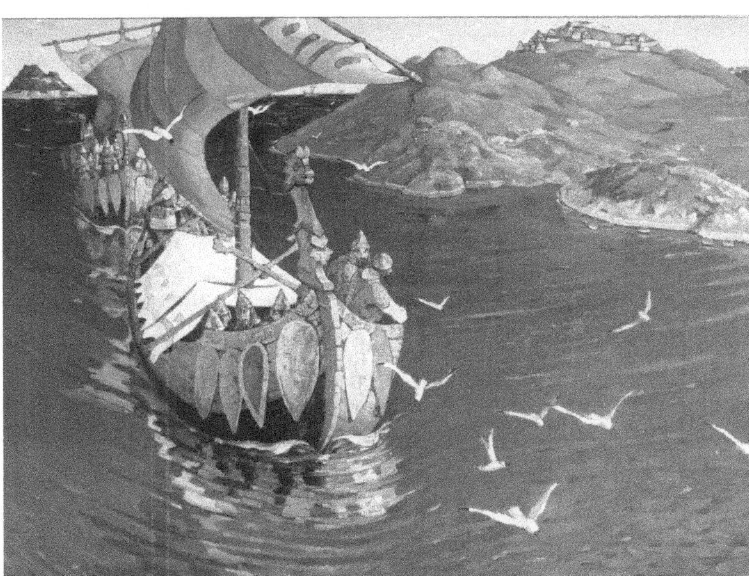

FIGURE 5.1 Nicholas Roerich, *Guests from Overseas* (1901)

according to the *Primary Chronicle* (c. 1113 CE), was invited by Slavic and Finnic tribes to "[c]ome reign and rule over us." The legend goes, then, that the Rurikids introduced the "civilizing" State onto "backward" Rus' (see Figure 5.1).[156] As a result of this privileged lineage, the Volkonsky family owned thousands of serfs and maintained an intimate relationship with the Romanov dynasty.[157]

Like Lev Nikolaevich's contemporary Peter Kropotkin—whose family in like fashion claimed descent from the Rurikids, who corresponded with Tolstoy, and who also became a radical anarcho-Populist—Sergei Grigorievich had graduated from the elite *Corps des Pages* military academy before embarking on a career that would involve distinction in the Napoleonic Wars, including a stunning promotion to major general by age 24. Inspired by his encounters with the ennobling heroism of the peasant conscripts and partisans, as well as with liberal-constitutionalist political systems in Paris and London, Volkonsky became a leader in the anti-Tsarist Decembrist conspiracy of 1825.[158]

Despite Volkonsky's example, the legend of Rurik served Tsarism and landlordism in much the same way that other forms of statist indoctrination have sought to convince the People themselves oppressed by bureaucratic power that they have somehow consented to their subordination.[159] As a foundational myth idealizing popular servility and non-resistance before the State, the story around Rurik is consistent with the Eastern Orthodox fetishization of self-denial and powerlessness.[160] Therefore, both Bolkonsky and Tolstoy are faced with the challenge of seeking to live in such a way that lives up to the example of the writer's revolutionary relative, Sergei Volkonsky, while *also* negating the sadomasochistic legacy of another of his ancestors, Peter Andreevich Tolstoy, who was Tsar Peter I's "most trusted statesman."[161] In other words, they must overcome Russia's hegemonic culture of violence, which insists that one is either dominator or dominated.[162]

The beginnings of such a disavowal of despotism are reflected in Pierre and Prince Andrei's "fifth column" status in *War and Peace*.[163] Still, their positive regard for Napoleon ebbs over the course of the *poema*: whereas neither Bezukhov nor Bolkonsky's affinity for Bonaparte at the outset is very well explained, other than as a cipher of their erotic and republican desires, by the time the *Grand Armée* has invaded Russia, Napoleon is "no longer the man who had inspired the armies of the *sans-culottes* in their first steps eastwards for the abolition of serfdom, absolutism, and inquisition." Instead, he was by then an "emperor, spoiled by the adulation of the courtiers of all Europe and the worship of the masses": one who held that Europe could not "be at rest except under a single head who will have kings for his officers."[164]

Hence, the heroic male couple will come metaphorically to resemble the Greek soldiers of the battle of Thermopylae (480 BCE), who perish courageously defending the potential for democracy against the tyranny represented by the Achaemenid invasion: Bolkonsky, as an officer resisting the "charismatic terrorist" Napoleon at Austerlitz and Borodino, and Bezukhov as an exiled or executed Decembrist, standing up to the agrobureaucratic Tsarist despots, Alexander I and Nicholas I.[165]

Unfortunately, there is evident misogyny in Pierre and Andrei's encounter after the opening *soirée*, particularly in light of the coldness, resentment, and even hostility Bolkonsky expresses toward his wife, Lise. The latter insists that "the princess [... not] deprive me of the pleasure of spending the evening with you," meaning Pierre. For instance, when Elizaveta Karlovna first approaches the prince's study containing the two men, Tolstoy remarks how Andrei's "face assumed the look it had had in Anna Pavlovna's drawing-room."[166] The prince does not welcome this intrusion into the *andron*, a movement that simultaneously threatens his homosocial feelings of residence while emblematically challenging male dominance.[167] When Lise expresses fear over her pregnancy—ultimately reflecting the "omnipresence" of non-being and the resultant "universal anxiety" over the fear of death, thus foreshadowing her own end—Andrei utterly dismisses her *Angst*.[168] Lise responds by protesting against her husband's egotism, crystallized in her comment that he "treat[s] me like [...] a child."[169]

Then, left alone again with Pierre, Andrei re-establishes strict patriarchal norms by insulting all women, calling them "[s]elfish, vain, stupid, trivial in everything [...]."[170] Reflecting the author's sexist animus and Andrei's attempt to sublimate his homoerotic frustration into misogyny, such derogatory comments follow Tolstoy's statements in *Family Happiness* (1859) about a former partner, Valerya Arseneva, who is described as "sweet but, alas, simply stupid."[171] They further foreshadow Lev Nikolaevich's declaration in *The Power of Darkness* (1886) that "women are vile creatures! One can't say much for men either, but women!"[172]

This exchange between Pierre and Andrei thus epitomizes the at-times unfortunate intermixing of regressive *and* progressive views in Tolstoy's works—testifying to his art "both [as] an opposition *and* a reaction"—symbolized here by the couple's commitment to the ideals of the French Revolution, and its constituent parts' misogyny, respectively.[173] In his anger, Bolkonsky exhibits the toxic masculinity expected of the soldier, the heterosexual male, *and* the active homosexual partner. For his part, Stalin likewise would express hostility toward women out of one corner of his mouth, and overt or subliminal gay interest out of the other.[174]

In Sum: Major Themes and Motifs in *War and Peace*

Considering the vast length and large cast of *War and Peace*, we will explore Tolstoy's classic by dedicating five chapters below to its respective four parts (and epilogue), arranged by themes, many of which recur over the course of the novel. Before we pass to this chronicle of the *poema*, however, we shall summarize its main themes and motifs, and explore the writer's relationship to Carl von Clausewitz.

Some of the major themes addressed by Tolstoy in *War and Peace* include the following: a satire of Russia's social aristocracy, and an idealization of spiritual aristocracy; a critique of war, its parallel labor, and the authority principle; a critique of the compulsory sadomasochism (or authoritarianism) of hierarchical social organizations; an exploration of the psychosexual process of coming out; an anarcho-Populist interpretation of history which emphasizes the "flow" of nations and peoples rather than the individual wills of "great men"; a predominant internationalism at times offset by resurgent Slavophilism and Russian communitarian chauvinism; sympathetic portrayals of resistance and non-cooperation; critique of the abuse of animals; examinations of the relationship between life and death; an avowal of harmonic or circular reason, alongside *Verstand*/разум (scientific or intuitive reason) and *Vernunft*/сознание (metaphysical reason, or consciousness); and recurrent homoeroticism and misogyny.

Lev Nikolaevich furthermore employs recurring motifs connected to these themes, such as the delirium brought on by loss and the internalization of hierarchical domination, and its supersession through the Kantian exercise of reason, as well as the motif of the door, symbolizing the transition from life to death—or from peace to war. In "On Life" (1911), the prose poet remarks that the "'exit doors' of death are the same as the 'entrance doors' we passed through at birth," and in an 1878 piece he similarly envisions death as a state into which we "enter again."[175] Furthermore, the writer weaves the hydrological motifs of bodies and flows of water into the narrative as metaphors both for the passing of time—the Buddhist concept of *anitya*, or impermanence, and the core Proudhonian concept of movement—and for the human mind, and humanity's collective action, which manifest the divine life within us, through which history is made.[176] In keeping with the traumatic centrality of maternal loss in Tolstoy's life and art, the prose poet's incorporation of hydrological imagery also suggests a sustained fixation on embryonic life and the mother. Lastly, the swarm motif is inseparable from the artist's naturalistic and metaphysical anarcho-Populist vision, which posits collective unity as a human ideal.[177]

Tolstoy and Clausewitz

Broadly speaking, *War and Peace* is an anti-war art-work. Tolstoy's normative critiques of combat and statecraft, which dovetail with the prose writer's "emotional existential" approach to warfare, predominate over any detached sense of harmonic reason.[178] In this, ironically, the author closely echoes the young Carl von Clausewitz, who early on likewise advanced an existential view of war, and so critiques the better-known elder Clausewitz, who advocated an instrumentalist and legitimizing philosophy that stresses the amorality of States wielding *Gewalt* (violence) and *Kampf* (struggle) in the pursuit of their material and political interests. Clausewitz famously argued that the military which acts most ruthlessly will reap the most benefits, assuming its opponents do not do the same. Significantly, General Clausewitz's approach anticipates the "realist" school of international-relations theory, which fetishizes State sovereignty, power politics, and the performance principle.[179] It grimly portends Bolshevik military specialist Mikhail N. Tukhachevsky's cruel suppression of the Kronstadt Commune in March 1921, which would prepare the ground for Stalin's subsequent takeover of the Soviet Communist Party.[180]

On the eve of the battle of Borodino (August 26, 1812), Tolstoy depicts Generals Clausewitz and Wolzogen, who along with 30 other officers had abandoned the Prussian military to fight Napoleon's forces alongside the Russians, as discussing their inhumane, "realist" proposals for strategy. Deliberating in German, they agree that the "war must be extended widely," and that "one cannot take into account the loss of private individuals."[181] Overhearing this dialogue as he discusses the prospects for the battle with Pierre Bezukhov, Prince Bolkonsky will paradoxically affirm this very same idea—that in combat, the most consistently sadomasochistic party will prevail—while also denouncing the German generals' insensitivity to the *actual lives* of concrete human beings, such as those of his family at Bald Hills. Metaphorically, such commentary can be taken as a repudiation of the objectification of human life inherent in *Gewalt* and warfare, and a reflection of the intimate links Tolstoy sees between political absolutism and the practice of total war.[182]

That being said, the poet does at times express common anxieties with the general about the destructiveness of the so-called mob, as his treatment of the peasants at the Bolkonskys' Bogucharovo manor reveals. This lapse, in turn, speaks to the contradictions in the writer's fidelity to his own ideals, as well as his experiences with serfs at Yasnaya Polyana who had resisted his plan for emancipation, as detailed in "A Landowner's Morning" (1856).

While it is unclear whether Lev Nikolaevich ever read Clausewitz himself, his apt critique of the Clausewitzian wielding of instrumental reason in war does appear to overlook the respect both he and the general commonly had for the material and psychological realities of combat. Although the German theorist is known for his objectifying view of warfare, military theorists Daniel Moran and Andreas Herberg-Rothe insist that this comprises but one dimension of his approach: unlike Bonaparte, depicted as he is as a malignant narcissist in *War and Peace*, Clausewitz sympathetically "recognized the impact of fear, danger, confusion, and fatigue on men in battle, and wrote about them with unusual candor."[183] Moreover, in examining the essential themes of Clausewitz's *On War*, we see several commonalities with Tolstoy's themes in *War and Peace*: namely, as Moran summarizes,

> that the essence of war is violence, which knows no natural limit; that war "does not consist in a single blow," but involves protracted interaction between opposing wills; that every attack loses its impetus as it proceeds, until it reaches a culminating point where it no longer exceeds the strength of the defence that opposes it; that war is dominated by chaos and chance [...;] that the only means in war is combat; that war is merely a continuation of policy; and so on [...].[184]

This first theme Tolstoy integrates into the "Sevastopol Sketches," *The Cossacks*, and *War and Peace*. The *poema's* length, in point of fact, speaks to the second theme, about a "protracted interaction." Moreover, as we shall see in Chapter 8, the battle of Borodino illustrates the third principle on momentum, which sketches the *Grand Armée*'s deceleration injury, evincing Isaac Newton's third law of motion and the postulated "superiority of defense to attack."[185] Tolstoy fully acknowledges the utter chaos of combat, and brings this to bear not only in his illustrations of historical battles from the Napoleonic Wars, but also in his exploration of the war's effects on non-combatants. Prince Andrei appositely describes the meaning of this chaos to his diplomatic officer counterpart, Bilibin, in an exchange made during the Russian army's retreat after the Austrians' disastrous defeat at Ulm in October 1805. When Bilibin asks why the army couldn't "capture one, just one, marshal," Bolkonsky responds drily: "Because not everything happens as one expects with the smoothness of a parade."[186]

Notes

1 Tolstoy 2017: 2.
2 Orwin 2012b: 98; Bartlett 2011: 106.
3 Kropotkin 1991: 117.
4 Emerson 8.
5 Morson 2002: 65; Clay 216; Maude 1987a: 311; Harris; Orwin 1993: 99; Kropotkin 1991: 128.
6 Gustafson 1986: xii–xiv; Shcherbakov 82; Love 2007: 127.
7 Gustafson 1986: xii, 203–4; Kropotkin 2018: 339; Habermas 1981: 167; Reitz 63; Benjamin 184–6; Eisler. Apropos, "[m]uch of what is central to Tolstoy seems embarrassing to Western critics" (Gustafson 1986: xiii).
8 Orwin 1993: 5–7, 106–21; Orwin 2002b: 222; Berdyaev 2009: 176–7.
9 Maude 2010: xvii; 1987a: 421; Gettone.
10 Samet 162, 216n5; Clay 209.
11 Ungurianu 41; Forrest 71.
12 Orend (emphasis in original); Emerson 8.
13 Harris 84; Chodorow 1999: 239.
14 Freud 1953: 426.
15 Tillich 56–66, 120–40.
16 Becker 272–5.
17 Orwin 2002b: 2; Bartlett 2001: 88.
18 Tolstoy 1987: 12.
19 Figes 2002: 89–91, 141; Tolstoy 1987: 12.
20 Schonfeld and Chang 10; Freud 1953: 424–7.
21 Berdyaev 1966; Yousef.
22 Tolstoy 2010: 1268.
23 Bartlett 2011: 368–9.
24 Kentish 15.
25 Bakunin 1867; Berdyaev 1966: 77.
26 Chekhov 235, 279.
27 Sloane et al. 59–61.
28 Newlin 367.
29 Maude 1987a: 300.
30 Feuer.
31 Newlin 372–9; Bartlett 2011: 62–98. Perhaps the most notorious Imperial monument was the Cathedral of Christ the Savior, first constructed on Alexander I's orders using the forced labor of 20,000 serfs, and featuring the massive embezzlement of funds that would inspire Nikolai Gogol's *The Government Inspector* (1836). Its site would be relocated by Nicholas I nearer to the Kremlin, completed in 1882, and then razed by Stalin's regime in 1931 (Figes 2002: 137–9).
32 Berlin 1978: 33; Grodetskaya 100.
33 Kropotkin 1991: 129.
34 Polosina 55.
35 Orwin 2012a: 3.
36 Emerson 1; Maude 2010: xi–xv; Sloane 2005: 106; Morson 2012: 82; Gustafson 1986: 228; Figes 2002: 361; Wachtel.

37 "Tolstoy was violently opposed to academic philosophy and theology and their technical languages" (Gustafson 1986: 89).
38 Bartlett 2011: 3–48, 121; Maude 1987a: 139; Foster J 197.
39 Maude 1987a: 224; Love 2011: 37.
40 Berlin 1978: 30 (emphasis added).
41 Maude 2010: xiii.
42 Chekhov 1999: 305.
43 Shlapentokh 500; Tolstoy 2010: 1005; Wilson J 2021.
44 Berdyaev 1966: 13–14; 2009: 17–20, 149–50.
45 Kropotkin 1991: 116.
46 Figes 2002: 157, 363–71, 391–426.
47 Love 2007: 126.
48 Berdyaev 2009: 172–80.
49 Compare Maude: "the depression resulting from the age-long failure of unorganized individualist effort to grapple with this gigantic problem [i.e., the economic question] is even more detrimental than an excessive devotion to the practical work of organization" (Maude 1987b: 111).
50 Bartlett 2011: 24–85.
51 Zorin 33–6; Sloane et al. 61–2.
52 Currie 254.
53 Kropotkin 1991: 290.
54 Bakunin 2005: 38.
55 Berdyaev 1966: 13; Foster J 22, 213n11; Love 2007: 126.
56 Berdyaev 1966: 16; Figes and Kolonitskii 14–27.
57 Tolstoy 2004: 234–45.
58 Shafer.
59 Morson 2002: 68–9; Berdyaev 2009: 179. Tolstoy's lack of optimism for the future is one characteristic difference between him and his Marxist contemporaries (Berdyaev 2009: 198).
60 Peterson 39n3. Golz is a Russian general and Republican commander of Hemingway's invention.
61 Figes 2002: 114.
62 Forrest 73.
63 Maude 2010: xvii; 1987a: 119; Orwin 2012b: 100.
64 Figes 2002: 134–5.
65 Lieven 2012: 18; Figes 2002: 135.
66 Figes 2002: 72–85; Bartlett 2011: 12.
67 Figes 2002: 75.
68 Stites 1989; Figes 2002: 76–118.
69 Jansen.
70 Evtuhov et al. 362–3. Nikolai Berdyaev interprets *sobornost'* as a more explicitly anti-authoritarian collective relatedness. The South and East African concept of Ubuntu, "the belief in a universal bond of sharing that connects all humanity," appears very similar (Berdyaev 2009; Kitonga).
71 Donaldson 1990b; Pietikainen 17; Berdyaev 2009: 203; Karlinsky.
72 Figes 2002: xxvi–xxxii, 44, 81–100.
73 Bartlett 2011: 254; Maude 1987a: 370–1.
74 Berdyaev 1966: 15–22; Evtuhov et al. 302–10; Bartlett 2011: 2, 99; Martin 44; Yarmolinsky; Stites 1990: 15; Borshchevskaya.
75 Evtuhov et al. 322.
76 Berdyaev 2009: 171–6; Gustafson 1986: 410)
77 Maude 1987a: 184; Bartlett 2011: 122, 247; Zorin 37–8; Venturi; Poole; Reitz.
78 Fuchs 3–15.
79 Rousseau 448.

80 Cruise 196; Gustafson 1986: 343; Tolstoy 2010: 16–8. The "Drubetskoys" are a thinly veiled parody of the Trubetskoy family, going back to Prince Dmitri Trubetskoy (d. 1625?), who had been a contender for Tsar during the seventeenth-century Time of Troubles (Evtuhov et al. 153–7).
81 Kropotkin 1991: 78; Wilson J 2021.
82 Figes 2002: 42–3; Fuchs; Honneth 64–5; Browne; Abromeit.
83 Evtuhov et al. 372.
84 Bartlett 2011: 21.
85 Shlapentokh 490; Reitz 27, 143; Pasternak 545.
86 Wittfogel 297–9; Figes 2002: 410–11; Chekhov 1999: 224; Berdyaev 1966; Clark 2019.
87 Tolstoy 2005: 98.
88 Chernyshevsky 75.
89 Tucker 90.
90 Salem.
91 Proudhon 90; Maude 2010: xv; Orwin 1993: 128; Tolstoy 2010: 489.
92 Maude 2010: xv; Emerson 1. In fact, Anatole and Natalya are near-anagrams (Orwin 1993: 123–6).
93 Gustafson 1986: 349–52.
94 Zorin 72–9.
95 Tolstoy 2010: 601–32; Emerson 7; Bekiempis.
96 Tolstoy 2010: 220, 718, 900.
97 Emerson 5.
98 Tolstoy 2010: 5.
99 Zorin 115; Evtuhov et al. 322–3.
100 Tolstoy 2010: 1221, Evtuhov et al. 311–19.
101 Bondarchuk; Evtuhov et al. 313.
102 Gerth and Mills 212; Ludwig; Terras 14; Berdyaev 2009: 196.
103 Evtuhov et al. 314–18; Figes 2002: 84.
104 Evtuhov et al. 313, 320–5; Ludwig.
105 McLean 2008: 83.
106 Mole 7.
107 Tolstoy 2010: 9–10 (my translation).
108 *Ibid* 11; Gustafson 1986: 72–3; Foster J 71.
109 Rancour-Laferriere 1989: 43–4; Love 2012: 85.
110 Bartlett 2011: 143, 170; Maude 1987a: 223.
111 Berlin 1978: 55, 65–6; Sorel 78, 242 (emphasis in original); Sternhell 99.
112 Sternhell 106.
113 Tolstoy 2010: 31.
114 Gustafson 1986: 62; Rancour-Laferriere 1985: 301–6; Tolstoy 2010: 15–16.
115 Orwin 2012b: 106; Zorin 18.
116 Gustafson 1986: 62.
117 Orwin 1993: 179.
118 Evtuhov et al. 73.
119 Alliez and Lazzarato.
120 Kropotkin 2018: 329–44; Waltz 100.
121 Borshchevskaya; Shkurenok; La Botz.
122 Love 2007; McLean 2008: 87n3.
123 Gustafson 1986: 40.
124 Stites 1989: 125.
125 Balan 464–7.
126 Orwin 1993: 129.
127 Love 2012: 85.
128 Bartlett 2011: 3; Orwin 1993: 130.

129 Tolstoy 2010: 483; Orwin 1993: 130–2. As an aside, this primacy of fantasy in Pierre's emotional life may suggest an autism diagnosis, which might help us better understand the character—and author (Békés et al.).
130 Taylor; Zorin 73–9.
131 Figes 2002: 223; Tolstoy 2010: 74–80. In this, as in the scene depicting the wounded Prince Andrei being carried to a field hospital by serfs, which we will analyze in Chapter 8, Tolstoy uncannily anticipates his death, and the conflicts between Chertkov and his family over his will.
132 Tolstoy 2010: 57; Figes 2002: 48.
133 Tolstoy 2010: 163; Orwin 1993: 105–8; Sloane 2005: 104; Kinna 2020b.
134 Orwin 1993: 5, 126–31, 162.
135 Sloane 2005.
136 Berdyaev 2009; Stites 1989: 19; Bondarchuk; Bartlett 2011: 23; Frank.
137 Tolstoy 2010: 1319–1320n3; Kant 1991: 102–5 (emphasis in original); Heller 130.
138 Reitz 105; Maude 1987b: 35.
139 Tolstoy 2010: 10–11, 21.
140 *Ibid* 21, 389, 575; Shafer 18.
141 Yarmolinsky; Figes and Kolonitskii 7.
142 Moyse and Porter; Gustafson 1986: 404; Hall 138.
143 Abromeit 376.
144 Tolstoy 2010: 23, 1262; Fuchs 25.
145 Fuchs 13; Dynes 1990a; Dynes 1990k; Hekma.
146 Figes 2002: 44–5.
147 Tolstoy 2010: 25–6; Percy 1990c. The Code Napoléon (1810) upholds the French Constituent Assembly's 1791 decision to exclude "sodomy" from the list of sexual crimes (Johansson 1990k). Although part I of *War and Peace* takes place in 1805, the evident homoerotic atmosphere in this scene may in part connote accordance with this landmark reform.
148 Rancour-Laferriere 1985.
149 Tolstoy 2010: 27 (emphasis in original).
150 Ulam 509.
151 Johansson 1990h.
152 Mole 9; Kant 1784.
153 Along the same lines, "Count Lev Tolstoy [...] never had to work for gainful employment" (Gustafson 1986: 434).
154 Zorin 25.
155 Johansson 1990l; Newton.
156 Zorin 8; Evtuhov et al. 13; Tolstoy 2010: 108.
157 Zorin 45.
158 MacLaughlin; Figes 2002: 72–85.
159 Kinna 2020b.
160 Rancour-Laferriere 1995.
161 Bartlett 2011: 277.
162 Troianovski.
163 Tolstoy 2010: 133.
164 Kropotkin 1991: 133; Fournier 250.
165 Johansson 1990i; McCall.
166 Tolstoy 2010: 27–9. Indeed, this tension may allude to Pushkin's lines in the poem "To Chaadaev" (1821): "You know, my dear, we're all free men now / We keep away from society; don't mingle with the ladies" (Figes 2002: 77).
167 Benjamin 187.
168 Tillich 45; Becker 21.
169 Tolstoy 2010: 29.
170 *Ibid* 31; Benjamin 187.
171 Maude 1987a: 161.

172 Tolstoy 2019: 60.
173 Malia 287.
174 Rancour-Laferriere 1988: 102.
175 Rancour-Laferriere 1998: 33–4.
176 Newlin 381–2; Tolstoy 2010: 1273; Kinna and Harper; Gustafson 1986: 178.
177 Rancour-Laferriere 1995: 190; Gustafson 1986: 96–7.
178 McPeak 116; Herberg-Rothe 142.
179 Herbert-Rothe 142–5; Waltz 206; Dunne and Schmidt.
180 Croll; Bookchin.
181 Moran 208; Tolstoy 2010: 830.
182 Herberg-Rothe 152.
183 Moran 208.
184 *Ibid.*
185 Herbert-Rothe 151. Newton's third law proposes an "equal and opposite reaction" to every action.
186 Tolstoy 2010: 165.

6

WAR AND PEACE, BOOK ONE

"Andrei Bolkonsky"

In the first book of *War and Peace*, which constitutes almost a fourth of the text, Tolstoy advances three major themes: a humanistic critique of war, its parallel labor, and the authority principle; followed by a general critique of the compulsory sadomasochism (or authoritarianism) of hierarchical social organizations; and a satirical portrayal of the vast worlds of privilege built through the systemic plundering of the peasantry. In the Russian Empire, the power of the landed aristocracy, Church, and State depended on this parasitical relationship. As an experimental tour of imperial history through the vast Winter Palace (now known as the Hermitage Museum), Alexander Sokurov's 2002 film *Russian Ark* starkly exhibits the architectural looting, ostentation, and "inequality carved in masonry" on which Tsarism based itself.[1] In contrast to Sokurov, whose reactionary nostalgia centers elites, States, and empires, Lev Nikolaevich Tolstoy presents an anarcho-Populist interpretation of history in *War and Peace* which emphasizes the movement of nations and peoples in social reproduction and the (re)construction of reality.

In this chapter, we contemplate Tolstoy's critiques of war, labor, and hierarchy in *War and Peace*, and trans-historically apply them to our own day. We focus in on the queerness of the *poema*, especially as relayed through Prince Andrei Bolkonsky's journey of psychosexual self-discovery in conditions of combat, and find that same-sex attraction often conveys bell hooks's concept of the "anarchism of love": namely, the idea that "[w]hen love is present the desire to dominate and exercise power cannot rule the day."[2]

War and Peace: Tolstoy's Populist, Anti-Authoritarian Perspectives

For the subversiveness he promotes in *War and Peace*, Tolstoy came under figurative fire from General Mikhail Dragomirov (1830–1905), who nevertheless gave credit to the artist for his insights into the psychological dimensions of war, despite

DOI: 10.4324/9781003328964-6

disagreeing with his criticism of military hierarchies. Other Russian officers who fought in the Napoleonic Wars accused Lev Nikolaevich less charitably of being a "killer" of history.[3] To an extent, though, many such veterans resented that Tolstoy had refused to integrate their memoirs into his research for the novel.[4] Being himself an apologist for militarism, General Dragomirov would object most strongly to the prose poet's portrayal of regimental flags as mere "pieces of cloth on sticks," the novelist's contempt for tactics and strategy, and the author's portrayal of battles not as sites of heroism and brilliance, but of "mindless carnage and confusion."[5]

That being said, as Orwin rightly argues, Tolstoy's elucidation of a Populist vision reveals one of the shortcomings of this approach: namely, a relative minimization of class struggle within feudal Russian society, especially upon Napoleon's invasion, and an insistence that members of the gentry, "the main actors in the novel," are part of the *Narod*, just as much as the peasants and merchants.[6] The historian Catherine Evtuhov and her colleagues describe how such a model of the "Russian people" follows Tsar Alexander I's close adviser Mikhail Speransky's proposed reorganization of the previously existing five *soslovie* ("estates") categories into the three categories of gentry, working people, and middle classes.[7] In other words, in his *poema*, Tolstoy runs the risk of contradicting anarchism by envisioning an authoritarian, anti-capitalist national revolution.[8]

The limitations of Populism and Tolstoy's focus on the gentry notwithstanding, it cannot be denied that Lev Nikolaevich greatly satirizes the Russian social aristocracy in his novel. Bondarchuk's film adaptation of *War and Peace* (1966–1967) strikingly traces the vast scale of the architecture of artifice, irrationality, exploitation, and waste involved in the existence of the aristocratic ruling class. Yet, rather than celebrate such ostentation, as Sokurov's film does, Bondarchuk contrasts the absurdity of aristocratic social gatherings with the realities of impending war and death. The 1972 *BBC* serialization begins with three minutes of a house serf setting Count Rostov's dinner table. Art thus imitates the real-life expectations of Count Andrey Ivanovich Tolstoy (1721–1803), the author's great-grandfather, who would expect to dine on fresh sterlet from the White Sea and oysters imported from Holland.[9]

Hunting expeditions such as those organized by Russian diplomat Lev Izmailov (1685–1738), involving some 3,000 hunters and 2,000 hounds, presupposed "ownership of vast serf armies," the monopolization of "virtually all the land," and the mass-exploitation of wildlife and domesticated animals.[10] In "Peasants" (1897), Chekhov reports on how "whole wagonloads of game [hunted by agricultural workers] used to be sent to Moscow for the young masters."[11] Even the preparation of Natasha Rostova's beautiful appearance at the St. Petersburg ball where she and Prince Andrei will meet presupposes a great amount of alienated and forcible labor on the part of servants, who are certainly more peripheral to the plot than the aristocratic protagonists.[12] Pierre, for his part, is oblivious to the existence of the house serfs' quarters in the back of his father's estate until the elder Bezukhov is on his death-bed. In reality, he enters the *poema*'s world without having a clear idea of what is happening.[13]

Shaken by his confrontation with the passing of his old friend Bezukhov, Prince Vasili Kuragin experiences a crisis of identity and vocation, as his conventional consciousness is temporarily disrupted.[14] He reflectively remarks to Pierre, "How often we sin, how much we deceive, and all for what? [...] All will end in death." When Princess Katerina Semënovna, Pierre's cousin, confesses that she "ha[s] a wicked heart" and cries that she "knew that [she] could expect nothing but meanness, deceit, envy, intrigue, and ingratitude [...] in this house"—referring to the Bezukhov mansion, where she has been colluding with Prince Vasili to secure the dying Bezukhov's inheritance—she passes such judgment not only on her own particular family, but on the privileged classes in general.[15]

Anatole Kuragin is introduced as a rowdy, toxic male who enslaves a young bear, "Bruin," for the purposes of his entertainment, aping the precedent set by Tsar Ivan IV ("the Terrible").[16] Diverging radically from the Kuragins, Princess Marya Nikolaevna Bolkonskaya's "spiritual and reasonable" character is based on Tolstoy's own mother before her marriage, just as his paternal aunt Tatiana Alexandrovna Ergolskaya served as the inspiration for Sonya Rostova, Natasha's cousin.[17] Though passionately attracted to Count Nikolai Tolstoy, Lev's father, "Toinette" sacrificed erotic satisfaction to allow her would-be partner to marry the heiress Marya Volkonskaya instead. Sonya does precisely the same in *War and Peace*, hence affording Rostov the chance of settling his debts, as of enjoying a life of luxury, through appropriation of Princess Marya's dowry, which in real life included 800 serfs and the Yasnaya Polyana estate.[18]

Along similar lines, in a resounding affirmation of her (and Tolstoy's) preference for Christian over erotic love, Princess Marya utterly rejects Anatole's courtship.[19] Plus, in keeping with Tolstoyan Slavophilism, the marriage between Pierre and Princess Hélène Kuragina, both of whom bear French names, is evidently insipid and contrived. Hélène, in fact, resembles Napoleon due to her egotistical, careerist interests, such that Pierre's own wife simultaneously brings to mind the beloved *and* the enemy.[20] In short, their marriage is sadomasochistic. By coming to "possess" Hélène's great beauty, and so integrating this alluring "object" into a self-object relation reminiscent of early infantile life, Pierre considerably inflates his self-esteem, all the while losing personal autonomy and entrapping another in the process.[21] Tolstoy makes a point of associating such symbiosis with delirium and self-forgetting.[22] Even in the *poema*'s finale, Peter Kirillich repeats similar regressive patterns in his second marriage, with Natasha Rostova, after having advanced more closely to understanding love as mutual recognition under his mentor, the "holy fool" Platon Karataev, as we shall see.[23]

Tolstoy's perspective, then—here, as elsewhere—is complex, at times contradictory, and syncretic. For all that, *War and Peace* stands out in its condemnation of militarism and conquest. Many of its most poignant anti-war scenes have echoes elsewhere in Tolstoy's works. For instance, the effective family-separation involved in military conscription, and the suffering of the soldiers' families which results, as seen in Princess Marya's weeping at Andrei's departure to the war in 1805, is repeated later in Tolstoy's *The Kingdom of God Is Within You* (1893), a tract that elaborates the author's critique of violence, coercion, and statism.[24] Such sequences are funereal in tone, given that conscription regimes were effectively death-sentences that typically lasted a quarter-century.[25] In terms of literary allusions, the plaintive scenes in which Lise and Marya lament Andrei's departure recall classical partings from Homer's *Iliad*.[26] After all, in the years before his marriage (1862), the count had read Plato's *Phaedo* and *Symposium*, as well as Homer's *Iliad* and *Odyssey*, with great interest.[27] Besides this, the *poema* resembles the Bible in many ways, considering its numerous parables and scores of biblical allusions that reflect its author's faith, not to mention its often prophetic-messianic tone.

As Andrei departs for combat in *War and Peace*, the "door motif" is first introduced. Whereas Marya seeks to demonstrate a "thoughtful, kindly, and unaccustomed brightness" to her brother at what could well be their final meeting, "he was not looking at his sister but over her head towards the darkness of the open doorway."[28] In this manner, Andrei anticipates his own death due to injuries suffered while awaiting orders behind the front lines at Borodino. The author's realistic depiction of the violence of war, particularly at the battle of Schön-Grabern in Austria[29] between Russian and French troops (November 4, 1805), stunningly recalls the brutal realism of the "Sevastopol Sketches"—as well, it must be mentioned, as the numerous ongoing wars of our own day.

As in the "Sketches," Tolstoy's critical attitude toward warfare is manifested in the graphic yet authentic presentations of suffering, disability, and death on the battlegrounds. Lev Nikolaevich has a certain Prince Nesvitsky exclaim, upon witnessing the first deaths in combat, that "[i]f I were Tsar I would never go to war."[30] The central themes of "The Death of Ivan Ilych" (1886)—finitude, death-anxiety, and existential shock therapy—are relived constantly among Tolstoy's troops at Schön-Grabern, who are haunted by an "unseen line" dividing the living from the dead, such that "the question [of] whether they would cross it or not, and how they would cross it, agitated them all."[31]

In turn, the prose poet refers to this dividing line of mortality in the theater of war as a "mysterious domain of smoke" and a "universal disaster" suggestive of Armageddon.[32] The narrator of Bondarchuk's film version aptly channels Tolstoy's humanistic and messianic critique of militarism by commenting in the following way on preparations before the battle of Austerlitz, otherwise known as the "battle of the three emperors" (Napoleon, Alexander, and Francis), where the French will inflict great devastation: "Men were not brothers, but both the implements and victims of death."[33] Doubly so, in light of the Austrian Emperor Francis' proposed separate peace with Bonaparte.[34]

Tolstoyan Meditations on War, Labor, and Hierarchy

Consistent with his anarcho-Populism and Christian anarchism, Tolstoy presents his elaborations of war, armies, and militarism in ways that both illuminate and defamiliarize hierarchical power and decision-making structures. The writer's critique may be visualized schematically by imagining pyramids, with the numerically large popular base of humanity subordinated to various levels and systems of power and domination that are reified, or made falsely "objective."[35] In pyramidal societies, "those who occupy the pinnacle [...] determine the social life of those at the base."[36] In the same way, "management is about control": etymologically speaking, the verb manage is either derived from the word "*manus* (hand) or *maeggiare* (to handle, especially horses)."[37] Just as circus handlers break captive elephants by wielding bullhooks, managers of labor assume the power to dominate subjugated workers, coercing them to forget about fantasy and obey orders.[38] In this sense, management's totalitarian hatred of democracy follows from the imperative of seeking to maximize profit.[39]

Historically, the merchant and war galleys that were propelled for millennia in the Mediterranean Sea by regimented human labor served as prototypes for modern factories, which were first established by Portuguese slavers in West Africa.[40] Charles Fourier, therefore, was not wrong to call factories "mitigated jails."[41] As functional means of domesticating *dikost* (iconoclastic creativity) and maintaining "order," the hierarchical arrangements of modern bureaucratic institutions are fundamentally and involuntarily sadomasochistic, in that any resistance to imposed circumstances of powerlessness is severely punished.[42]

As if to illustrate the brutality of constituted power, in *Palace Walk* (1956), the first volume in *The Cairo Trilogy*, the Egyptian author Naguib Mahfouz (1911–2006) renders homage to Prince Andrei's trance at the battle of Austerlitz using a verbal image whereby the youthful Fahmy is killed at a protest against British colonial rule, but not before he regards the peaceful sky and thinks of his forbidden love.[43] In *Red Cavalry*, Babel portrays Army commander Semën Budënny likewise threatening to shoot anyone who deserts.[44]

Like traditional workplaces in class society, armies function on the basis of a false sense of superiority of officers relative to soldiers, a fallacious sense of inferiority on the part of rank-and-file troops vis-à-vis their commanders, and a false mutual dehumanization of self and Other on the battlefield. In similar fashion, if a child is brought up by sadistic parents who deny the place of human freedom, she will confront vast pressures to surrender her will.[45] By accepting the imposed "need" for sacrifice, conscripts—like their fellow laborers—affirm the symbolic political order that ostensibly renders meaning to their disfigurement and death, all the while *perpetuating* these same losses through their obedience.[46]

In like manner, the combination of strict hierarchy and the emphasis on loyalty and the wielding of power (власть) in medicine constitute strong risk factors for abuse. These can explain but never excuse the collaboration of junior and senior physicians alike in atrocities such as the Holocaust.[47] The *Lancet* Commissioners on Medicine and the Holocaust, who came together in 2021, are right to observe that "[m]edicine during the Nazi period and the Shoah (Holocaust) is not a matter of the distant past."

> Historical evidence documents that the reasoning, values, and activities of health-care professionals and biomedical researchers in this context represented extreme manifestations of potential problems inherent in medicine more generally [...].[48]

Accordingly, there is a need to examine "the behaviour of physicians [and other healthcare workers/professionals] when tempted or pressured by those in power or providing financial resources," together with the reproduction of racism, sexism, traditionalism, workplace hierarchy, abuse, and social paternalism within the healthcare system, in the absence of community accountability.[49] To this day, medical school and the clinical environment emphasize conformity and mastery.[50] The dependence of junior doctors on their senior counterparts leads the former to wield their power typically to obey, and to affirm the established order. Along these lines, the German medical establishment has been reticent to fully confront its legacy of Nazi collaboration. It thus forgets the courage of the anti-fascist medical students of the White Rose, who were executed in 1943 for protesting Hitler's regime.[51]

In this sense, Jean-Paul Sartre's observation of a sort of "complicity between the oppressor and the oppressed" echoes Immanuel Kant's recognition of the surrender of conscience and consciousness before political and clerical powers, and so may complement Tolstoy's critique of the intoxicating self-surrender before State and capital.[52] After all, in masochistically accepting one's subjection through voluntary obedience, the worker, soldier, or serf does violence to oneself, perpetuating oppression and the myth of unfreedom, and so threatening self-destruction.[53] In turn, the encouragement of "self-determination, agency, and social change" may point to a way out.[54] As suggested by Hegel's idea of the master-slave dialectic or Freud's analysis of sadomasochism, the resistance undertaken by those compulsorily subjected to domination may ultimately point toward the dissolution of hierarchy, statism, and militarism altogether.[55]

Courage for Tolstoy means precisely this: the steadfast resistance of the individual and collective against such evils as suffering and death, especially in war.[56] His conception therefore anticipates the arguments of the Christian existentialist Paul Tillich, who asserts poignantly that "[c]ourage is self-affirmation 'in spite of,' namely in spite of nonbeing," as of his fellow Christian anarchist Nikolai Berdyaev, who contends that individual personality is defined by a continuous refusal of enslavement.[57] Certainly, there is plenty of negation and dehumanization in Russian history, which has spanned at least six epochs: namely, Kyivan Rus', Russia under the Mongol yoke, Muscovite Russia, the Tsarist Empire, the Union of Soviet Socialist Republics (USSR), and the post-Soviet context.[58] Indeed, the Kremlin bound the vast majority of peasants for centuries as serfs; actively enshrined patriarchal despotism against women; and reconstituted serfdom in the post-revolutionary context of the USSR through militarism, forcible collectivization, brutal industrialization, and the GULAG system, all the while employing a "lexicon of battle" to feign that the Soviet Union was pursuing social justice.[59] With reference to the twenty-first century, the writer Vladimir Sorokin observes that President Putin's crumbling "pyramid of power" hearkens back to medieval times, before the Enlightenment.[60]

Despite this, Tolstoy illustrates resistance as self-affirmation through various thought-images in his *poema*, hence strongly contesting inherited Russian customs of masochistic habituation to despotism. In this way, he develops a position close to that espoused by his fellow anarchist Sébastien Faure (1858–1942) at a youth peace congress held in Bierville, France, in August 1926. In his address before the congress, Faure declares the authority principle underpinning capital and the State "on the one hand, [to] caus[e] conflicts to emerge, and on the other" to only know how to "resolve them, through force, pressure, [and] violence," thus resulting in shooting wars.[61]

In his *poema*, Lev Nikolaevich considers combat first from the vantage points of Napoleon and Kutuzov, shifting from the headquarters of the general staff to the front lines, and descending through the ranks from commanders "down to lowly privates."[62] In this sense, just as Rick McPeak observes that the novelist wishes to convey that "war [is] an extension of the duel," we can add that Tolstoy is furthermore suggesting that war-making is akin to the exploitation of labor—or conversely, that labor-exploitation is akin to war.[63] On the battlefield, conscripted workers, serfs, and servants risk life and limb, and very often end up sacrificing themselves altogether, at the behest of commanders, adjutants, and generals who face far less risk. This is similar to how workers, peasants, and slaves are overworked, disabled, and even killed by their labor, which by definition disproportionately benefits the capitalist-feudal bosses. By all means, through obeying the officer class, conscripts in the Tsar's army reproduced the expected submission of peon before landowner.[64]

Using naturalistic metaphor, Tolstoy likens the working majority to the worker bees of a hive colony, and the State and ruling class to the "drones," otherwise known as "robber-bees."[65] To extend this metaphor, these conscripted "bees" would face considerable risk, if they were to rebel against their circumstances. For instance, in 1892, the Tolstoyan peasant conscript Nikolai Iziumchenko was sentenced to two years in an Imperial penal battalion, and a subsequent three years' exile in western Siberia, for conscientiously objecting to military service for the Tsar.[66]

Reproducing authoritarian social dynamics through obedience and conformity, peasants, workers, soldiers, commanders, and bosses alike seek to overcome their isolation, fears, frustrations, and relative powerlessness by either dominating others through the psychical phenomenon known as authoritarian aggression, or by accepting their own domination, as in authoritarian submission.[67] It is telling in this sense that Erich Fromm and Jessica Benjamin define the exploitative, non-productive character orientation as sadistic, aiming to attack the body and transgress the boundaries of the Other. They add that the masochistic "consent" granted to such oppression in turn represents an abdication of human freedom.[68]

According to Kropotkin, the destructiveness of war includes not only the torment and slaughter of humanity, but also "the destruction of human labour," living and historical, "on a colossal scale." In comments that are especially apt, in light of the current devastation of Ukraine by the Russian military, he writes:

> Every war is the destruction of a formidable [amount of] material, which includes not only the war material itself but also things most necessary for everyday life, to society as a whole: bread, [...] vegetables, foodstuffs of all kind, dra[f]t animals, [...], coal, metal, clothing. All this represents the useful

> work of millions of [people] over decades; and all this will be wasted, burnt or scrapped in a few months.[69]

In this sense, warcraft is the ultimate expression of the State functioning as a "population machine" that treats humanity as cattle, or chattel slaves.[70] In an essay on religion published over three decades after *War and Peace*, Lev Nikolaevich observes in parallel that "the destruction of millions of human lives for the conveniences of the ruling minority is regarded as a most commonplace and necessary facet of living, and happens continually."[71] In his novel *Resurrection* (1899), the sage summarizes his criticisms of militarism and hierarchy illuminating the "Sevastopol Sketches" and *War and Peace* alike in the following terms:

> Military life in general depraves men. It places them in conditions of complete idleness, that is, absence of all rational and useful work; frees them from their common human duties, which it replaces by merely conventional duties to the honour of the regiment, the uniform, the flag; and, while giving them on the one hand absolute power over other men, also puts them into conditions of servile obedience to those of higher rank than themselves.[72]

Here, we find a humanistic reaffirmation of the anti-militaristic, anti-statist spirit that links the waging of war to labor-exploitation and social hierarchy. After all, the "shell shock" or "combat exhaustion" that plagues soldiers is also experienced by burned-out workers, particularly healthcare workers in the COVID-19 pandemic.[73] Still, the most obvious difference between war-making and other forms of alienated or forcible labor—whether as a serf, slave, or wage-earner—is that relations of subordination within combat typically lead to more immediate, devastating, and widespread disability, post-traumatic stress, and death than most other types of labor. With the exception of highly dangerous forms of work, such as in mining, fossil-fuel extraction, construction, prison labor, and "essential" services during COVID, non-military work tends to kill more slowly over time, as through "depreciation" and aging.

Then again, within the context of a given regional or global capitalist economy, workers and their families are fundamentally dependent on self-provisioning through labor for survival, since by definition there exist no commons, maroons, or *quilombos* to which one can escape in such settings.[74] The feudal master-servant laws that underwrote early capitalism, and that persist in contemporary labor law and managerial theory, obligate workers to debase themselves before owners, such that autonomy from the class system is by definition impossible for workers under bourgeois domination.[75]

A 2020 US study found that three out of four workers feel burned out, thus admitting to a condition that shares many features with major depression, and even "shell shock."[76] In parallel to the waves of soldiers used by commanders to win battles, the ruling classes compensate for labor's depreciation, exhaustion, and turnover by instituting the "general law" of capital accumulation. In rendering vast swathes of humanity effectively "surplus populations," this law ensures the reproduction of class society through the creation of an industrial reserve army. Such a reserve army of labor in turn depresses wages and disciplines workers into accepting exploitation out of fear of termination and attendant ruin, homelessness, and premature death, both for oneself and one's loved ones and dependents.[77] Individual and familial survival, then, depend upon one's precarious labor, which in turn presupposes the laborer's fatefully habituated submission to authority. Due to this coercive dynamic, today, "work, for many people, has come to feel like a battlefield, and daily life, including politics and life online, like yet more slaughter."[78]

Founded, therefore, in the systematic robbery of the surplus value produced by workers within conditions not of their own choosing, and against which they cannot protest or organize without fear of retaliation and ruin, capitalism is involuntarily sadomasochistic to its core.[79] By definition, workers are harmed while bosses benefit from the exploitation of labor, even if the contracts detailing their effective trafficking should be "consensually" agreed to, from a liberal or positivist perspective.[80] In light of the close organizational affinities between the military and the healthcare industry, the fact that hundreds of physicians and thousands of veterans die by suicide on an annual basis is an especially poignant illustration of the traumatic atrociousness of work, combat, and, ultimately, social hierarchy.[81] In reality, as the English sociologist Anthony Giddens describes, the division of labor and the attendant

> separation of the labourer from control of his [*sic*] means of production which Marx singled out as the most distinctive feature of modern capitalism is not confined to industry, but extends throughout the polity, army, and other sections of society in which large-scale organisation become prominent.[82]

Alienation is therefore universal under capitalism, and the State's appeal for (self) sacrifice, particularly through the idealization of the "masculine soldier," merely serves to underpin the perpetuation of the irrationality, brutality, and estrangement inherent to capitalism and bureaucratic authoritarianism, as Theodor W. Adorno recognized.[83] A few examples from the class struggle in recent years may help to illustrate this point. According to striking miners at the Kryvyi Rih Iron Ore Plant in Ukraine—who remained underground in a work-stoppage for 43 days, from early September to mid-October 2020, to protest their labor conditions—management treated them like "slaves." They did so by actively derogating them as lacking interests or value altogether, through subjecting them to dangerous work, deprived of the proper equipment; withholding wages; and inviting State security services to harass the miners once they had collectively decided to strike.[84] After labor and management came to an agreement to suspend the work-stoppage, which had spread to three other mines and involved over 400 miners, the bosses turned around and decided to sue the union for ostensibly "illegal" strike activity. Viktor Stoyanovsky, chair of the Independent Trade Union of Miners of Ukraine, Oktyabrska branch, has condemned this "despotism and dictatorship [...] being carried out even at the enterprise level."[85]

Likewise in California's Central Valley, the agricultural corporation Primex Farms fired dozens of workers in July 2020 after they struck to demand two weeks' paid sick leave following the deadly propagation of COVID-19 through the workforce.[86] Undocumented agricultural workers laboring outside in Coachella Valley in extreme heat during a viral pandemic voice that they feel like "chess pieces that politicians move around."[87] Frontline healthcare workers, thousands of whom have perished due to COVID-19, rightly perceive that management considers them disposable.[88] Hence, it is no exaggeration either to liken the expected labor-capital relationship to organized crime, or to point to the continuities between criminal trafficking and everyday life under capitalism. This is so, considering that rebellious self-assertion in one's individual or collective interest runs the risk of one's being killed or ruined in retaliation, whether at the hands of the vindictive State, bosses, or their hired hands, or due to resulting privation from unemployment and/or black-listing, whether formal or informal.[89]

Strikingly, inequality in the US is at its highest levels in the century that has passed since the Battle of Blair Mountain raged in West Virginia (1921), when a racially integrated army of thousands of unionized miners fought the hired guns of King Coal, the police, and the National Guard to free striking fellow miners and their families, whom the bosses had imprisoned, and were starving into submission.[90] In short, wage-labor remains forced labor.[91]

Paradoxically, then, it is evident that *both* being subjected to a lifetime of alienated labor and being without a job in the contemporary capitalist economy are "forms of *living death*," and that sadomasochistic social relationships tend toward mutual destruction.[92] In like manner, the bosses strive to deny their own mortality, perpetual insecurity, and dependence on subordinates by asserting dominance through an "endless pursuit of elusive power."[93] Through their separation from and domination over the less privileged, administrators fundamentally exhibit disrespect for persons. As Chernyshevsky asks rhetorically, "Who dares possess another person?"[94] Berdyaev's answer is that a "free [person] does not desire to lord [...] over anyone."[95] Rejecting class society on the basis that everyone should be considered a noble, and existence should be made interdependent, this personalist socialist reinterprets capitalist sadism and proprietor despotism as multifaceted forms of dependency in the following way:

> The bourgeois is always a slave. He is the slave of his property and of his money, he is a slave of the will to enrichment, a slave of bourgeois public opinion, a slave of social position, he is the slave of those slaves he exploits and of whom he lives in fear.[96]

Of late, monopoly capital has imposed onto laborers total work, a term defined by its inventor Josef Pieper (1904–1997) as an insidious process whereby workers' lives are reduced to and utterly dominated by their labor, which is designed to be ceaseless. Total work leads to "restless, agitated activity, anxiety about the future, a sense of life being overwhelming, nagging thoughts about missed opportunities, and guilt connected to the possibility of laziness." It exacerbates the basic *dukkha* of servitude: namely, the one-dimensional colonization of existence by suffering, frustration, and dissatisfaction, and the concomitant suppression of contemplation, reflection, art, sensuality, and love.[97] Such drudgery has also been called "hustle culture," or "bullshit jobs."[98] Commenting on the societal imposition of alienated labor under conditions of general market dependency, in the absence of organizing efforts inspired by visions of humanistic social reconstruction, Fromm observes that "[a]ll [one] can do is fall in step like a marching soldier."[99]

Fundamentally, then, the experience of instrumentalization and dehumanization, of being "degrad[ed] to the level of an appendage of a machine," is common to workers, peasants, servants, *lumpenproletarians*, prisoners, soldiers and veterans, and people with disabilities, as well as racial, gender, and sexual minorities—especially so at the intersections among these realities and identities.[100] As B. R. Ambedkar, W. E. B. DuBois, Martin Luther King, Jr., and Isabel Wilkerson have recognized, the brutality of the Hindu caste system is replicated in the US racial-caste system.[101] Despite significant theoretical differences, these thinkers and activists share with Tolstoy and Marx a Kantian concern for the objectification and domination of human life, one that is common to the Buddhist, Christian, and existentialist traditions as well.[102] This remains the case, despite the fact, on the one hand, that Marxist-Leninist regimes have instrumentalized human labor and considered the individual as a mere "brick" for the Taylorist construction of state capitalism, and that, on the other, many European existentialists have preferred Dostoevsky for his emphases on evil, alienation, and psychopathology—echoing the late-nineteenth century introduction of capitalism into the Tsarist Empire—over any engagement with Tolstoy's avowal of Christian love.[103]

As if emblematically to anticipate this latter divergence, Lev Nikolaevich characteristically observes that "coercion is used only from [...] lack of respect for human nature."[104] In reality, the basic psychodynamic tendency of sadism is to instrumentalize the Other, while in masochism, it is to "make a pipe of oneself."[105] Moral and political despotism accordingly overlap, inhibiting self-determination.[106] Within the economic sphere, humanity's "commodity-dependency" as objectified labor ensures the persistence of poverty and inequality.[107] As if to illustrate this dynamic, in *Cannery Row* (1945), John Steinbeck links the industrial exploitation and would-be "canning" of marine and amphibious wildlife with the exploitation of labor and femicide.[108]

According to Achille Mbembe, following Giorgio Agamben, State sovereignty is fundamentally based on the power to decide who is disposable, and who is not.[109] Hierarchy, in short, facilitates abuse, whether in the military, workplace, school, or interpersonal relationships.[110] In this sense, the persistence of bourgeois society to date speaks to the truth of Jürgen Habermas's notion of the "refeudalization of the public sphere," as rooted in the highly selective rationalization processes imposed by capital.[111]

Although the existentialist Martin Heidegger (1889–1976) would achieve fame by publicly agonizing over the reification of social life in capitalist modernity—for which he actually served as an apologist, given his explicit Nazism—it requires clarifying that he appropriated the very concept of reification (*Verdinglichung*) from the Hungarian Marxist György Lukács (1885–1971).[112] Along similar lines, this German ultra-rightist took many of his most famous concepts precisely from Tolstoy: in Walter Kaufmann's opinion, "Heidegger on death is for the most part an unacknowledged commentary on *The Death of Ivan Ilyitch*."[113] In that novella, Lev Nikolaevich demonstrates just how a mechanical, conventional existence is akin to death-in-life.[114] Therefore, considering Heidegger's avowal of a "joyless" and loveless "existence, overshadowed by death and anxiety," as Herbert Marcuse observed late in life, it is unsurprising that the author of *Being and Time* (1927) would have sided with Hitler.[115] Günther Anders (1902–1992), another student of Heidegger, denounces his "*Idealism of unfreedom*," which neglects human sensual needs, ignores friendship and love, disappears class struggle, naturalizes isolation and terror, and promotes private and collective forms of nihilism.[116] In this sense, it goes without saying that Heidegger's death-cult values fundamentally clash with Tolstoy's anarchist principles.

Considering how Fromm diagnosed the widespread internalization among workers of the compulsory sadomasochism imposed by capitalism, or "automaton conformity," as a defense mechanism against domination by a false, mechanical society (*Gesellschaft*) which in turn reproduces that very society; that Berdyaev perceived that "[a]cquiescence in slavery diminishes suffering," while "refusal increases it," averring that "the choice is either God-man or automatic humanity, machine-humanity"; and that the Martinican revolutionary Frantz Fanon (1925–1961) found in the dehumanization of psychiatric patients and in the colonial relationship between master and slave nefarious endeavors to reduce humanity to a machine, it is remarkable to contemplate that the word "robot" is etymologically related to работа, the Russian word for labor, which is derived in turn from раб ("slave").[117] In *Rossum's Universal Robots* (1921), a variation on Mary Shelley's *Frankenstein* (1818), the Czech artist Karel Čapek envisions humanoid "robots," or mechanized slave workers, replacing human laborers and soldiers, only to rise up and destroy humanity.[118]

Within late capitalism, observes the critical theorist Agostino Cera, the categorical imperative—rather than amounting to the Kantian call to treat others and oneself as ends rather than mere means—becomes that one "make a *Bestand* [standing-reserve, or stock] of everything, including the self."[119] Considering that *ständisch* can be translated as "feudal," and that the term "human capital" is derived from the Nazi term *Menschenmaterial*, former President Donald Trump's adviser Kevin Hassett's announcement on CNN in May 2020—in other words, at the very outset of the COVID-19 pandemic—that "[o]ur [*sic*] human capital stock is ready to go back to work" helps us complete the circle of domination.[120]

Although Tolstoy's *War and Peace* is set in the early nineteenth century, as feudalism evermore gave way to capitalism or was combined with it, the basic organizing principle of social hierarchy is a continuity shared by both systems, together with military and State bureaucracies, then as now. In Kim Stanley Robinson's speculative *Red Mars* (1993), the protagonist John Boone announces this very point to his fellow exilic pioneers from atop Olympus Mons, the largest known volcano in our solar system: "this system we call [capitalism] is just feudalism all over again."[121]

Tolstoy's Anarchist Anti-Militarism

In book one of *War and Peace*, hierarchical differentials of privilege, power, and suffering are illustrated during the retreat eastward of the Russian military, whose commanders and rank-and-file soldiers alike were shocked by the unprecedented collapse of the Austrian army led by General Mack before Napoleon's forces at the October 1805 battle of Ulm. The Russian officers "stan[d] together out of range of the shots" in their escape along the Danube River, while conscripts are afforded no such luxury, as the *Grand Armée*, which outnumbers its Russian counterpart by a factor of three, bears down on them.[122] On both sides, troops advance out of fear of the whip, following the orders handed down by officers, who in turn fear being considered cowards by both their superiors and underlings.[123]

Analogously, before bidding farewell and opening the door to Andrei *en route* to the theater of war, General Prince Nikolai Bolkonsky insists that his "son need not serve under anyone *if he is in disfavour*," simply because of his name and family background. The implication here is that no mere serf would have the luxury of so resisting an unjust overlord in the military or penal service.[124] In keeping with such feudal privileges, as well as the inter-generational homophilic bond he has forged with the Russian commander-in-chief, Andrei will land a prestigious position as adjutant to General Kutuzov without having any actual combat experience.[125]

On a typical day during the Napoleonic Wars, according to Tolstoy, common soldiers must work throughout the night after having marched 30 kilometers, while officers plan and scheme—just as the labor of "tired footmen and cooks" facilitates the *soirées* of the ruling class.[126] In this light, the only checks on those privileged by feudal-bureaucratic and involuntarily sadomasochistic hierarchies appear to be necessity, or fate.[127] Giving voice to a paradoxically aristocratic anti-elitism he sees as regenerative, Tolstoy will present the hussar Count Nikolai Rostov's grievance about the divergent experiences of "men who have been under the enemy's fire," compared with those of the "fellows on the staff who get rewards without doing anything."[128] Dialectically, Rostov's frankness in the presence of his commanding officer Prince Andrei risks provoking a duel between them, which Bolkonsky dismisses in light of the "greater and more serious duel" with the *Grand Armée* which awaits them at Austerlitz.[129]

In the canvass of retreat along the Danube painted by Tolstoy, an evident verbal image can be discerned which contrasts idealized nature with a corrupted, martial humanity. Count Rostov internally remarks on the great beauty, tranquility, and glory of celestial bodies and ecosystems: "*there* is so much happiness; but here… groans, suffering, fear, and this uncertainty and hurry."[130] Such spontaneous meditations on life and the biosphere build off Tolstoy's earlier expressed view that "the true, the beautiful, and the good were truly the same, […] embodied in both nature and the soul," mirroring his interest in a possible unification of the self with nature, and his belief in the essential goodness of human nature. All of these feelings in turn are arguably rooted in the transference of emotional meaning of pre-individuated life in symbiosis with his mother, Marya Nikolaevna Tolstaya, and later, with his aunts Aline and Toinette.[131] War, then, is a dystopian violation of the ideas of the *kalokagothon*, the synthesis of ethics with beauty, as well as of harmony, union, and residence.

Dramatically, Prince Andrei will experience a similar, more sustained epiphany while lying wounded at the battle of Austerlitz, as his symbolic self and physical body separate, in a surreal experience of Kantian transcendental idealism.[132] Similarly, two weeks before Russia's resounding defeat at Austerlitz, during the battle of Schön-Grabern, Rostov is injured, as his horse, Rook, is killed by an artillery shell. Feeling dazed, the hussar naïvely disbelieves that his French counterparts seek his death: "He remembered his mother's love for him, and his family's, and his friends', and the enemy's intention to kill him seemed impossible."[133] As the count experiences mortality-salience, he appreciates his existence deeply and ecstatically, connecting with the biophilia and human love which tie him to nature and society. In turn, his reverie confirms the framing of terror management theory, which suggests that self-esteem promotes resilience and so protects us from death-anxiety, just as his immediate reaction provides evidence of another instance of the mind taking protective flight into a traumatic neurosis.[134] Through fantasy and delirium in response to this near-death experience, Rostov anticipates, if only as a flash, a matriarchal future, without war and oppression, characterized by cooperation, love, and mutual aid, in a world without borders.

While Tolstoy seeks consciously to challenge the "great man" theory of history—also known as the "Napoleon myth," which privileges the "individual level of analysis"—by counterposing his anarcho-Populist views in *War and Peace*, this bold effort is not without its contradictions. We have already mentioned Tolstoy's controversial inclusion of officers and aristocrats within the ranks of the *Narod*.[135] That being said, in his depiction of the battle of Schön-Grabern, Lev Nikolaevich illustrates how much more crucial is the commitment and action of the unyielding mid-level artillery officer, Captain Tushin, compared to any higher-ranking commander.[136]

Highlighting the important role that a militant minority can play, presaging the revolutionism of the Communards of Paris and the Kronstadt sailors in the Russian Revolution, and symbolizing the Gramscian "war of position," the soldiers in Tushin's battery heroically hold the French at bay in the wake of Mack's unexpected defeat by maintaining a fierce barrage, despite a total lack of covering troops, and in defiance of two orders to retreat.[137] Exemplifying the concept of the "fog of war," the French delay attacking the battery "because [they] could not surmise that anyone could have the effrontery to continue firing from four quite undefended guns."[138] As if in a trance, the artillery company finds residence together in its joint struggle, and so turns the tide of history.[139]

In an after-action review at which the commanding officer, the Georgian Prince Peter Ivanovich Bagration, chastises Tushin for having abandoned one of the cannons in question, Prince Andrei parries Bagration's unreasonableness with a homoerotic flourish. Responding to this unstated threat, Bolkonsky stands up to defend his comrade and platonic love, personifying an erect phallus.[140] He insists to Prince Bagration that the Russians' victory was due "chiefly to the action of that battery and the heroic endurance of Captain Tushin and his company."[141] Be that as it may, the commander cannot believe that a single unit could have accomplished so much.[142]

Equally importantly, although Schön-Grabern can be considered a formal victory, given that it successfully shielded the Russian army's retreat, the battle definitely involved much human loss, too—as Bondarchuk's cinematic portrayal makes plain. Tolstoy comments that a "frightful" number of soldiers were wounded at Schön-Grabern, foreshadowing Rostov's bearing-witness to vast death and disability on the battlefield of Austerlitz.[143] Both at Schön-Grabern and later at Borodino, many horses were similarly exploited and killed, recalling the gruesome *venationes* of the Roman Empire, whereby "exotic" animals would be ritualistically exhibited and slaughtered in the Colosseum to satisfy the emperors' bloodlust.[144] Likewise in *Red Cavalry* (1926), the Tolstoyan reporter Isaac Babel laments the widespread killings of horses in war.[145]

Critically, then, Lev Nikolaevich's emotional-existential perspective reminds us that "[v]ictory requires victims," and that "each war is a tragedy."[146]

Tolstoyan Queerness as Human Relatedness

As a manifestation of human sex-love and unity, homoeroticism features prominently in *War and Peace*. Reflecting group cohesion, tenderness, courage, horizontalism *and* verticalism, and collective heroism, emergent homophilic and homosexual relationships are evident within key military sequences of the *poema*, including the battles of Schön-Grabern and Borodino, as well as during troop-reviews made by General Kutuzov and Tsar Alexander I. These verbal icons conveying equality, solidarity, and erotic ecstasy likely hearken back to Tolstoy's experiences during the Crimean War, when the artillery officer first fought alongside serf-soldiers. The phenomenon of "comrade-love" or "military comradeship" practiced among Russian soldiers and officers in defiance of the official ban on sodomy renders homage to the Dorian-Greek and Samurai exaltation of male homosexuality as a central aspect of war, art, honor, attachment, and education.[147] Indeed, in his historical review, *Sexual Hegemony* (2020), Christopher Chitty finds the institutions and motifs of "a democratic army, nude exercises, homoerotic art and literature, baths, intense male friendships and bonding" all to be related.[148] Freud similarly observes that male homosexuality facilitates group ties, and that sublimated homoeroticism plays a central role in collective and collaborative forms of labor.[149]

At the well-known *Symposium* held at the poet Agathon's home in Athens in 416 BCE, attended by Socrates and later recorded by Plato, Phaidros praises Eros as the "most ancient of all" and by all means the highest good, with the "most power to provide virtue and happiness" to humankind.[150] According to Agathon's word at this drinking banquet, Eros "flies in full flight away from the Old Age," anticipating collective liberation by arousing experiments beyond war, separation, and the gendered division of labor.[151] Love comes "from a different world," entering this one to proclaim "infinite subjectivity" and "the world of freedom." At best, it moves beyond the "possible" and breaks through to the realm of existential time, imparting one's identity and vocation.[152] In this sense, King Henry V's "St. Crispin's Day Speech," as rendered by Shakespeare on the eve of the upset English victory over the French at the battle of Agincourt (1415), marries the collective cause of a "band of brothers" with the ambitious goal of social leveling.[153]

In parallel, in Tolstoy's portrayal of the battle of Schön-Grabern, there is plenty of evidence of spontaneous and ecstatic comrade-love, which imparts Berdyaev's sense of Russians' anarchic and "natural dionysism." This can be seen both in Tushin's battery—wherein the captain takes "delight" in the "every movement" of a "handsome drunkard" he calls uncle, who commands the second cannon—as in the emergent relationship between Bolkonsky and Tushin, whose figure Andrei finds "quite unsoldiery [...] but extremely attractive."[154] As with the character Yeroshka in *The Cossacks*, Tolstoy's euphemistic use of "uncle" here to designate an endeared elder of the same sex mirrors the *tetki*, or "aunties," of St. Petersburg, who were known to seek out junior partners among students, peasants, cadets, and other soldiers.[155] When first encountering the captain during battle preparations, Bolkonsky immediately finds Tushin's voice and words pleasant, and intimately familiar. In turn excelling in his duty by holding the French imperialists at bay, after having openly declared to his comrades just before the battle that "we know there is no sky [or heaven]; only the atmosphere," the philosopher-captain Tushin provokes erotic wonder in Andrei Nikolaevich.[156]

Like Turgenev's *alter ego* in the 1878 lyrical poem "The Realm of Azure," Prince Andrei hence unexpectedly encounters "words and poems filled with wondrous beauty and inspired force fl[ying] from someone's lips."[157] In this scene, Bolkonsky visits a gay world, and finds himself in a meeting of the minds with an Other who is alike yet different.[158] While under fire, experiencing conditions threatening oblivion, during which the male soldier is expected to behave in a typically "masculine" manner, it is the novelty of Tushin's queer presentation which provokes Bolkonsky's ecstasy.[159] Intuitively, Andrei detects Tushin's camp, or so-called "intermediate" gender/sexuality and social character, as revealed through the captain's androgynous presentation, and the latter's passion and skill in covering the retreating Russian army.[160] As Freud might say, Andrei's attachment is to "someone who combines the characteristics of both [male and female] sexes [...]."[161] Through his spontaneous arousal, Bolkonsky is engulfed by a world of queer attraction, which anticipates a different future, and a non-appropriative meeting between self and Other.[162] At the battle's conclusion, the captain weeps "for some unknown reason" upon taking leave of his "dear fellow" Andrei. Bolkonsky, too, appears to lament having to take leave of Tushin, and so break this shared pleasure of mutual presence, alluringly promising, "Well, till we meet again..."[163]

Although such tears and heartache may be expected releases, secondary to the great trauma of combat, and/or the manifestation of pride in a job well done, they may equally convey the author's association of the death-anxiety to which soldiers are constantly exposed in combat with an opening to the reality of their poly-morphously-perverse sexuality and "true" queerness, which otherwise might be suppressed. Intuitively, both Tushin and Bolkonsky lament the loss of their human bond, and sense, "I am not [with] that other, but I could be."[164] In defiance of the heteronormativity that has dominated much of the world for over two millennia, this platonic couple briefly experiences the "great practical principle" and "the axis on which revolves the history of the world": namely, that humans should love one another.[165] Through ecstatic arousal and mutual recognition in the light of fusion, the characters dissolve hegemonic affective solidarities and step outside convention in order to find their true selves and relate freely with each other: an "I" with a "Thou."[166]

Like the revolutionary soldiers and sailors who in February 1917 wore their caps tilted to one side, exposed themselves by unbuttoning their uniforms, and tore off the epaulettes of officers to symbolize liberation, it is Tushin's ineffable queerness which binds Andrei to him.[167] Certainly, Andrei's attraction toward Tushin, echoing Tushin's captivation by "uncle," transmits the Tolstoyan ideals of communion, belonging, and "striving toward union" as expressions of the immanence of love and the realm of the divine.[168] Such bonds of religious enthusiasm, psychic integration, and mutual sympathy reveal the depth of partnership power and the identity of "God [as] the self-consciousness of [hu]man[ity] freed from all discordant elements."[169] Indeed, the following saying (*hadith*), attributed to the Prophet Muhammad (c. 570–632 CE), may help to illustrate the erotic dynamic: "I saw my Lord in the shape of a beautiful young man with his cap askew."[170]

Likewise, the Persian Sufi poet Sa'adi (c. 1213–1292) believed that male beauty serves to evince the divine.[171] Still, as Berdyaev declares, beauty "is not contemplation only." Rather, it presupposes "creative victory and conflict with the slavery of the world," and it "speaks of the co-operation of [hu]man[ity], of the joint action of [humankind] and God." Accordingly, Tushin and Bolkonsky's approximation belongs to the realm of freedom, anticipating the socialist transformation of society.[172] As their bodies release adrenaline, oxytocin, and dopamine, strengthening their bond and "creat[ing] new meanings out of nothing," the captain and the prince experience a Marcusean sense of libidinal reason and so activate bell hooks's theory of the "anarchism of love," thus undermining hierarchy through sociability.[173] They both intensely feel the virtue of Eros, according to Audre Lorde, which overcomes separation through integration.[174] The Greek playwright Aristophanes might not have disagreed, considering his remark in the *Symposium*, that "when one [...] meets his own proper half, [...] then they are wonderfully overwhelmed by affection and intimacy and love."[175]

Inspired to protect the vulnerable Russian army by his muse and the phallic nature of the cannons he is commanding (one of which is called a "unicorn," another of which is remarkably "large"), Tushin takes after Cleomachus, the seventh-century BCE Greek warrior who led a rout of the Eretrians in the Lelantine War after receiving the kiss of his beloved junior male partner (*eromenos*). He also mimics Achilles the *eromenos* after the literary death in battle of his *erastes* (elder male lover) Patroclos in *The Iliad*.[176] In much the same way, Socrates and Alcibiades fought jointly at the start of the Peloponnesian War (431–404 BCE), with the latter *eromenos* praising his *erastes*' courage in combat and tender dedication, considering that Socrates risked his life to carry the wounded Alcibiades to safety.[177]

Just as Don Quixote draws on his "platonic and continent" cross-class love for the peasant Dulcinea del Toboso in his adventures, and as medieval knights were driven to heroic deeds as sublimation for their desired attachments to certain ladies *or* given squires, Tushin is "spurred [on] to his deeds of bravery" by love "for the [elder] comrade who stood beside him in the ranks."[178] The artillery company's collective success in shielding the larger collective's retreat illustrates Phaidros' faith in the limitless potential of "an army [being] made up only of [male] lovers and beloved," and Agathon's belief that "in courage 'not even Ares [god of war] stands up against Love [Eros].'"[179]

The Roots of Bolkonsky and Tushin's Bond

In light of the pervasiveness of homoerotic and non-binary imagery and motifs in *War and Peace*, and the positive regard in which Tolstoy generally presents queer desire, it is plain that the prose poet is celebrating unity in diversity through such expressions of non-normative sexuality and gender fluidity, all the while artistically sublimating his own gay lust. As such, the writer resists what the feminist poet Adrienne Rich condemns as "compulsory heterosexuality." He does so by challenging the repressive social ideologies that look down upon same-sex attraction and non-binary presentations, limiting gender and sexual freedom, then as now.[180] In reveling in queerness, Tolstoy presents a thought-image that prefigures his anarchist "vision of a transfigured universe of all together," enjoying a "real existence" marked by "an infinite, reciprocally compensating variety."[181]

Developmentally, as well, he may be celebrating the reflection of the "past in the present," engaging in ancestor worship, and exhibiting his residence through the extolment of his own non-traditional sexuality and that (presumably) of his maternal grandfather, Nikolai Sergeivich Volkonsky, a man who loved plants, flowers, music, and aesthetics, who abhorred hunting, and who never remarried after a partnership of convenience to Princess Ekaterina Trubetskaya (1749–1792).[182] This Volkonsky is the prototype for General Prince Nikolai Bolkonsky in the *poema*, who shares a tender moment with his son Andrei not only as the junior officer leaves Bald Hills to face off with Napoleon, but also just as news of Lise's death breaks.[183]

Tolstoy's father, Nikolai Ilych, on whom Count Rostov is based, may have had queer tendencies as well, in light of his artistic sensitivities, and his evident attachments to Bashkir horsemen, as well as to his male serfs, Petrusha and Matyusha. These "strong, handsome men" never married.[184] As the historian Dan Healey has shown, in Tsarist Russia, men privileged by the feudal hierarchy would often rely on their less powerful same-sex counterparts for erotic satisfaction. Beginning in 1882, one Prince Obolensky treated two brothers who served him as coachmen,

Peter and Fedor Filonovsky, to luxurious food, drink, and living arrangements, in exchange for sex. Peter Tchaikovsky's partners in Moscow included male servants. Students, peasants, young workers, and clerical novices would often be propositioned by their male elders and/or superiors, in keeping with long-established pederastic master-slave relations.[185]

Considering the formal ban on same-sex love in the Russian military, Prince Andrei's attraction to Tushin as a "most unmilitary military man" is decidedly part of Tolstoy's exaltation of the rebellious heroism evinced by the captain and his soldiers, whose vital-sexual energies emanate precisely as ineffable alternatives to heterosexist hyper-masculinity.[186] By so establishing a homogenic, seemingly mutual attraction between Bolkonsky and Tushin mediated by courage (*andreia*) and virtue (*arete*), Tolstoy imparts this relationship as channeling the mythological Apollo, another classical Greek god arousing same-sex love, together with Anteros, the god of mutual love.[187]

We suspect that Bolkonsky/Tolstoy's focus on Tushin may be related to the writer's twin rejection of the values of militarism and toxic masculinity, which besides having philosophical and erotic dimensions, also include developmental and autobiographical elements, especially in light of the trauma the poet himself experienced in combat. The scene disclosing Tushin and Bolkonsky's spontaneous love-bond is likely a variation on one of Tolstoy's own verbally accessible memories from his time fighting in Transcaucasia, and/or during the Crimean War.[188] Reflecting a deeper "past unconscious," the author's relative Sergei Grigorievich—the future Decembrist—was drafted into the Tsar's military as a child soldier, and his family on both sides politically rejected Tsarist absolutism.[189]

Sadly enough for this would-be gay couple, however much Bolkonsky and Tushin's encounter activates transference and mutually erotic ecstasy in the pair, there is no follow-up to this initial expression of a desire for merging in the remainder of the *poema*, beyond the protective attitude that Andrei evinces toward the captain while defending him against Bagration's questions in the after-action review following the battle of Schön-Grabern. The support Prince Andrei provides Tushin in this retrospective scene is consistent with what was often expected of the older male (*erastes*) in a classical gay relationship, as the *erastes* took pride in the successes of his *protégé* (or *eromenos*), cultivated virtue and citizenship in him, and sought to initiate him into society.[190]

While this chaste same-sex bond defies easy classification, in that it combines pederastic and androphilic dimensions (despite that both characters are grown men), it features a combination of the erotic love which ascends and the compassionate or caritative love that descends.[191] For all that, the transience of the bond between Tushin and Bolkonsky distinctly reflects Tolstoy's masochistic ambivalence about queer relationships and eroticism as a whole in his own life. In fact, the comrade-love evinced between Tolstoy and William Frey during the latter's five-day visit to Yasnaya Polnaya in 1885 closely echoes the homoerotic approximation between Bolkonsky and Tushin, in that no further intercourse would take place between these two real-life men after this seemingly mutually satisfying encounter.[192]

Lesbianism, Hermaphroditism, and Drag

A similarly tantalizing dynamic will govern the lesbian attraction between the characters Marya Bolkonskaya and Julie Karagina, who love each other intensely, but at a distance, in an expression of the author's own anxious-insecure attachment style.[193] In truth, the debate between Marya and Julie on conforming to straight marriage evinces the self-defeating sexual pleasure vs. guilt conflict, which contributes to the frustration of erotic needs and the perpetuation of unhappiness.[194] The content of their letters is suggestive of Tolstoy's own conversations in 1856 with a long-standing gay love interest, Dmitri Dyakov, about his wedding Valerya Arseneva.[195] In turn, in her novel *Thirty-Three Monsters* (1907), Lidia Zinovieva-Annibal portrays a suicide-inducing loss of love between a lesbian couple, as one of the partners relents and makes herself available to the eponymous 33 male suitors.[196]

Like the frustration experienced by Bolkonsky and Tushin, the failed relatedness between Bolkonskaya and Karagina exhibits the overall gratification inhibition conflict that grips masochists, undermining self-efficacy in the pursuit of desired goals and relationships.[197] Some lesbian feminists might view Princess Marya's resistance to Julie's advances as a reflection of false consciousness, and/or an unheroic capitulation to hegemonic lesbophobia.[198] At the same time, Tolstoy's exploration of this relationship involving Marya, the literary equivalent to his mother, may implicitly telegraph the author's own queerness.

Beyond this, Jennifer Wilson cogently emphasizes the androgyny of the protagonists Pierre Bezukhov and Princess Marya, particularly as manifested in the latter's observation of *noblesse oblige* toward the so-called "God's Folk"—being itinerant indigent pilgrims, some of whom are physically and/or mentally ill, and who at times defy the gender binary—whom she receives at the Bald Hills manor, against the wishes of her father and brother.[199] In the sympathy he expresses for these "Folk," Tolstoy channels the kind example of his aunts Aline and Toinette, his surrogate mothers, who received and gave to the itinerant poor, embodying Christian love.[200] He also imitates the paternalistic altruism expressed in a revolutionary sense by Chernyshevsky in his radical 1863 novel, *What Is to Be Done?*[201]

While both Pierre and Prince Andrei tease Marya and some of the visiting "God's Folk," following from their Jacobin-male points of view, Pierre will act contrite afterward and claim to "understand them so well and have the greatest respect for them."[202] As a pacifist and a soon-to-be Freemason, Bezukhov constitutes an androgynous, even queer character, who empathizes with Lise Bolkonskaya's fears over pregnancy and childbearing, agrees with her opposition to war, and endures General Prince Bolkonsky's criticism of his anti-militarism as "old women's nonsense."[203] In this sense, the novelist Margaret Atwood might consider him a "gender traitor."[204] Indeed, on Peter Bitsilli's reading, "Pierre fulfills the role of 'life-giver' in the novel."[205]

For her part, Princess Marya seeks to desire to transcend the limitations imposed onto women by patriarchal custom. She attempts to do so through philanthropic commitment to her "*people*," and by observing the idea of chastely living to serve others in need, rather than her father or Anatole Kuragin.[206] In reality, once

Rostov "rescues" Marya Nikolaevna from the peasants of Bogucharovo, whose rebellion against the landlords contains misogynistic overtones, she becomes enchained to a conservative-authoritarian, traditionally masculine count, who brutally beats his serfs and affirms Orthodoxy and autocracy.[207]

Earlier in the text, in an illustration of the Christmastide ritual involving the annual visit by serfs to their lords, whereby peasants would cross-dress, put on animal costumes, and/or present in fancy clothes to ridicule their social exclusion and oppression, Count Tolstoy presents a "people's epic" and "festival of freedom." During this celebration, Nikolai Rostov dresses up as an "old lady in a hooped skirt," and his erstwhile love-interest Sonya Alexandrovna disguises herself as an "extraordinarily becoming" Circassian male.[208] According to the philosopher Mikhail Bakhtin (1895–1975), laughter and the concept of Carnival allow for the at least temporary integration of utopian desire with reality, through imagined social leveling, the desacralization of the constituted authorities, and the attendant overcoming of one's fears of custom, repression, and power.[209] Likewise, David Graeber and David Wengrow assert that popular festivals nurture political self-consciousness by opening the possibility that Carnival might become "the new reality."[210]

Through such playful inversion, attesting to the instinctive rootedness of queerness within the human condition, Sonya momentarily feels liberated to actively pursue her attraction to Rostov, in a way that might not otherwise have been possible for an early nineteenth-century noble Russian woman, of whom timidity, modesty, and passivity were expected.[211] Nikolai in turn accepts Sonya's advances in drag ecstatically, merging (again, temporarily) with her in profound happiness, and telegraphing a sort of authentically queer partnership that would eschew a union agreed to for the purposes of perpetuating privilege—a characterization that would, in fact, fit the future marriage between Nikolai and Princess Marya.[212]

Plus, during the *poema*'s wolf-hunt, Count Ilya Rostov, who lets the she-wolf go, is accompanied by a "buffoon" in drag who goes by Natasya Ivanovna. (For more about this notorious hunt, see the next chapter.) Afterwards, in the rustic cabin of her uncle, a "holy fool," Natasha Rostova enjoys a platonically lesbian relationship with Anisya Fëdorovna, her uncle's peasant mistress, whose sensuousness is conveyed through her excellent cooking skills.[213]

Authentically sharing her husband's openness to non-normative sexualities, Countess Sofia Tolstaya, in her story "Whose Fault Is It?," will depict her *alter ego* Anna as experiencing a passionate lesbian attraction for the "tall, attractive Lyubasha," who ardently kisses the protagonist on the lips after she reads Christ's passion aloud to peasant girls.[214] Happily, Sofia and Lev's youngest daughter, Alexandra Tolstaya (1884–1979), may have enjoyed a loving lesbian partnership with her mother's secretary, Varvara Mikhailovna Feokritova (1875–1950).[215]

A Tale of Two Troop-Reviews

In parallel, if we examine General Kutuzov's entrance early on in *War and Peace*, when the commander-in-chief will review a battalion of Russian troops occupying

Austria, "burdening the inhabitants on whom they were quartered," we find the ironically festive atmosphere to be palpably queer.[216] First of all, Kutuzov's entourage includes several men (including the adjutant Andrei) who are described as handsome, and all of his subordinates make conscious aesthetic efforts to please the supreme commander, who is partially blind, as though they were participating in a beauty contest.[217] Reveling in the array of men, even while lacking full vision, Kutuzov proceeds through the review slowly, enjoying his sensuality. Likely recalling the experiences of the author as a sub-lieutenant, as well as possibly alluding to Richard Burton's theory about the "Sotadic Zone" (see Chapter 2 above), the general encounters an old comrade from his campaigns against the Ottoman Empire, and, praising his counterpart's bravery, suggestively projects that "[w]e all have our weaknesses [...]. He used to have a predilection for Bacchus."[218]

While this comment may refer to alcoholism, considering the importance of drinking in Bacchanalian revelries, it may equally amount to a classic example of camp, in light of Dionysus's homosexual connotations. Along these lines, the troop-review will conclude with a climactic spectacle of song and dance, performed primarily for the "simulated and unconsummated" pleasure of the senior general. The scene conveys the soldiers' and officers' dialectical consciousness of unity and a state of regimentation as they embody *sobornost'*.[219] This "communally based, psycho-acoustic" interplay of freedom and necessity reminds us of early life, in cooperative unison with our (allo)mothers, as well as of our own basic residence within the universe, which was "born out of sound and amounted to one big party of constantly, intensely vibrating atoms."[220]

Continuing in a ludic vein, Tolstoy depicts Count Rostov's intoxicated attachment to Tsar Alexander I's person, whom the junior officer encounters at a grander review of troops in Olmütz before the battle of Austerlitz—that of the three emperors, which takes place on the one-year anniversary of Napoleon's self-coronation.[221] This bond is deeply homoerotic, reflecting enthusiasm for the Tsar, an affirmation of the intersection between hierarchy and collective belonging, and an enunciation of the perennial Russian phenomenon of "naïve monarchism." According to this latter concept, the *Narod* would project its desires for liberation onto the Tsar's person, who is reinterpreted as well-meaning but politically ineffective, and view persistent State oppression and exploitation as resulting from the machinations of the nobles and the "little father's" irremediably corrupt ministers and advisers. As though to illustrate the staying power of this myth, even after the abolition of the Romanov dynasty over a century later, in February 1917, many peasants simultaneously celebrated the Revolution while calling for a "good Tsar" or "peasant king" to be elected.[222]

To a certain extent, continuing the precedent established at Kutuzov's entrance, the review of the Austrian and Russian troops presents a timeless scene that connects the classical Greek associations between Apollo and athleticism with the LGBTQ+ Pride marches of our day. While Pride marches have been held in a number of Ukrainian cities in recent years, especially since the popular ouster of Kremlin-oriented Viktor Yanukovych in 2014, such demonstrations are illegal in

Russia, which has banned "gay propaganda" toward minors since 2013.[223] At the same time, the "Pride" shown at Olmütz conveys an authoritarian collectivism that diverges from the insurgent spirit of the "original" Pride at Stonewall in 1969. Defying official homonegativity, Tolstoy revels in dancing, twirling, and wheeling soldiers, "smartly dressed bandsmen," and a "quiver[ing]" cannon.[224] He expresses that "[e]very [Russian] general and every soldier was conscious of his own insignificance [...] and yet at the same time [...] of his strength as a part of that enormous whole." He remarks at the collective strength of the Russian army: "the men themselves were awed by their multitude and the immensity of the power they constituted."[225]

In the face of the terror posed by death and defeat in war, the army's homoerotic rituals function to promote individual, collective, and national survival.[226] Such psychosexual feelings of collective identification vindicate Tolstoy's invocation of swarm theory, which emphasizes how masses and multitudes cooperate to overwhelm their enemies. More recently, swarm theory has been applied to so-called "open-source warfare."[227] In naturalistic terms, the review before Austerlitz is reminiscent of avian symbolism, which can have queer and metaphysical connotations, as of Kropotkin's description of the mass-flights of butterflies and dragonflies in Indonesia and Amazonia, invariably for the purposes of copulation, reproduction, and group cohesion.[228] During the nineteenth century, sperm whales used social learning to adapt to the threats posed by whalers, often opting to escape by swarming upwind rather than mobilizing in their typical defensive formations.[229] Certainly, sperm whales have employed a diversity of tactics to resist hunting, with the sinking of over a dozen whaling ships attributed to the enormous Mocha Dick—Melville's muse—two centuries ago.[230]

Both at the individual and collective levels, the amassed Russian forces—from the generals "with their thin or thick waists" to the "elegant, pomaded officers," "freshly [...] shaved" soldiers with "clean and polished" weapons," and even the well-groomed horses—respond erotically to the appearance of Tsar Alexander. In the troops' willingness to please their lord, the scene even takes on aspects of the burlesque. The narrator describes how, "[t]ill the Tsar reached it, each regiment [...] seemed like a lifeless body," but then became alive upon encountering their leader, with "tensely passionate attention," as though aroused. By idealizing Alexander as at once omnipotent and sexually attractive, the soldiers express their submission to his despotism, paradoxically affirming toxic masculinity, but also paradoxically compensating for their helplessness in the face of death in combat.

Count Rostov is shown to experience a "feeling of tenderness and ecstasy such as he had never before known" for Alexander, and to sense a fanatical willingness to die "for his Tsar!"[231] To be sure, the narrator claims that, at the review in Olmütz, "nine-tenths of the men in the Russian army were then in love [...] with their Tsar and the glory of the Russian arms." Rather like Buddha outside the palace walls, the Tsar is idealized as lamenting, "What a terrible thing war is," after encountering a dying soldier at the battle of Wischau (November 25, 1805). Count Rostov's "internal defensive ecstasy" is such that he believes the Tsar to "underst[an]d everything."[232]

In both entrance scenes for the supreme leaders of the Russian military, the writer confirms Carpenter's hypothesis about the great importance of homogenic love in society.[233] "What if he gave me a place near him?" Rostov asks, fantasizing about Alexander. "Oh, how I would guard him, how I would tell him the truth, how I would unmask his deceivers!"[234] In his depiction of the review at Olmütz, Tolstoy may mean to mock the hussar's self-subordination to the Tsar as an affirmation of corrupted love and authoritarian political communication, whereby humans suspend their consciences and "deliver them[selves] over to seducers who simply make their chains heavier."[235] On such a reading, the scene serves to satirize the "administrative" or "panegyric utopia," which celebrates majesty, militarism, and mechanistic dehumanization.[236]

On the other hand, an alternate possibility is that Rostov's attraction to Alexander I derives implicitly from the latter's education in republican and constitutional ideas, his youthful commitment to liberal reform of the State, his meetings with the utopian socialist Robert Owen to redesign society, and the false hopes he had raised regarding the possibility of abolishing serfdom.[237] According to Sofia Andreevna Tolstaya, Lev Nikolaevich felt indebted to Alexander II (r. 1855–1881), who had freed Volkonsky and his wife from Siberian exile.[238] As well, Tolstoy's contempt for the hypocrisy of Swiss republicanism and British parliamentary imperialism is well-known, though that does not rule out sympathy with the constitutional cause, in keeping with the author's interest in the baron of Montesquieu (see the next chapter).[239]

To what degree Tolstoy means to uphold or satirize such naïve views of Tsarism in book one of *War and Peace* is ambiguous. His critic, the Formalist Viktor Shklovsky, charges that Lev Nikolaevich depicts Alexander as an "ideal monarch," whereas the military historian Elizabeth Samet interprets the writer's portrayal of Rostov's "self-forgetfulness" as intended to be critical, reflecting the poet's anarchism.[240] Extending Jennifer Wilson's analysis of Tolstoy's creative explorations of "sexual alterity" and social critique, we believe that Tolstoy meant to include Tsarism as one of the primary obstacles to societal *and* sexual liberation in his *poema*.[241] Perhaps, in his treatment of the relationship between Emperor and soldier, master and slave, Lev Nikolaevich is dialectically recording, celebrating, *and* critiquing the "Orthodox and monarchist loyalties" that motivated many Russians in the war against Bonaparte.[242]

Accordingly, he presents here a verbal icon disclosing the dialectical image of residence and estrangement—human harmony and unity achieved through reciprocal, communal bonds of erotic and compassionate love, being mediated paradoxically by "absolute and coerced belonging."[243] If this be Pride, it is pride in servitude. Still, such intermixing of Eros and Thanatos has an enduring history. Like Tsars Paul, Alexander I, and Nicholas I, who were possessed by "paradomania," Stalin enjoyed compelling his male subordinates to dance for him.[244]

If we compare Kutuzov with Tsar Alexander, we see that the first appearances of both of these supreme commanders are marked by hierarchical displays of mass-homoeroticism. At the same time, considering their differences in personality, we may be encountering an implicit verbal image expressing Tolstoy's judgment on what anarchists sometimes call "justified" vs. "unjustified" hierarchies. Assuming that Kutuzov is a Daoist sage, Bodhisattva, or charismatic warrior leader leading the Russian "band of brothers" to victory and self-overcoming through "spiritual federalism," Alexander's "spiritual centralism" demands erotic submission, thus amounting to a cult of personality.[245] After all, Alexander views his male subjects as little more than human toys or instruments.[246] If Alexander is an authoritarian, then Kutuzov is an ethical leader.[247] To extend the metaphor, Kutuzov is a "good" gay—Alexander, a "bad" one.[248]

That being said, regardless of the flatter hierarchy between Kutuzov and his men, compared to that between the Tsar and his subordinates, the army's expressions of affective solidarity and benign group narcissism run the risk of becoming destructive and reactionary, considering the "short step" from identificatory love to bondage. The context of competing, warring States only worsens the risk that the strong passions associated with in-group identity will result in atrocities.[249] Paradoxically, then, in this scene, horizontal collectivism facilitates vertical collectivism.[250]

As a consequence, the Tsar's emotional bond with his male underlings in the face of death serves to "imprison the subject in a disabling fixation," and reify charismatic authority and "national unity." This reality in itself illuminates the continuities between Tsarism and Caesarism, or Bonapartism, developing the veiled dual critique which we find in *War and Peace* from the start.[251] By means of such thought-images, Tolstoy subtly relays a critique of false forms of human society—despotism, enthrallment to power, estrangement, enslavement, and the mechanical *Gesellschaft*—while affirming more humanizing ones, such as humanism, residence, and a new community, or *Gemeinschaft*.[252]

Undoubtedly, later in his career, the queer sage would become Tsarism's greatest public critic. The State's religious censor viewed the French translation of Tolstoy's *The Kingdom of God Is Within You* (1893) as the "most harmful foreign book" it had ever banned, and Konstantin Pobedonostsev (1827–1907), Chief Procurator of the Holy Synod, despaired at the "terrible infection of anarchy and atheism" Tolstoy was "spreading [...] throughout the whole of Russia!" Correspondingly, Tsar Alexander III (r. 1881–1894) considered that the count had to be stopped in his tracks.[253]

Indeed, there is no ambiguity as to why the Tsars might think so. Tolstoy's treatment of Alexander II during a cameo in *Anna Karenina* (1875–1877) is evidently hostile: in contrast to the pomp and circumstance surrounding Alexander I at Olmütz, Alexander II in *Anna Karenina* appears with his "whole court" as spectators of a steeplechase, during which Count Vronsky will kill the lovely mare Frou-Frou from exhaustion and over-exploitation, in a bid to out-compete his fellow Horse Guards and impress the Tsar.[254] Even more boldly, in a 1902 letter to Nicholas II, written under the impression that his death was imminent, Tolstoy exclaims that "Tsars may be and have been *monsters and maniacs*." In "I Cannot Be Silent" (1908), the artist openly chastises the State for its mass-executions of the protagonists of the 1905 Revolution.[255] In a 1904 diary entry, the writer contrasts the present with a "time when anarchy was unthinkable," considering that "the people no longer worship, [...] and no longer put up with power [власть], but want freedom, *complete freedom*."[256]

Eros and Authority, Part II: Whither LGBTQ+ Unions?

Let us return to Olmütz once again. Does Tolstoy mean to disparage Rostov's self-surrender before Alexander, as Wilson implies, or rather, bless communitarian and Populist expressions of in-group sentiment among the Russian soldiers, officers, and Tsar? The answer may be suggested in the passionate, spontaneous homoeroticism conveyed in an exchange by Count Rostov and his German landlord in the interim between Kutuzov and Alexander's troop-reviews:

> "And hurrah for the whole world!" [...]
> "And long live the whole world!"[257]

Beginning with the landlord praising the Austrians and Russians before Rostov replies by proclaiming humanist internationalism, this pair's exchange anticipates how late-nineteenth century revolutionary Ukrainian students would respond with "Glory to all the earth!" to the slogan "Glory to Ukraine!" (*Слава Україні!*) Using this phrase, which is now a battle-cry against Russian imperialism, the poet Taras Shevchenko (1814–1861), who never married, concludes his famous "To Osnovyanenko" (1840).[258] In this sense, the banter between Rostov and his landlord may allude to Tolstoy's queer anarchism, and thus tap into the cosmopolitan-internationalist desires for free love and collective liberation which the author fashions in *War and Peace*.[259]

Ideally, Eros, residence, and ecstatic belonging will expand outward in a productive sense, incorporating all of humanity and creation with love, but the intoxication of in-group sentiments can also be mobilized thanotically for aggression.[260] This is especially true when hyper-masculine homoeroticism holds sway.[261] In a similar vein, if nationalism overpowers humanism in the scene at Olmütz, then we should consider Adorno's parallel anxieties about the fascist utilization of male bonding, homophilia, and sublimated homosexuality, especially among the essentially all-male far-right paramilitary groups and death cults that were active during the Weimar Republic (1918–1933), including the Nazi Party and the Hitler Youth.[262]

Disconcertingly, the *Sturmabteilung* (SA, brownshirt) leader Ernst Röhm (1887–1934), who was gay, argued that it was due to a strong homoerotic sense of belonging that the Nazis defeated their rivals, the Social Democrats and Communists, and put an end to Weimar-era liberalism.[263] This is not, of course, to give credence to Adorno's reductive homonegativity, paranoia over an ostensible "Nazi-Soviet gay conspiracy," or the related oppressive Stalinist delusion about queerness being a counter-revolutionary or "fascist perversion," as Justice Commissar Nikolai Krylenko and Maxim Gorky would claim, respectively, in a *kowtow* to Stalin and his deputy secret police chief, G. G. Yagoda (1891–1938).[264]

On Stalin's orders, Gorky penned an ill-named essay on "Proletarian Humanism" for *Pravda* and *Izvestia* as a public response to the challenge privately raised in 1934 by the British Communist Harry Whyte to the USSR's ban on the "bourgeois degeneracy" of same-sex relations. In this article, Gorky notoriously declares, "Destroy the homosexuals—Fascism will disappear."[265] In parallel, the Marxist psychoanalyst Wilhelm Reich (1897–1957), who appropriated Otto Gross's theories of sexual revolution while ignoring his predecessor's openness to non-normative eroticism, viewed homosexuality as "deeply rooted in fascist ideology."[266]

Undoubtedly, Stalin's doctrine on "social fascism," together with the pyramidal organization of the social-democratic and Communist opposition to the Nazis, facilitated Hitler's rise to power in 1933. The anarcho-syndicalist Rudolf Rocker considered the "cult of [Ernst] Thälmann," German Communist leader, and the "corpse-like obedience" that Marxist parties had propagated in the labor movement to have been "fascist element[s]."[267] In Italy, it did not help that Fascists and revolutionary syndicalists shared an economic program based on the partial expropriation of the capitalist class and the corporate integration of hierarchically organized syndicates.[268] For their part, Stalin and Hitler, megalomaniacal allies and seeming would-be suitors, paradoxically imitated each other's heteronormative proclamations. When Stalin recriminalized and medicalized same-sex relations in 1933, a decade and a half after his Party had decriminalized them—and following the example of criminalization in the Soviet republics of Azerbaijan, Uzbekistan, and Turkmenistan in the 1920s—Hitler would do the same a year after seizing power.[269] In this sense, the mobilization of social hatred and "social cleansing" against homosexuals under Stalin's regime, leading to the conviction of between 25,000 and 60,000 men, complemented the despot's reimposition of patriarchal norms and codes, thus rolling back the utopian-feminist currents and legislative advances of the early post-revolutionary period.[270] Likewise in Nazi Germany, SS leader Heinrich Himmler founded the Reich Central Office for the Combating of Homosexuality and Abortion in 1936.[271]

As uncovered by historian Anna Hájková, the case of a possible lesbian relationship in the Auschwitz death camp between SS guard Anneliese Kohlmann and Helene Sommer, a pseudonym for a Czech Jewish woman, may crystallize the continuities *and* contradictions between the basic human desire for relatedness and the corrupting effects of imposed institutional and ideological imperatives.[272] The testimony of Sommer's anonymous fellow Holocaust survivor, who reports having borne witness to this relationship, suggests it may have been platonic—thus reflecting the indistinct boundaries between sexual consent and sexual harassment, even in an environment so extreme as this one.[273] Hájková cites witnesses who report that they slept together, but concedes she does not know who initiated the relationship, and "whether or to what extent Kohlmann coerced Sommer," without losing sight of the context of camp society. She frames the bond as one that Kohlmann saw as love, and that Sommer saw as "sexual barter." In other words, the Auschwitz prisoner secured survival, protection, and resources for herself and her mother by providing sex and/or affection for her female camp guard.[274]

Lest it be forgotten, months after Hitler's seizure of power, in May 1933, Nazi students destroyed Berlin's Institute of Sexual Science, a haven for the LGBTQ+ community, together with its archive. The Institute had been directed by Magnus Hirschfeld (1868–1935), a prominent sexologist, gay activist, and inventor of the term transgender.[275] In June 1934, Hitler signed off on the mass-liquidation of the SA, which contained many gay members, after having used the paramilitary group to seize power, and he criminalized and mass-murdered sexual minorities at the same time as he perpetrated the Holocaust. Between 5,000 and 15,000 gay men ended up in Nazi concentration camps, where they were often subjected to medical experimentation, while other queers would be summarily executed or sent on suicide missions. The death rate among these prisoners was approximately two-thirds.[276] Stalin's Great Terror, in turn, expanded on his counterpart's purge of Röhm and company, whereas the Soviet despot's identification with and attraction to Hitler fatally led him to minimize the possibility of betrayal and invasion by the *Wehrmacht.* In psychodynamically provoking paranoia, his sublimated gay partnership with Hitler led Stalin to masochistically prepare for defeat by annihilating 90 percent of high-ranking military officers a year or two before the start of World War II.[277]

Consequently, while Alexander I is not Hitler, nor is Caesarism the same as fascism, Tolstoy and Adorno remind us that—alongside heterosexual abuse—same-sex attachment and/or trafficking have played important roles in upholding authoritarian-bureaucratic, militarist, and patriarchal institutions throughout history, until the present day.[278] Movements as varied as nationalists, Zionists, socialists, Communists, and Fascists have encouraged same-sex intimacy as "cadre training" to promote loyalty to their causes. In addition, from the Mamlukes of the Middle Ages to gangs in the republican city-state of Florence during early modernity and the Afghan *mujahideen* and Taliban of the twentieth and twenty-first centuries, "bad gays" have competed violently to sexually exploit boys. In modern Europe, charges of "sodomy across hierarchies of age and status" were indelibly tied to domination within the phenomenon of apprenticeship. Concurring with Cesare Beccaria, we can say that these abusive dynamics follow from the very existence of class, "dependence[,] and servitude."[279]

In sum, the State, the capitalists, and the clergy mobilize not only compulsory heterosexuality, but also our polymorphously perverse sexuality to advance their necrophilic goals. Such projects fundamentally contradict the human freedom and union sought by Eros and ecstasy, which at their best, oppose and bind aggression to ensure survival.[280] Through his Dionysian affirmation of sexual pluralism and productive homoerotic love, and his warnings about the homoerotic lure that reproduces hierarchical authority instead of provoking mutual recognition, Lev Nikolaevich provides a transhistorical critique that equally targets Tsarist and Marxist-Leninist heterosexist oppression, together with both systems' fetishization of the authority principle, while belying Michel Foucault and Chitty's pessimism about the revolutionary potential of gay liberation.[281]

Internationalism on the Battlefield

Returning to the opening scene of *War and Peace*, we see that Anna Pavlovna Scherer calls Napoleon a "murderer," while the Russian diplomat Bilibin refers to him, in parallel, as "Usurper and Enemy of Mankind."[282] Is Tolstoy suggesting that the Tsar Alexander is any different? As we have discussed, his romantic idealization of Rostov's "love and devotion to the sovereign" and his Slavophilic distortion of the Tsar's personality may either be satirical, *or* point to a contradiction in Tolstoy's thought. After all, the novelist's depiction of protests among officers against high-ranking German commanders may betray a degree of Great-Russian chauvinism.[283] For instance, Tolstoy's presentation of the Russian army's strategic retreat into the Empire's vast geographical interior during Napoleon's invasion as being unplanned and chaotic is misleading and ahistorical. The reality is that the Baltic German Field Marshal General Prince Andreas Barclay (1761–1818) ordered the execution of this strategy.[284] For all that, both in Tolstoy's telling, as in Bondarchuk's cinematic adaptation, the Tsar's impetuousness and predilection for instrumentalizing human life are plainly exhibited in his pressuring General Kutuzov to begin combat at Austerlitz, even before all the Russian units are ready.[285] "We are not on parade and not on the Tsaritsyn Field,"[286] replies Kutuzov, in an express repudiation of the Emperor.

Tolstoy's internationalist and anarcho-Populist framing of society and warfare is one of the classic's major themes, however much it may be undermined at times by declarations of Russian in-group communitarianism. Though he is himself an adjutant to General Kutuzov—much like Tolstoy was himself an officer and a landlord—Prince Andrei is represented as experiencing an almost instinctual revulsion for the Austrian Minister of War and his own adjutant: "Away from the smell of [gun]powder, they probably think it easy to win victories!" remarks Andrei to himself. In an epochal parallel to an argument held between the Mexican anarchists Ricardo Flores Magón (1873–1922) and Praxedis Guerrero (1882–1910) on the eve of the latter's departure to fight in the Mexican Revolution in late 1910, wherein Guerrero would fall in battle, Tolstoy outlines Bolkonsky's principled rejection of Bilibin's entreaty that he acknowledge that, being "*un philosophe* [...], your duty [...] is to take care of yourself."[287] Instead, Prince Andrei will fight on and die, defending his country.

Prince Andrei is driven by dreams of "completely transform[ing]" Russia, particularly its military, which he describes not as "an army," but rather, "a mob of oppressed disciplined slaves who have submitted to robbers and mercenaries."[288] Although the author's proposals are motivated by a kenotic sympathy with soldiers and contempt for many fellow officers, and despite consisting of proposals for improved training, tactics, strategy, conditions, and morale, they will inevitably be frustrated by existing hierarchies, much as was his initiative to organize a Society for the Education of the People (1860). This dynamic of disappointment followed by direct action will mirror Lev Nikolaevich's own lifelong journey of political and sexual self-discovery, self-radicalization, and coming out.[289]

Witnessing his army's pillaging of local populations, Bolkonsky recognizes, at least to himself, the limitations of nationalism: "*Voilà le cher* [dear] Orthodox Russian army."[290] This honest acknowledgment suggests echoes in the writer's memory of having witnessed the looting and burning by Cossacks and Russian infantry of a Chechen *aul* during his first outing as a "volunteer" fighter in a punitive raid in the Caucasus in 1852.[291] These crimes are continuous with the destruction and massacres the Russian military has carried out more recently in Syria and Ukraine. Indeed, Prince Andrei's acknowledgment registers the depth of White-Russian brutality, marking the gap from Don Quixote's proud declaration, that "I am not in the habit [...] of despoiling those whom I vanquish."[292] Furthermore, such vindictive plundering can be considered a violation of the internationalist "hurrahs" raised to the world by Count Rostov and his short-lived German landlord during the 1805 campaign.[293]

Despite all this negativity, queer anarchism can provide a positive remedy. On the front lines, the subversive, comradely banter between Cossacks and French soldiers exemplifies a humanizing and homoerotic example of mutuality which threatens to put an end to the war effort altogether:

> peals of such healthy and good-humoured laughter from the [Russian] soldiers [came] that it infected the French involuntarily, so much so that the only thing left to do seemed to be to unload the muskets, explode the ammunition, and all return home as quickly as possible.[294]

In this thought-image, Tolstoy unites internationalist mutiny with gay orgasm. The anarchist message conveyed here has its parallels in the concepts of mutual recognition and the general strike, as in the calls made both by Tolstoy and Faure in 1909 and 1926, respectively, for soldiers and youth to refuse mobilization orders and desert the armed forces.[295] Historically, French and Russian soldiers engaged in fraternization during the siege of Sevastopol in the Crimean War, and German, British, and French troops declared a Christmas Day truce in 1914 in the Belgian trenches during World War I, according to the slogan, "live and let live."[296] Likewise, seeking to spread the good news of the February 1917 Revolution, militant soldiers performed the "Marseillaise" on the Russian-German front in the early days after Nicholas' abdication.[297] In parallel, in his memoirs, the Tolstoyan peasant-intellectual Dmitri Morgachëv (1892–1978) recalls the humanizing tenderness with which he tended as a conscript to a dying Austrian counterpart across the line of control. In like fashion, his comrade Yakov Dragunovsky discusses his first-hand experience of a spontaneous Easter truce in 1916 consensually agreed to by ordinary Russian and German soldiers, despite opposition from officers on both sides.[298]

In *War and Peace*, rank-and-file Russian soldiers are rendered as fighting at the mercy of the officer class, which "wandered about in the fog" without giving timely orders during the battle of Austerlitz. The cruelties of combat are seen portrayed realistically, in that only 18 of the Horse Guards survive a charge on the French; in the "distressing screams and groans" of the injured and dying heard by Rostov as he searches desperately for the Tsar; and in the partisan Fëdr Dolokhov's witnessing of a hellish stampede of desperate men "disfigured by the fear of death" who, under artillery fire, try to flee across a frozen pond, only to drown *en masse* as the ice collapses under their weight.[299]

Prince Andrei's Trance at Austerlitz: Living Reason and Psychosexual Self-Discovery

Bolkonsky's near-death experience at Austerlitz presents the reader with a juxtaposition between the atrocity and artificiality of war, power, and glory on the one hand, and the beauty of nature and social existence, rightly ordered, on the other. For Tolstoy to have included this moment of truth imparts his "openness to absorbing and self-altering experiences," "involv[ing] at least a temporary suspension of metacognitive critique of fantasies or sensations."[300] The scene is metaphysical, surreal, even psychedelic: ironically, given the violent context, it conveys a considerable enhancement of Bolkonsky's openness to experience.[301] As he lies bleeding on the battlefield after having been shot while taking up the Russian standard in an effort to rally the troops, Andrei reflects on the sky:

> How was it I did not see that lofty sky before? And how happy I am to have found it at last. Yes! All is vanity, all falsehood, except that infinite sky. There is nothing, nothing, but that.[302]

In essence, as the hour of his death nears, Prince Andrei encounters Kantian transcendental idealism, or "the doctrine that all appearances are regarded as mere representations, not as things in themselves."[303] The sky symbolizes nature's representation as "living reason," connecting Bolkonsky to the emblematic associations made among light, the color yellow, and the concept of *Vernunft*, or metaphysical reason, by the bisexual writer Goethe, who was influenced by Kant and the Persian poet Hafez (1315–1390).[304] As he lies dying, he sees infinity in the sky, and "takes off" into the light representing the Kantian moral

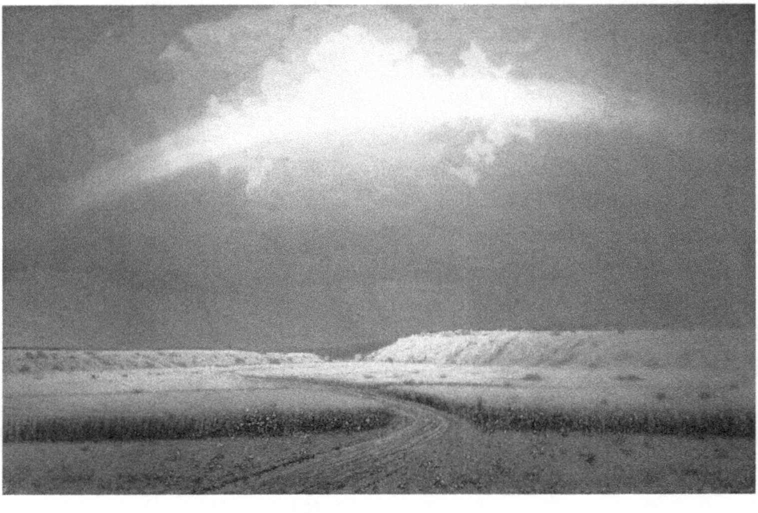

FIGURE 6.1 Arkhip Kuindzhi, *Rainbow* (1905)

law, signifying his residence within nature, and his hopes for a better future (see Figure 6.1).[305] Through existential ascent and the experience of wonder, he intuitively senses the need for a radical break with the past, connects with Eros and the Kingdom of God, and flies into another world, freed of nationalism and material wealth.[306] In Eastern Christianity, as a matter of fact, light is suggestive of the presence of the divine essence, and prayer presupposes that the world is full of meaning. Plus, the allusion to vanity references the Orthodox renunciation of the world's wickedness, from the battlefields to the *salons*.[307]

Likewise, in the 2019 feature documentary *For Sama*, named for the Syrian video-journalist protagonist Waad al-Kateab's newborn daughter, Sama (whose name means "sky" in Arabic), the infant child and the upper atmosphere alike stand for the regulative ideals of peace and tranquility, contrasting with ethical nihilism and the suffering of war perpetrated by the Syrian regime and its Russian and Iranian allies: "the sky we want, without aircraft, bombings—with sun, clouds, birds."[308] As Mel Campbell observes, the "upward gaze" may constitute "an escape into another dimension of feeling—away from the relentless forward momentum of modernity," just as myriad artists have viewed the tranquility of the Eurasian steppes as inducing contemplation and symbolizing hope.[309] Nature writing, in this sense, reconfigures ecosystems not as warehouses, property, or killing fields, but rather, as the "continuation of community."[310] For Adorno, indeed, the image of "lying on water and looking peacefully at the sky" is intimately connected with the hopes for the "fulfilled utopia" characterized by "perpetual peace."[311]

By all means, Count Tolstoy may intend to associate Prince Andrei's paradoxical near-death experience of calm and joy at the sight of the "immeasurably lofty" sky while lying wounded at Austerlitz—an example of "true prayer"—with a sudden metaphoric encounter with the self, his connection to "Heavenly" Aphrodite Urania, and a "queerpiphany."[312] His trance quietly complements sexual alterity as a "standing critique of the entire society and its illnesses."[313]

> "What's this? Am I falling? My legs are giving way," thought he, and fell on his back [...]. Above him there was now nothing but the sky [...]. "How quiet, peaceful, and solemn, not at all as I ran," thought Prince Andrei "—not as we ran, shouting and fighting [...]: how differently do those clouds glide across that lofty infinite sky."[314]

This contrast between heaven and earth, ideal and base, parallels Pausanias' differentiation in the *Symposium* between common and divine love, only the latter of which, on this account, impels virtue.[315] Equally, Lev Nikolaevich will restate this duality by affirming that "[w]e who live after Kant cannot get away from the distinction he indicated": namely, between the earthly-sensual and moral-spiritual realms—*Sinnlichkeit* (sensibility) vs. *Vernunft*/сознание (metaphysical reason), respectively.[316] This juxtaposition is reiterated in a diary entry from October 1879 which contrasts "worldly" and "winged" people:

> There are worldly people, heavy and wingless. Their sphere is down below. There are strong ones among them: Napoleon. They leave terrible traces among men and cause an uproar, but it is all on the earth [...]. There are those whose wings grow equably and who slowly rise and fly: monks. There are light people, winged, who rise easily from among the crowd and again descend: good idealists. There are strong-winged ones who, drawn by carnal desires descend among the crowd and break their wings. Such am I.[317]

Likewise in Tolstoy's *Youth* (1857), while awaiting the arrival of a beloved woman, the protagonist Nikolenka looks up into the night sky:

> But the moon would rise higher and higher, brighter and brighter in the sky, [...] and as I would gaze upon and listen to it all, *something would tell me that even she with her bare arms and passionate embraces was far, far from the only bliss*, and the more I would look at the high full moon, did true beauty and bliss seem to be higher and higher, purer and purer, nearer and nearer to Him [...].[318]

As with Andrei's epiphany while lying wounded, regarding the atmosphere's light blue (голубой) color—with голубой having gay connotations—Tolstoy's self-representation as a "winged one" torn among monasticism, idealism, and eroticism; his fantasies of flight through the heavens contrasted with his earthly sins; and his intuition that bliss rests "above" his elusive female lover signal veiled acknowledgments of his own "polymorphous-perverse" sexuality.[319] After all, Freud interpreted dreams of birds and flight as reflecting the desire for erotic satisfaction.[320] The motif of "wings" alludes to Socrates's dialogue with Phaidros, wherein the renowned thinker tells his interlocutor that philosophers and gay lovers are linked to the divine realm.[321] Moreover, the Tolstoyan researcher Nina Nikitina links the writer's use of lunar symbols with an implicit acknowledgment of "the tragic impossibility of arranging his personal life with the help of only female love," while the Russian sexologist Igor Kon supports the idea of emblems of the moon reflecting desires for same-sex intimacy.[322] For her part, Le Guin associates moon-gazing with lunacy and visionary insight.[323] Along these lines, Turgenev appears to pay tribute to Bolkonsky's trance in his lyrical poem "The Realm of Azure" (1878), wherein the speaker visits a "realm of azure, light, youth, and happiness" in a dream-state of homoerotic union:

> We were together, a few guys, in a tattered little boat [...]. I did not know my comrades, but in all my soul I felt that they were as young, light-hearted, and happy as I! But I didn't even notice them. I beheld all round me one boundless azure sea, dimpled with scales of gold, and overhead the same boundless sea of blue, and in it, triumphant and mirthful, it seemed, moved the sun. And among us every so often rose laughter, ringing and gleeful, like the laughter of the gods![324]

Turgenev envisions his comrades and himself embarking on a collective psychosexual odyssey involving discoveries of gems, flowers, and "rainbow-colored birds":

> We came on islands—enchanted islands, translucent with the prismatic lights of precious stones: of amethysts and emeralds. Odors of bewildering fragrance rose from the rounded shores; some of these islands showered on us a rain of roses and valley lilies; from others, rainbow-colored birds of long wings suddenly arose.[325]

Notably, Mikhail Alekseevich Kuzmin (1872–1936) would use similar heavenly imagery to openly communicate his queerness in his groundbreaking autobiographical novel *Wings* (1906). Like Prince Andrei in *War and Peace*, though less indirectly and more explicitly, this memoir tells the story of a young man coming to terms with his non-traditional sexuality.[326]

Following his survival of this near-death experience at Austerlitz—ironically enough—Prince Bolkonsky continues his psychosexual processes of self-discovery and self-determination, striving to satisfy his needs for fulfillment, meaning, and mirroring with Others within the boundaries of Eros and death.[327] Like Don Quixote, Andrei opts to become a knight-errant of sorts, "whose profession it is to assist the needy of every kind," and to "forgive the humble and punish the arrogant; [...] to succour the wretched and destroy the cruel."[328]

Through his coming-out process, linked to mutual liberation of self and society, Andrei will transition from being predominantly heterosexual, with a suppressed homosexual element, to embracing a subtly queer-anarchist heroism that sublates the legacies of Dorian Greece and Japanese Samurai without fetishizing warfare or reproducing class stratification. After Austerlitz, Bolkonsky withdraws from the military to live on his Bald Hills manor, where he improves the lot of the serfs bound to him. Then, when the *Grand Armée* invades Russia, the prince abandons the general staff to serve with the soldiers on the front-lines. Considering that the prince's life-partner ends up being Natasha Rostova, Bolkonsky's tragic death does fall far short of Kuzmin's ideal, as expressed in *Wings*.[329]

While contemplating the heavens, the semi-conscious Andrei actually comes face-to-face with Napoleon, his former "hero," and the "new Caesar," as the emperor reviews the battlefield.[330] In a reflection of his newfound queer anarchism, the dying Bolkonsky takes little interest in the statesman, and cannot see him as anything more than a "small insignificant creature." Peering into his eyes, Andrei comes to realize the "*insignificance of greatness*"—much as Pierre later recognizes Napoleon as a "wretched comedian."[331]

Suddenly, Bonaparte orders Andrei and his fellow surviving Russian officers to be attended to by his own surgeons, ensuring their survival. Although this act may be at variance with the Emperor's established narcissism, cruelty, and desire for glory, and thus perhaps suggestive of an anomalous humanism and observance of the military concept of honor—reflecting Lev Nikolaevich's efforts to find human dignity in *everyone*—it also serves Napoleon's instrumental goal of intelligence-gathering about his enemy, thus re-entrenching authority, war, and estrangement.[332] The scene is therefore dialectically consistent with Tolstoy's presentation of Napoleon as an "impassive automaton" and a "criminal lunatic," who is "driven only by lust for power and indifferent to the massive suffering he has inflicted." As well, it suggests a twist on the real historical precedent, whereby a Russian officer attended to the wounds of his injured French counterpart after an ambush near Krasnoe by directing him expeditiously to the company surgeon.[333]

Notes

1 Stites 1989: 128.
2 Sokurov; Mureithi.
3 Lieven 2012: 12–13; Forrest 72.
4 Orwin 2012b: 99.
5 *Ibid* 104–7; Lieven 2012: 16; Forrest 72.
6 Orwin 2002d: 52.
7 Evtuhov et al. 325.
8 Sternhell 248.
9 Schama; Bartlett 2011: 19.
10 Figes 2002: 107; Colling 22.
11 Chekhov 1999: 336.
12 Tolstoy 2010: 484–7.
13 Gustafson 1986: 340.
14 *Ibid* 411.
15 Tolstoy 2010: 79–80, 92.
16 *Ibid* 32–9; Colling.
17 Rancour-Laferriere 1998: 50–1.
18 Zorin 14; Bartlett 2011: 21–43; Maude 1987a: 8.
19 Tolstoy 2010: 99–102, 246–7; Orwin 1993: 128; Bartlett 2011: 166.
20 Tolstoy 2010: 228; Gustafson 1986: 286–7.
21 Rancour-Laferriere 1989: 41–6. By entering symbiosis with Natasha Rostova, Bezukhov merely conforms to the stipulation set forth in the Imperial Law Code for a husband to consider his wife "as his own body" (Bartlett 2011: 242).
22 Gustafson 1986: 346–7.
23 LeBlanc 2007: 120.
24 Tolstoy 2010: 100, 105.
25 Evtuhov et al. 375.
26 Vinitsky 80.
27 Maude 1987a: 176.
28 Tolstoy 2010: 115; Vinitsky 80.
29 German for "beautiful graves."
30 Tolstoy 2010: 157, 192–4.
31 Yalom 160; Tolstoy 2010: 199.
32 Jackson 29.
33 Bondarchuk; Foster J 43.
34 Tolstoy 2010: 167, 1326n167.
35 Reitz 142.
36 Ken 147.
37 Parker et al. 31.
38 Colling; Stites 1989; Hardt and Weeks.
39 Klikauer.
40 Chitty 83, 99; French.
41 Marx 1976: 553.

42 By law, the death penalty would be applied against a soldier who struck a superior officer in Imperial Russia, and severe punishment was meted out for insulting the Romanov family (Maude 1987a: 308; Figes and Kolonitskii 37).
43 Foster J 175–7; Fontesse et al.
44 Babel 71.
45 Benjamin 36.
46 Becker 246.
47 Reis et al.
48 Roelcke et al.
49 *Ibid.*
50 Ballou and Landreneau 75.
51 Hyde.
52 Reitz 84–5; Sartre 338.
53 Gerth and Mills 194; Remley 130, 242n27.
54 Dong and Temple 174.
55 Freud 2016: 71–2; Chancer 1992: 58–63; Clark 2019: 198.
56 Orwin 2002c: 224.
57 Tillich 66; Berdaev 2009.
58 Berdyaev 1966.
59 Rancour-Laferriere 1995: 1–2, 55; Figes and Kolonitskii 183–90.
60 Sorokin.
61 Faure 255–9.
62 Clay 212; McLean 2008: 84.
63 McPeak 112.
64 Smith L.
65 Bartlett 2014: 13–14.
66 Donskov 137.
67 Chancer 1992: 15–19; Adorno et al.; Fischer et al.
68 Fromm 1947: 108–11; Benjamin 53–5; Becker 249.
69 Kropotkin 2018: 340–1.
70 Cunliffe.
71 Tolstoy 1987: 101.
72 Tolstoy 2004: 42.
73 Schonfeld and Chang 10–12, 219–25; Berger.
74 Chancer 1992: 15; Polanyi.
75 Shantz and Williams 112–14; Klikauer.
76 Lepore; Hillman 28.
77 Marx 1976: 782–94.
78 Lepore.
79 Chancer 1992: 33–5, 94–7.
80 Furner; Fudge; Giammarinaro.
81 Wible; Kaplan et al.
82 Giddens 158.
83 Racy.
84 Stamenova; Burdyga.
85 КВПУ; Burdyga.
86 Ho.
87 Thompson G.
88 Huetteman.
89 Chancer 1992: 122, 204; Hardt and Weeks.
90 Keeney.
91 Marx 1983; Berdyaev 2009.
92 Dinerstein (emphasis in original); Benjamin 65.
93 Chancer 1992: 108–9. Compare Becker (210; emphasis in original): "in some way [the worker] must pay with life and consent daily to die, to give oneself up to the risks and

dangers of the world, allow oneself to be engulfed and used up. Otherwise one ends up *as though dead* in trying to avoid life and death. This is how modern existentialist psychiatrists understand depression […]."

94 Gustafson 1986: 397; Chernyshevsky 76.
95 Berdyaev 2009: 62.
96 *Ibid* 183, 215.
97 Taggart.
98 Griffith; Graeber.
99 Fromm 1994: 131–2.
100 Marx 1976: 799.
101 Wilkerson; Ramnath.
102 Clark 2019: 204; Tillich 138–52; Furner; Hudis; Berdyaev 1966.
103 Berdyaev 1966: 153; Hall; Medzhibovskaya 2004.
104 Maude 1987a: 253.
105 Fromm 1969: 165; Maude 1987b: 298.
106 Medzhibovskaya 2004.
107 Reitz 36.
108 Steinbeck 1–34, 99–116.
109 Mbembe 2003.
110 Maude 1987b: 43–5.
111 Habermas 2014; 1981: 180.
112 Reitz 145.
113 Irwin 15.
114 Sokoloski; Danaher.
115 Marcuse 2005: 169–170. Even so, Heidegger's life ironically resembled that of Ivan Ilych.
116 Dawsey 9–22 (emphasis in original).
117 Chancer 2020; Durkin; Khayar; Berdyaev 2009: 28–46.
118 Lowe.
119 Cera.
120 Habermas 1981: 171; Lennard; Klikauer and Campbell.
121 Robinson 380.
122 Tolstoy 2010: 132–3, 145, 156–9.
123 Orwin 2002c: 224.
124 Tolstoy 2010: 117 (emphasis added); Zorin 25.
125 Orwin 2012b: 108.
126 Tolstoy 2010: 74, 119, 223.
127 Chancer 1992: 214.
128 Tolstoy 2010: 259. Incidentally, Tolstoy consciously alters the historical record to accommodate the narrative by depicting the Pavlograd Hussars, Nikolai Rostov's unit, as fighting in the battle of Ostrovno (July 25, 1812), when in reality they were part of General Barclay's First Army, stationed near Kyiv at the time (Ungurianu 2012: 35).
129 Tolstoy 2010: 259; McPeak 117.
130 Tolstoy 2010: 158 (emphasis added).
131 Orwin 1993: 30, 125, 181; Rancour-Laferriere 1998: 180; Chodorow 1999.
132 Becker 218; Kant 2007: 342.
133 Tolstoy 2010: 201.
134 Solomon et al. 47–55; Schonberg and Chang 10.
135 Welch 176.
136 Kropotkin 1991: 131.
137 Balan 465; Samet 167.
138 Tolstoy 2010: 203.
139 Gustafson 1986: 358–9; Orwin 2002c: 231.
140 Rancour-Laferriere 1985.
141 Tolstoy 2010: 212.
142 Samet 168.

143 Tolstoy 2010: 213, 305; Bondarchuk.
144 Colling xiv–xvi.
145 Babel 121–2, 146.
146 Hillman 35; Herberg-Rothe 159.
147 Bartlett 2011: 118–19; Carpenter 1919: 86–122; Fone 11; Johansson 1990i.
148 Chitty 58.
149 Freud 2016: 60–1; Rancour-Laferriere 1985: 342.
150 Plato 2015: 79–81.
151 Carpenter 1919: 171–2.
152 Levinas 261; Berdyaev 2009: 234–65.
153 Shakespeare 165.
154 Berdyaev 1966: 8, 65; Tolstoy 2010: 184, 205.
155 Healey 31–41.
156 Orwin 2002c: 230–5; Carpenter 1919: 27, 117; Ziarek 44, 60; Tolstoy 2010: 189.
157 Turgenev 1878b.
158 Ginzberg 82–7; Benjamin 32–53.
159 Carpenter 1919; Gustafson 1986: 339.
160 Dynes 1990f; Johansson 1990f; Carpenter 1912: 31–2.
161 Freud 2016: 64.
162 Ziarek 45.
163 Benjamin 31–40; Tolstoy 2010: 206.
164 Ginzberg 84–6; Hall 220.
165 Gilman-Opalsky 71; Feuerbach 271; Berdyaev 2009: 51.
166 Ferguson 186; Benjamin 23; Berdyaev 2009: 181.
167 Figes and Kolonitskii 32–3, 52–4.
168 Gustafson 1986: 97–102, 359–69.
169 Reitz; Benjamin; Feuerbach 67–98.
170 Shively 1990b: 515. Another version of this *hadith* is as follows: "I fell asleep, until I woke up, and there, in front of me, was my Lord, under the most beautiful form" (Williams W 448).
171 Schild.
172 Berdyaev 2009: 43, 243.
173 Marshall; Никитина 88; Erwin-Jansen; Gilman-Opalsky 211; Healey 80, 187.
174 Ginzberg 73–4.
175 Plato 2015: 93.
176 Tolstoy 2010: 205–6; Miller; Plato 2015. Patroclos' death arguably represents the turning point of *The Iliad*, as it provokes Achilles's consequent rage, and so portends the Trojans' ultimate defeat.
177 Gilman-Opalsky 82.
178 Cervantes 701; Carpenter 1919: 121.
179 Plato 2015: 79–80, 98.
180 Chancer 1992: 207; 2020: 101.
181 Gustafson 1986: 401; Feuerbach 158.
182 Chodorow 1999: 45; Bartlett 2011: 26.
183 Tolstoy 2010: 116–18; Bondarchuk.
184 Bartlett 2011: 23–45; Miri 87–94; Gustafson 1986.
185 Healey 22–31; Chitty.
186 Love 2012: 94–5.
187 Carpenter 1919: 124.
188 Schonfeld and Chang 224.
189 Figes 2002: 119; Chodorow 1999: 45; Maude 1987a: 14.
190 Carpenter 1912: 80–1; Carpenter 1919: 119–36; Fone 14; Benjamin 29. In this sense, compare the etymological closeness of *paideia*, or education for citizenship, and *paiderastia*, or love of male youth.
191 Dynes 1990o; Johansson 1990m; Benjamin; Berdyaev 2009: 55–7, 237.

192 Maude 1987a: 158; 1987b: 166–73.
193 Carpenter 1912: 27–8, 48, 66–7.
194 Békés et al.; Freud 1995.
195 Tolstoy 1985: 105.
196 Healey 102.
197 Békés et al.
198 Ginzberg 76.
199 Wilson J 2014: 33; Tolstoy 2010: 417–20, 1329n417.
200 Bartlett 2011: 41–3.
201 Katz and Wagner 7.
202 Tolstoy 2010: 421.
203 Wilson J 2014: 36–8; Tolstoy 2010: 27.
204 Jones O.
205 Harris 81.
206 Wilson J 2014: 33 (emphasis in original); Stites 1990: 70.
207 Figes and Kolonitskii 14–16.
208 Bartlett 2011: 45–6, 206; Tolstoy 2010: 561; Figes and Kolonitskii 33, 45.
209 Clark 2019: 300; Hall 6–7, 158–61; Figes and Kolonitskii 14.
210 Graeber and Wengrow.
211 Carpenter 1912; Wilson J 2014: 31; Edwards 97.
212 Wilson J 2014: 31–2.
213 Tolstoy 2010: 532–4, 545–8.
214 Tolstaya 2014b: 85–6.
215 Parini 90–2.
216 Tolstoy 2010: 119.
217 Dynes 1990c.
218 Chitty; Dynes 1990h; Tolstoy 2010: 124.
219 Tolstoy 2010: 127–8; Houser 292; Gustafson 1986: 270, 347–8.
220 Benjamin 27; Lawrence.
221 Tolstoy 2010: 290.
222 Figes and Kolonitskii 3, 138–41.
223 Ahmed; Kondakov.
224 Tolstoy 2010: 260; Carpenter 1919: 123–4.
225 Tolstoy 2010: 260–1.
226 Solomon et al. 78–81.
227 Sloane 2005: 107; Samet 172.
228 Dynes 1990d; Freud 1961b: 86–7; Kropotkin 2009: 235.
229 Hoare.
230 Colling 64–6.
231 Tolstoy 2010: 260–2; Dynes 1990c; Benjamin 100–7; Lanzieri and Hildebrant.
232 Tolstoy 2010: 271–2, 273, 283; Yalom 130.
233 Carpenter 1912: 67–71.
234 Tolstoy 2010: 283. Compare the letter Tolstoy sent to the new Tsar Alexander III in March 1881, requesting mercy for the assassins of his father, Alexander II. He promises that, if his ruler were to spare their lives, "I, poor subject, would be your *dog* and your *slave!* I should weep with emotion every time I heard your name [...]" (Maude 1987b: 63, emphasis added).
235 Fuchs 13; Gilman-Opalsky 282; Rousseau 405.
236 Stites 1989: 19–24.
237 Tolstoy 2010: 1224; Evtuhov et al. 320–1; Berdyaev 1966: 23.
238 Parini 4.
239 Tolstoy took Charles Dickens' comment in *Hard Times* (1854) about Parliament being the "national dust-yard" seriously. On his visit to London in March 1861, Lev Nikolaevich listened to Prime Minister Lord Palmerston's three-hour speech on naval strategy in the Houses of Parliament, but found it tiresome (Maude 1987a: 48;

Bartlett 2011: 142). Closer to life's end, at 80 years of age, Lev Nikolaevich wrote that "the work of the senator, the minister, the monarch, and the leaders of political parties is just as base, vile and alien to human nature and, perhaps, even worse than the task of the executioner or spy, since it is just the same, but covered in hypocrisy" (Tolstoy 1987: 218).

240 Ungurianu 37; Samet 171–2.
241 Wilson J 2014: 30. In parallel, for C. L. R. James, Melville's critical portrayal in *Moby Dick* of the regimentation of labor in the whaling industry, and of Captain Ahab's megalomania, anticipated the totalitarian "leader principle" (Johnson).
242 Solomon et al. 121; Lieven 2012: 17.
243 Gustafson 1986: 12, 109, 348–62; Triandis; Berdyaev 2009: 161.
244 Stites 1989: 19; Rancour-Laferriere 1988: 100.
245 Berdyaev 2009: 204; Benjamin 6; Hall 155.
246 Stites 1989; Scott 18; Sorel 167.
247 Levitin.
248 Staples.
249 Thompson M 38–9; Benjamin 145; Ferguson 182.
250 Triandis.
251 Hall 127; Racy; Bell.
252 Reitz; Ken; Berdyaev 2009.
253 Bartlett 2011: 252, 343–65.
254 Tolstoy 2018: 128–9.
255 Maude 1987b: 423, 450 (emphasis added).
256 Tolstoy 1985: 378; Толстой 2021 (emphasis added).
257 Tolstoy 2010: 136. Translation by the Maudes.
258 Yuzich.
259 Chitty 59.
260 Gustafson 1986: 368–9.
261 Lanzieri and Hildebrant.
262 Berdyaev 1966: 21; Adorno 45–6; Dynes 1990e; Rancour-Laferriere 1985; Buruma and Margalit.
263 Johansson 1990b; 1990o.
264 Rancour-Laferriere 1988: 103–4.
265 Healey 188–91.
266 Oosterhuis 238–42.
267 Bernardini 8–9.
268 Sternhell 177–86.
269 Johansson 1990b; Percy 1990a; Mogutin; Karlinsky; Healey 182–6; Mole 3.
270 Healey; Stites 1989.
271 Mergier.
272 Batty 2020a; Gustafson 1986.
273 Batty 2020b; Williams et al.
274 Hájková 112, 123–5.
275 Mergier.
276 *Ibid*; Carlo.
277 Rancour-Laferriere 1988: 103–5; Evtuhov et al. 673.
278 Donaldson 1990a; Bell; Carpenter 1919; Homer 16; Dynes 1990j; Museu Marítim de Barcelona.
279 Gerth and Mills 175; Mondloch; Staples; Chitty 29–30, 47–51, 80, 169.
280 Benjamin 66–74; Freud 1995.
281 Karlinsky; Chitty 153.
282 Tolstoy 2010: 5, 267.
283 *Ibid* 283, 288–9.
284 Lieven 2012: 14.
285 Tolstoy 2010: 294–5.

286 This reference to the "Tsaritsyn field" is most likely an allusion to the location of a decisive Tsarist victory over the forces led by the Cossack rebel Yemelyan Pugachëv in 1774 (Evtuhov et al. 288).
287 Tolstoy 2010: 162, 175; Lomnitz 259–65.
288 Tolstoy 1985: 83; Bartlett 2011: 112.
289 Tolstoy 2010: 173–5; Zorin 30; Bartlett 2011: 111–13; Maude 1987a: 239–57.
290 Tolstoy 2010: 176.
291 Tolstoy 1982; Bartlett 2011: 206.
292 Cervantes 169.
293 Tolstoy 2010: 136.
294 Tolstoy 2010: 188.
295 Berdyaev 2009: 162; Tolstoy 1960: 583–91; Faure 2019: 258.
296 Forrest 71; McPeak 118; Johns; Smith L; Singer 46.
297 Figes and Kolonitskii 64.
298 Morgachëv 128; Dragunovsky 191–3.
299 Tolstoy 2010: 289, 302–9.
300 DeYoung 69.
301 Schiffman; Moberg.
302 Tolstoy 2010: 299.
303 Kant 2007: 342.
304 Percy 1990b; Adib-Moghaddam.
305 Orwin 1993: 126–38, 203–4; Stites 1989: 170.
306 Lopez; Ziarek 161; Stites 1989.
307 Gustafson 1986: 64, 450–1; Jay; Berdyaev 1966: 45; Berdyaev 2009: 25–53, 225; Freud 2013: 23.
308 Al-Kateab and Watts.
309 Campbell; Figes 2002: 409.
310 Lopez.
311 Adorno 157.
312 Plato 2015: 81–9; Gustafson 1986: 326–7, 455; Johansson 1990r; Blais 13–14; Lee.
313 Warfield et al. 125.
314 Tolstoy 2010: 299.
315 Plato 2015: 81–6.
316 Maude 1987b: 264.
317 *Ibid* 18.
318 Gustafson 1986: 36 (emphasis added).
319 Dynes 1990g; Dynes 1990j; Gustafson 1986: 213.
320 Freud 1961b: 86–8.
321 Plato 360 BCE.
322 Никитина 96–7; Кон.
323 Le Guin 335.
324 Turgenev 1878b.
325 *Ibid.*
326 Johansson 1990g; Karlinsky.
327 Durkin 9; Zorin 70; Poole; Benjamin 19.
328 Cervantes 743, 840.
329 Dynes 1990e; Healey 101.
330 Tolstoy 2010: 312; Stroganov 56.
331 Tolstoy 2010: 312, 576 (emphasis added).
332 *Ibid* 310–313; Orwin 2012b: 109; Orwin 1993: 6; Fuchs 14.
333 Taylor; Herberg-Rothe 150; Forrest 67.

7

WAR AND PEACE, BOOK TWO

"Natasha Rostova"

In book two of *War and Peace*, known as "Natasha Rostova," Tolstoy focuses mainly on matters of "peace," away from the international battlefields. As a foil to Napoleon, the youthful Natasha experiences self-doubt and deceit around her coming of age. The Slavist Caryl Emerson knowingly associates Natasha, who symbolizes Imperial Russia, with the "emotional cluster 'love-beauty-happiness-spring-spiritual renewal.'"[1]

In this book, Rostova is shown to be happiest during her courtship with Prince Andrei, which is made possible by the death of Lise Bolkonskaya in childbirth. After they agree privately to engagement, however, Natalya Ilyinichna is misled by the base Anatole Kuragin, who conspires with Dolokhov to abduct her during Andrei's long absence, both emotional and physical. Within the heteropatriarchal and sexually repressive ruling-class culture of early nineteenth-century Tsarist Russia—which alarmingly persists today—Natasha is effectively punished for "inviting" Kuragin's sexual propositions. That her planned union with Bolkonsky had remained a secret is part of the problem for Natasha: confronted with a hyper-masculine male such as Anatole, she might have been able to refer to her engaged status to ward him off, though in the reality of the text, she cannot do so. The result is criminal patriarchy: Kuragin pursues her and lays waste to her reputation, leading her to attempt to die by suicide. Tolstoy thus lays bare a critique of masculinity and sexual abuse, though not without including some victim-blaming.

In this section of *War and Peace*, Tolstoy features his thematically critical portrayal of the Russian social aristocracy and his critique of class hierarchy. At an extravagant nationalist celebration of Tsar Alexander I, where the 300 guests are seated "according to their rank and importance," Pierre arbitrarily challenges Dolokhov to a duel based on an anonymous note he had received, suggesting Dolokhov and his wife Hélène had been having an affair.[2] Despite a lack of evidence, Pierre feels humiliated, such that he will need to "restore" his honor through challenging this

DOI: 10.4324/9781003328964-7

man whom he suspects of cuckolding him, and Dolokhov's machismo will prevent a simmering of tensions.[3] The latter's unrelenting need to defeat his male challenger leads him to dismiss the very idea of de-escalation: "No apologies, none whatever."[4] Such mindless brinkmanship noticeably mirrors the petty conflicts which often lead to war among states.[5] It also recalls Tolstoy's brazen challenging of his mentor Turgenev to a duel in 1861, shortly after having offended him by falling asleep during a reading of his new novel, *Fathers and Children*, not to mention the duel which tragically cut short the life of Pushkin, Tolstoy's distant cousin, at age 37.[6]

In this duel, despite not knowing how to wield a firearm, Bezukhov incredulously wounds and nearly kills Dolokhov, who then misses Pierre altogether.[7] The course of the duel illustrates how Clausewitzian elements like chance, injury, and reduced visibility can lead the underdog to prevail in combat.[8] Fortunately, Dolokhov will survive his gunshot wound. Then again, soon after recovering, he will pivot to financially ruin Rostov through gambling. This course of events echoes Tolstoy's own gambling-away in 1854 of the ancestral family home at Yasnaya Polyana, which he personally had inherited, together with 300 serfs, while playing *shtoss* for two days and nights straight with fellow officers in Crimea.[9] The amount lost by Rostov in the *poema*, 43,000 rubles, amounted at the time to the "combined annual salaries of fourteen provincial governors or forty-one infantry colonels."[10]

All of this wastefulness and loss, and for what? Hyper-masculinity and manipulation, in both cases. When Hélène confronts Pierre about his numerous missteps in the case of the duel and their own marriage, Bezukhov silences her—to which she responds, "Why shouldn't I speak? I can speak as I like [...]." He then abruptly threatens to kill her using a broken marble slab.[11] Thankfully, Hélène flees, and Pierre demands separation instead. Though he does not commit femicide, he will come close. Reduced to a spectral "bad breast," the "marble beauty" of his wifely mother-icon has been smashed.[12]

Count Pierre Bezukhov as Freemason

Soon after threatening and mandating separation from his wife, Pierre will encounter the Russian Freemason Iosif Alexeevich Bazdeev, who is based on the historical Freemason O. A. Pozdeev. Bazdeev illuminates Bezukhov's life of deceit and fraud, based on an idleness secured through the exploitation of "tens of thousands of slaves."[13] Taken aback by his interlocutor's frankness, Pierre will begin to consider the possibility that the divine is immanent in the life-world. These mental shocks reflect the author's own experiences, which galvanized him to trace Pierre's path, from transitioning from living a life akin to that of the Kuragins, to one dedicated to political struggle and Christian anarchism.

Such defamiliarization will lead Pierre to synthesize his Enlightenment idealism and Christianity with Freemasonry's own ostensibly freethinking, internationalist ideology and join the homosocial Masonic Order—and so become a Resident.[14] After all, Freemasons preach liberty, equality, and solidarity. Bezukhov envisions

Freemasonry as the "*fraternité* [brotherhood] and equality of men who have virtuous aims": namely, to subvert and ultimately overthrow the global *ancien régime*.[15] Along similar lines, Berdyaev and Kropotkin consider Freemasonry to have been the "first form" of self-organization and political thought in the Russian Empire.[16] After all, two years after banishing Alexander Radishchev to Siberia for his literary critique of serfdom, Catherine II imprisoned the Freemason Nikolai Novikov for his satires likewise denouncing feudal slavery.[17]

Of the seven core Masonic principles, the following five resonate the most with Peter Kirillich: "*courage, generosity, morality, love of mankind, and* especially *obedience*." Foretasting the title and basic idea of Tolstoy's 1893 seminal text on the Kingdom of God, the Freemason who is seen accepting Bezukhov's application stresses to him that "[t]he source of blessedness is not without us *but within…*" Then, in the Masonic Lodge, the Grand Master warns against "making any distinctions which may infringe equality." As a result of the anti-hero's new commitments, it will not be long before Pierre's standing will have "sunk greatly in the esteem of [the high] society" of which he incongruously remains a part. At the same time, he takes immediate measures to commence the manumission of the serfs of his estate—though Andrei, following his friend's example, will carry this project out more faithfully upon his return to the Bald Hills estate, after his wife Lise dies, giving birth to their son Nikolenka. By taking advantage of Tsar Alexander's 1803 "law on free agriculturalists," which formally allowed landowners to free their serfs and provide them land, Pierre and Andrei will establish schools and hospitals for their feudal slaves.[18]

Explaining his newfound philosophical commitments and enthusiastic sense of purpose to the mournful and estranged Andrei on a visit to Bald Hills, Pierre animatedly describes Freemasonry as "the teaching of Christianity freed from the bonds of State and Church, a teaching of equality, brotherhood, and love." At last having come to align with Abbé Morio, or Kant, Bezukhov announces to Bolkonsky that "a time would come when there would be no more wars."[19] Whereas, in accordance with Kant's analysis, the modern age is currently far from enlightened, Tolstoy/Bezukhov view the hegemony of despotism as necessarily bounded by space and time. For this reason, they avow Enlightenment to destabilize autocracy and prepare the ground for a free republic. In so declaring himself, Count Tolstoy, like Herbert Marcuse, discloses his concordance with Kant's educational philosophy, which poses the improvement of the human condition through autonomy as the goal of Enlightenment.[20]

In the same way, it is plain that, in presenting Pierre's commentary on Freemasonry, Tolstoy means to advance his *own* anarchist interpretation of Christianity, and likewise to experiment with his own queer impulses, through sketching male-bonding within an erotic-political subculture.[21] Bezukhov is shown as "suspect[ing] that Russian Masonry had taken a wrong path and deviated from its original principles," such that he argues to his "brothers" that they must act to change the movement's direction.[22] In reality, his proposals are rejected for being excessively republican-constitutionalist, and therefore dangerous to the future of the organization. In parallel, the Russian Freemasons unsuccessfully tried to distance themselves from Radishchev's radicalism in the wake of the publication, and immediate confiscation, of this *philosophe*'s dual condemnation of serfdom and Tsarist despotism—such that Tolstoy may be linking Bezukhov (and therefore, himself) with the iconoclastic Radishchev.[23]

After all, Tolstoy's focus on "the possibility of active brotherly love among men," and Pierre's evidently burgeoning longings for union with Bazdeev, as the anti-hero's marriage with Hélène breaks down further, likely constitute sublimated expressions of the author's own homoerotic desires. Just as Bolkonsky escapes from his marriage to explore his polymorphously perverse sexuality in the military campaign against Napoleon, Bezukhov does the same in the Freemason movement. For instance, whereas the entries in the dream diary of the Russian Freemason P. I. Titov (1758–1818) served as Tolstoy's source for Pierre's own diary of dreams, it is obvious that the prose writer adds gay imagery not found in the original, such as the "throbbing heart" (or phallus) with which Pierre awakens one morning, thinking of Bazdeev.[24] Peter Kirillich's homophilic attachment to Bazdeev, as revealed through dreaming consciousness and fantasy, helps clarify his identity and vocation: namely, that his bond with Bazdeev is one with his commitment to humanity.[25] Hence, such ties confirm Feuerbach's humanistic interpretation of religion as "nothing but the belief in human dignity":

> The love of God makes me loving; the love of God to man [*sic*] is the cause of man's love to God; the divine love causes, awakens human love [...]. What, then, is it that I love in God? Love: love to man. But when I love and worship the love with which God loves man, do I not love man; *is not my love of God, though indirectly, love of man?*[26]

In accordance with Feuerbach, Bezukhov/Tolstoy sublimate their homoerotic urges into a generally humanitarian, or Christian, sense of love. This redirection of libidinal energies is in keeping with Carpenter's view about the intimate associations between philanthrophy, art, and queerness, as well as the English anarchist's faith in the "immense capacity of emotional love" within the Uranian, or gay-male, temperament.[27] In similar fashion, the Tolstoyan communard Dmitri Morgachëv, who was imprisoned multiple times by the Bolsheviks for subversion, describes his life's motivation in his memoirs as advancing "the cause of drawing all people together in brotherly union on the basis of freedom, reason, and labor."[28] As the anarchist writer Lara Messersmith-Glavin observes, "[w]hat we learn in our bodies we can practice in community."[29]

The overlap that Lev Nikolaevich presents among progressivism, homoeroticism, and Freemasonry reflects the reality that Proudhon, Bakunin, numerous Decembrists, and several members of the revolutionary Mexican Liberal Party's inner circle were themselves Freemasons, just as the insurrectionist anarchist Luigi Galleani (1861–1931) transitioned to anarchism from republicanism.[30] Though a statist vanguardist, Auguste Blanqui (1805–1881) similarly developed his romantic-revolutionary theory, which centered atheism, direct action, and socialism, from a combined radicalization of republican principles and an idealization of the example of the ultra-left Hébertists from the French Revolution, whose leader, Jacques-René Hébert (1757–1794), had been executed by Robespierre.[31]

Furthermore, radical Polish officers foreshadowed the November 1830 popular uprising against Tsarist domination by self-organizing in masonic secret societies, whereas many militants within the International Workingmen's Association, or First International, were well-versed in Freemasonry.[32] Besides, after their leaders had held a disappointing meeting seeking conciliation with President Thiers in April 1871, numerous rank-and-file Freemasons in Paris joined the barricades of the Commune, and sacrificed themselves to defend it.[33] Plus, it was the Spanish Freemason Esteban Terrades (1883–1950) who sponsored Albert Einstein's 1923 lecture tour in Barcelona.[34] More recently, in the region of Valencia, following the death of despot Francisco Franco in 1975, a Christian Fraternity of Friendship emerged to agitate for the decriminalization of homosexuality, while the gay US activist Harry Hay (1912–2002) had originally planned to model the Mattachine Society, one of the first LGBTQ+ organizations in the US (founded in 1950), along masonic lines.[35]

Both despite, and perhaps because of, his participation in the Masonic Order, Pierre struggles to commit himself politically and socially. Echoing the thought of Arthur Schopenhauer and the call of asceticism, as well as reflecting the associations among impulsivity, creativity, and a fragmented identity, Peter Kirillich perceives an "evil and falsehood" entangling every endeavor and institution, which he believes to be governed by the "same pettiness, worldliness, and senselessness."[36] Bezukhov thus senses, like the pessimistic German idealist, that humanity is caught in a web of unfreedom.[37] As Ani Kokoboko observes, in parallel to Levin—one of the author's *alter egos* in *Anna Karenina*—Pierre "embrace[s] and discard[s] several life philosophies" before the novel's dénouement.[38] He must "undergo a long intellectual and moral development toward the radical ideas that would shape the novel."[39] In such light, Pierre's struggles to apply himself mirror the life experiences of the author.

Although Bezukhov remains true to Freemasonry's pacifism even during the climactic battle of Borodino, he will briefly consider raising a private regiment to fight the foreign invaders. Certainly, he clarifies identity and vocation when merging with the serf-soldiers, such that he imagines becoming one of them and "enter[ing] communal life completely." The problem is that a real commitment to anarcho-Populism and social leveling would require sacrificing his great wealth.[40] Whereas Prince Andrei Bolkonsky does not similarly become a Freemason, he does embark on a new life upon his return after Lise's death to Bald Hills, where he improves the serfs' conditions by reducing their rent and withdraws into a quiet life, "content to do no harm, and not disturbing himself or desiring anything."[41] By so retreating from society, Andrei Nikolaevich observes the Daoist practice of *wu-wei* (non-action), and mirrors the experience of many from the generation known as the "children of 1812," who would resign from military-civil service "with the aim of leading a more honest life."[42]

Certainly, Lise's death in labor will haunt Prince Andrei for some time. While Lise's fate recalls Tolstoy's childhood trauma over the death of his mother mere months after she bore his sister Masha, it may also convey the prose writer's subconscious guilt over having isolated his wife Sofia Andreevna in the countryside of Yasnaya Polyana, where obstetricians were far less readily available than in Moscow. Prince Andrei's period of mourning will last until he dances the *polonaise* with Natasha Rostova at a ball in St. Petersburg, in quintessential Imperial style, and listens to her singing, which moves him to propose marriage.[43] Through newfound union, both counterparts in the couple phase out as Strangers to become Residents.[44]

As a revitalized political Resident, Bolkonsky declares himself to be an admirer of the baron of Montesquieu (1689–1755), who was a critic of absolutism and agrobureaucratic despotism, and an advocate of the separation of powers and political accountability.[45] With this declaration, Tolstoy as author likely alludes to an assignment he had failed to complete for his law studies at Kazan University: namely, to compare and contrast Catherine II's *Great Nakaz* ("Instruction," 1767) with Montesquieu's *The Spirit of the Laws* (1748). This is a debate to which he would return in his diaries, holding that Catherine's *Nakaz* had personally benefited her more than it had Russia.[46] In addition, he may implicitly be conveying his interest in Montesquieu's ambivalence over pederasty and same-sex behaviors.[47] Indeed, the theorist of Enlightenment's apt observation—"give power to a man and they will use it"—underpins Tolstoy's anarchism.[48]

Further Denunciations: Of War, Artifice, and Hunting

Although book two focuses on "peace," war is not far away. Bilibin the diplomat writes to Andrei, lamenting how the "Orthodox" Russian army loots and devastates, leaving the local "inhabitants [...] totally ruined" and "famine [...] everywhere."[49] Hence, Bilibin restates Andrei's previously expressed concern for the Russian military's pillage, speaking to the continued *samsara* and *dukkha* of war, which persist to this day. In parallel, Rostov undergoes an internal conflict—which soon externalizes—upon encountering Napoleon and his beloved Tsar Alexander negotiating an alliance at Tilsit in 1807, as his conscience comes to contradict the introjected need to follow the established military hierarchy loyally and without question.[50] In this sense, the young count experiences acute moral injury, defined as a "strong cognitive and emotional response [...] following events that violate a person's moral or ethical code."[51] Demonstrating the associations found among moral distress, trauma, and suicidality, Rostov gripes and protests internally against the reified orders, made from above, which he must obey.[52]

Intuitively, he senses that the terms are a Russian capitulation, which they are. Alexander recognizes Napoleon as Emperor, acknowledges his puppet-regimes in Holland and Sicily, promises to mediate between Napoleon and England, and break off all British trade, thus furthering Bonaparte's imperialist aims.[53] Ultimately, although Rostov cannot stop thinking about the war-wounded when reflecting on the treaty's terms, he concludes that "[o]ur business is to do our duty, to fight and not to think! That's all..."[54] Such resignation, which Tolstoy implicitly ridicules, echoes the defeatism expressed from the "other side" in the queer poet Alfred Lord

Tennyson "The Charge of the Light Brigade" (1854), a work that describes the fatal attack of a British cavalry unit on Russian artillery in the Crimean War. Referring to the exploitation of soldiers by officers, Tennyson writes: "Theirs not to make reply, / Theirs not to reason why, / Theirs but to do and die."[55]

As if to illustrate the fundamental irrationality of hierarchy and the "administrative utopia," Prince Andrei's proposed new military laws are resoundingly dismissed by the Minister of War, Count Arakcheev. Although Bolkonsky is formally appointed, as a compromise, to the Committee on Army Regulations, his proposals are ignored in favor of an alternate set. Such informal process and bureaucratic arbitrariness will help uncover the implicit and logical solutions Tolstoy wishes to counterpose to our domination by such inhuman institutions: namely, self-determination, anarchism, and a transition away from the cities to agrarian life. "Let the dead bury their dead, but while there is life we must live and be happy," remarks Bolkonsky.[56]

Be that as it may, Tolstoy's allegorical portrayal of a wolf-hunt, which Natasha sadistically calls her "greatest pleasure," rebukes the exploitation and violence on which the very existence of the aristocracy depends, therefore tacitly repudiating the "bad infinity" which unites noble and serf.[57] In so reproaching the practice of hunting, Count Tolstoy implicitly voices a criticism of his father, Nikolai Ilych Tolstoy, who introduced him to the practice in childhood. The author also conveys his agreement with the loathsome view his possibly bisexual grandfather, Nikolai Volkonsky, took of such ritualized killing. As well, by extension, he may be blasting the Roman and English aristocracies for their common elevation of hunting to a status symbol.[58]

In effect, Lev Nikolaevich connects his critique of the violence of war and the exploitation of animals with the sadism expected of men, especially in the realm of (hetero)sexuality.[59] In parallel, this critical image anticipates feminist Carole Adams's advocacy of vegetarianism as a means of rejecting animal cruelty, sexual objectification, and male dominance all at once.[60] As such, Tolstoy contests the male-sadist view of the world as a universal "hunting grounds [...] in which nothing exists but prey."[61] Tenderly, Alexandra Tolstaya recalls in her diaries how her father in his older years would often invite her in the spring to go on "vegetarian hunt [s]" that would invariably involve mushrooming, and Valentin Bulgakov recalls his reflective elder welcoming the transformation in attitudes about hunting he had seen over the course of his life.[62]

As well, this scene may function as implicitly negative commentary on Russia's imperialist, depredatory eastward expansion into "Great Tatary" (Siberia), which involved the devastation of indigenous societies, wildlife, and ecosystems alike.[63] The aggressiveness and injustice of the hunt, whereby dozens of hounds and numerous horseback-riders harass and entrap a single she-wolf, symbolizes the violence that the ruling class imposes not only on the natural world itself—for which the wolf stands—but *also* the class and State oppression for which the wealthy are responsible, by coercing the working classes into performing such useless acts of violence. That the nobles' dogs kill five of the she-wolf's pups in this hunt, and that Count Nikolai Rostov terms the mother's successful capture as the "happiest moment of his life," speaks volumes to the baseness of aristocratic character. Not only is the she-wolf ensnared and her offspring killed, but the hounds also needlessly kill a fox and hare they come across—extending Tolstoy's metaphorical critique of hunting, which emblematically doubles as criticism of sexual predation.[64]

The author's thematic emphasis on the depravity of the rich and powerful provides continuity between the wolf-hunt and Anatole Kuragin's attempted seduction of Natasha. Following Andrei and Natasha's agreement to get married, Prince Nikolai Bolkonsky will stipulate that their term of engagement must last at least one year in length—in part, due to his impression that the countess is beneath his son. Rostova becomes anxious due to such artificial distance imposed by patriarchal custom between her and Andrei Nikolaevich, and she is shown managing her sexual frustration during the Christmas celebrations at her family's Otradnoe estate by "ordering the servants around"—and specifically, by asking the serf Nikita to fetch her a cock.[65]

This young noble woman, as a manager and an oppressor of labor, in turn is soon victimized, in an illustration of the volatility of sadomasochistic psychodynamics. By taking advantage of her youthful inexperience, erotic unhappiness, and narcissism, Anatole Kuragin provides Natasha with the attention she seeks in vain from Prince Andrei during their period of separation. Strikingly, as Sonya Rostova, Natasha's intimate friend, warns her, Anatole proceeds with his courtship surreptitiously, in contrast to Andrei, who had announced his intentions openly to her mother, Countess Natalia Rostova. That Kuragin had collaborated with Dolokhov on an elaborate plan to abduct and ravage Natasha, which is disrupted at the last moment, speaks to their vile, male-sadist character. Condemned as a "slut," Natasha attempts suicide.[66] Though she will survive, her relationship with Prince Andrei has been lost, and she has become a Stranger again.[67]

Notes

1 Stroganov 56; Emerson 7.
2 Tolstoy 2010: 332–8.
3 McPeak 116–17.
4 Tolstoy 2010: 337.
5 "In politics and particularly in international politics there is much that is delirious. People rush towards ruin, they subject themselves to fate [...]" (Berdyaev 2009: 222).
6 McPeak 111–12; Bartlett 2011: 37, 119, 144; Maude 1987a: 7.
7 Tolstoy 2010: 338–9.
8 McPeak 119–20.
9 Tolstoy 2010: 352, 362–4; Orwin 1993: 10; Bartlett 2011: 31, 82; Figes 2002: 140, 236; Maude 1987a: 117.
10 Martin 46.
11 Tolstoy 2010: 342–3.
12 Rancour-Laferriere 1989: 50.
13 Tolstoy 2010: 377, 1328n378.
14 Gustafson 1986: 73–4; Hekma.
15 Tolstoy 2010: 381; Johansson 1990c.
16 Berdyaev 1966: 23; Kropotkin 1991: 29–30.
17 Walicki 1979: 26.

18 Tolstoy 2010: 350–1, 382–3 (emphasis in original), 384 (emphasis added), 386, 389, 403–7, 447, 575, 772; Evtuhov et al. 321. In their actions, which function as verbal icons, Bolkonsky and Bezukhov anticipate the choices taken in life by Prince D. A. Khilkov (1858–1914), who resigned from the Imperial military and gave away most of his lands to proselytize non-cooperation. This was an offense for which he was banished to the Caucasus, and then abroad. Khilkov went on to participate in the Tolstoyan Colony in Purleigh, Essex, and then ultimately became a Socialist Revolutionary (Gustafson 1986: xii; Maude 1987b: 233–4).
19 Tolstoy 2010: 415, 421.
20 Heller 117; Reitz 73, 105.
21 Johansson 1990c.
22 Tolstoy 2010: 465–6.
23 Yarmolinsky.
24 Shcherbakov 70; Tolstoy 2010: 475.
25 Gustafson 1986: 326; Eisenberg.
26 Feuerbach 57 (emphasis added), 105.
27 LeBlanc 2007: 120; Carpenter 1912: 13, 107. Specifically, Carpenter speculates that ancestral queer men and women may have impelled the creation of religion, science, art, and literature by rebelling against the socially imposed gender roles of warrior and domestic laborer, respectively (1919: 58–60).
28 Morgachëv 177.
29 Messersmith-Glavin 47.
30 Grand Lodge of British Columbia and Yukon; Lomnitz 96–7; Kinna 2020a; Figes 2002: 85–6.
31 Shafer 16–20.
32 Evtuhov et al. 344; Lagalisse.
33 Shafer 81–2.
34 McHarg.
35 Moreira; Subrat; Johansson 1990c.
36 Tolstoy 2010: 577, 1189; Bulgakov 35; Fink et al.
37 Sloane 2005: 107.
38 Kokoboko 10.
39 Sloane et al. 64.
40 Tolstoy 2010: 804–6, 904.
41 *Ibid* 449.
42 Figes 2002: 78; Clarke.
43 Figes 2002: 274.
44 Gustafson 1986: 41–66.
45 Tolstoy 2010: 460; Wittfogel 1–8.
46 Bartlett 2011: 80–1; Maude 1987a: 36–7.
47 Chitty 116.
48 Willsher.
49 Tolstoy 2010: 401–2n1.
50 *Ibid* 444–6; Hall 148.
51 Williamson et al.
52 Gerth and Mills 285.
53 Evtuhov et al. 323–6.
54 Tolstoy 2010: 445–6.
55 Jones G; Tennyson.
56 Tolstoy 2010: 453–5, 463, 498, 500.
57 *Ibid* 529; Taylor; Figes 2002: 106; Adorno 339.
58 Colling.
59 Maude 1987a: 24; Bartlett 2011: 37. In this way, Tolstoy anticipates the 1885 booklet denouncing the cruelties of hunting written by his intellectual partner Vladimir Chertkov, with whom Lev Nikolaevich had an at least platonic relationship. This same year, Tolstoy

renounced hunting and smoking and, thanks to the influence of William Frey, adopted a plant-based diet (Maude 1987b: 163, 546).

60 LeBlanc 1993: 20–21n32.
61 Adorno and Horkheimer 6.
62 Parini 89, 103.
63 Figes 2002: 377–8.
64 Tolstoy 2010: 536–7, 538–43.
65 Orwin 1993: 159; Tolstoy 2010: 554.
66 Tolstoy 2010: 630.
67 Gustafson 1986: 40.

8

WAR AND PEACE, BOOK THREE

"The Year 1812"

Book three of *War and Peace*, the *poema*'s climax, reproduces the epic national-liberation struggle of the Russian People (*Narod*) against Napoleon and the *Grand Armée* following their invasion. This began "[o]n the 12th of June 1812," when "the forces of Western Europe crossed the Russian frontier and war began," initiating an "event [...] opposed to human reason and to human nature."[1] At the start of this incursion, the Russian army constituted approximately 200,000 soldiers and officers, and the *Grand Armée*, 600,000.[2] Of the latter, as the French Emperor acknowledges, only about one-third spoke French. The rest were mercenaries and conscripts from regions of Europe other than France, Belgium, and Switzerland which had been incorporated into the Empire.[3]

Bonaparte's hubristic confidence in securing a quick victory through the application of a "strategy of annihilation" would be belied by the resistance of the *Narod*, who would "total[ly] destr[oy] their enemy" while liberating their country from foreign occupation and thwarting Napoleon's bureaucratic designs to resurrect Caesarism.[4] Despite the *Grand Armée*'s final, resounding defeat at the battle of Waterloo (June 15, 1815), the legacy of Bonapartist imperialism would invigorate the Fascist Benito Mussolini, as well as numerous other nineteenth- and twentieth-century dictators and "revolutionary usurpers."[5] In light of the apocalyptic destruction and systematic looting of Moscow carried out by the French and allied soldiers, officers, and assorted kings and dukes accompanying the *Grand Armée* in 1812, the fate of the Russian capital at the edges of Europe mirrors that of so many other colonies desolated by Western imperialism. This confrontation thus evinces the "incipient post-coloniality in *War and Peace*," as seen in its critical portrayal of "booty capitalism" and the "doctrine of the divine right of white people to steal."[6] As Moscow is ravaged by fire and occupying forces, W. E. B. Du Bois' comment resonates: "This is not Europe gone mad; [...] this *is* Europe."[7]

DOI: 10.4324/9781003328964-8

Psychosocially, Tolstoy wants to know why more than half a million soldiers serving Napoleon would go along with such endeavors as the invasion of foreign lands, and the torture and plundering of their inhabitants. Why enable Bonapartist crimes by surrendering one's will to the Emperor? Lev Nikolaevich believes this dynamic follows from the mass-suspension of reason, and the forgetting of compassion. According to the Russian philosopher Semion Liudvigovich Frank, who under Tolstoy's influence espoused a new "living ethics" that would synthesize the realms of reality and potentiality, such suspension of moral reasoning is the consequence of an effective mass-hypnosis.[8] Lev Nikolaevich hence compares Napoleon's troops traveling "from west to east to slay their fellows" implicitly to the Mongol "hordes" who had "come from the east to the west slaying their fellows" in the Middle Ages.[9] Though Tolstoy does not mention him, the militant French nationalist Nicolas Chauvin—soldier and aide to Napoleon, and originator of the term *chauvinism*—fought and appears to have died in the *Grand Armée*'s Russia campaign.[10]

Two decades after *War and Peace*, in "The Kreutzer Sonata" (1889), Tolstoy will reduce music to its martial and bureaucratic applications, observing that, "[i]n China, music is a State affair," while asking, "How can one allow anyone who pleases to hypnotize another, or many others, and do what he likes with them?"[11] His anarchism, tinged with Orientalism, comes out clearly here, as he alludes to his later, sex-negative views, which echo Proudhon's Puritanism. Returning to the image of Tsar Alexander at Olmütz, we see that the intoxicating musical, homoerotic, and patriotic spectacle serves the interests of the State, in accordance with Plato and Socrates's view of instrumental music, by acting directly on the emotions.[12]

Whereas humanity lives for itself, presumably seeking its liberation, each individual contributes to the "historic, universal aims" ostensibly sought by the species, in spite of the aims of the authorities. Even so, history remains unconscious, so long as rulers lord over those they consider their subjects.[13] In other words, the theory of "so-called great men" in history is part and parcel of this history of domination, as the "Napoleon myth" is all too readily wielded to rationalize "autocratic exercises of power."[14] Otherwise stated, the hubristic "insanity of self-abandon" is inseparable from the atrocities perpetrated by these "great men."[15]

In line with Paulo Freire's belief that oppressive social, political, and economic dynamics can be overthrown by those stifled by them, Tolstoy discloses that the fetishization of authority is based on fantasy and projection, voluntary obedience, and a mistaken sense of self-derogation.[16] Rather than history progressing through the wills of "great men," its course is shaped by the human collective—the "coincidence of the wills of *all* who take part in the events" of moving humanity evermore forward toward self-perfection.[17] According to the Slavist Patricia Carden, Tolstoy's view of the relationship between the individual and history therefore strongly echoes that of Herzen, the radical publicist whom the prose writer had met in London in 1861, and whom he admired, in light of their common passion for social change.[18]

Napoleonic Orientalist Expansionism vs. Russian and Spanish National Liberation

In keeping with his comparison of the French and their allies to the Golden Horde, Lev Nikolaevich depicts the invaders, upon crossing the Niemen River into the Russian Empire, as hailing and deifying their leader. They will even fantasize about Napoleon installing them as governors of India and Kashmir in the near term—considering that the *Grand Armée* had by then already taken "Vienna, Berlin, Madrid, Naples, Rome, and Warsaw," so that it seemed unstoppable.[19] Undoubtedly, such a haughty self-concept reflects the belief held by some of Bonaparte's soldiers that Eastern Europe, like Iberia, was more "backward" than central Europe and France.[20] "Scratch a Russian and you will find a Tatar," Napoleon is to have said. Demystifying Bonapartist ideology, Tolstoy clarifies that the French invaders are deceiving themselves by believing that they are republican "liberators" of peoples benighted by the legacy of Genghis Khan.[21]

> *Moscow, the Asiatic capital of that great empire, the sacred city of Alexander's peoples, Moscow with its countless churches in the form of Chinese pagodas*, this Moscow gave Napoleon's imagination no rest.[22]

In an illustration of the necropolitical nature of imperialism, Napoleon's troops are effectively led to believe that they have crossed into an "Eastern" world in which *Jus publicum Europaeum* (Western legal order) does not apply. Accordingly, they feel free to abuse the inhabitants as they see fit, all in the self-contradictory name of advancing Enlightenment and overcoming "Asiatic despotism."[23] For Napoleon, Moscow is akin to an "oriental [*sic*] beauty" who resists him. He envisions himself "civilizing" the Russians as a bureaucrat handing down "just laws" from the Kremlin—or a man "domesticating" his wife.[24] In this sense, we see that, for Bonaparte, the *Narod* is a passive sex object from which he demands total surrender.[25]

The French officers' dependence on their leader is so extreme that, even immediately following the drowning of dozens of cavalrymen in the Niemen River, a colonel and "some of his men" praise their Emperor upon reaching the other side. By so fetishizing "irrational hero-systems" and perpetrating symbolic and actual violence, these soldiers proclaim their lack of trust in and of knowledge of themselves, their authoritarian submission and devotional servitude, as well as their intoxication by history and convention.[26] Likewise, before the battle of Borodino, the *Grand Armée*'s troops model Fromm and Tillich's concerns for the surrender of freedom, the sacrifice of the self, and the escape into authority as means of confronting the anxieties of fate and meaninglessness. In response to their Emperor's "proclamation offering them, as compensation for mutilation and death," mere "words of posterity," they cry, "*'Vive L'Empereur!'* [...] just as they would have [...] at any nonsense that might be told them."[27] In this sense, Bonaparte's war-rally is quite similar to Alexander's troop-review at Olmütz.

Revealingly, as Napoleon's invasion commences, Tsar Alexander I is idly enjoying a festive dinner reception and ball at a landowner's estate in Vilna province (which is now Lithuania).[28] While this contrast counterposes artifice and hedonism with real threats to the "common life" of the *Narod*, Tolstoy continues to strongly suggest affinities between the two emperors. He does so by comparing one of Napoleon's generals, Davout, and Alexander's Minister of War, Arakcheev, to "wolves" of State, and by juxtaposing Alexander and then Napoleon occupying the very same army-headquarters in Vilna, just days apart.[29] As well, the parallelism in structure between the two armies—commanded by a single supreme leader on either side, who is advised by a high command comprised of marshals—*and* the similitude even of their tight-fitting uniforms suggest intimate commonalities between these ostensible enemies, and implicitly, a critique of the dual despotisms headed by Napoleon and Alexander.[30] To this point, it is plain that the conscription on both sides resembles "serfdom in uniform," with the Emperor and Tsar both functioning as bureaucratic despots.[31] In Bondarchuk's film adaptation (1966–1967), the unbroken continuum of imperialism and authority is starkly elucidated in scenes of the buffoonish Bonaparte governing from the Kremlin, following the Russian defeat at Borodino in August 1812.

Given their common enthusiasm for expansionism and the centralization of power, Alexander and Napoleon were not so radically different. Such affinities in State governance, even among enemies, remind us of the inter-imperialist dimensions of the Napoleonic Wars. Still, the authoritarian overlap between Tsar and Emperor does not mean that the causes of the armies fighting at Borodino were the same. As the Ukrainians now are, the Russians then were fighting in self-defense for national survival and liberation. In turn, we should not follow Tolstoy's lead in blocking out consideration of the rising tide of Great-Russian imperialism, after the *Narod* and "General Winter" joined forces to beat back the *Grand Armée*.[32]

In *War and Peace*, during negotiations with a certain General Balashov, whom Tsar Alexander has sent to stave off the invasion, Napoleon expresses a conspicuously instrumental view toward "the Poles," whom he has supposedly liberated from Prussian and Russian imperialism. He threatens to weaponize their loyalty by turning them against the Russians *en masse*.[33] Apropos, Bonaparte is reported to have made the following remarkable comment to his *aide-de-camp* Comte Narbonne in 1812: "I want a [military] camp in Poland, not a [democratic] forum."[34] Such outbursts betray Bonaparte's hostility to Poland's historical role as a conduit for European Enlightenment penetrating Russia after 1789. Indeed, they convey his sadism and megalomania.[35] In the text, Napoleon warns Balashov not to "stir up Prussia against me," for otherwise, he'd "wipe it off the map of Europe!"[36]

Although the French Emperor tries to humiliate Balashov numerous times during their dialogue, the fate of Napoleon's ill-conceived invasion plan is foreshadowed in the Russian's response to Bonaparte's query about the number of churches that exist in Moscow. When Balashov tells him 200, and Napoleon replies in Jacobin fashion that "nowhere in Europe is there anything like that," the general brings up Spain. This was another front of Napoleonic expansionism, wherein the Emperor's aims were not being met.[37]

Otherwise known as the "Spanish ulcer," the popular Peninsular War (1808–1814) against Napoleon's occupation and installment of his brother Joseph as king would not only bog down Bonaparte's military and invite a strategic offensive from the Austrians—these Spanish, Portuguese, and British campaigns against the French would also hearten the Russian resistance to the *Grand Armée*. In this light, Balashov's knowing comment suggests the unexpected inversion of majesty through devotion, as though to connect the resistance in Spain and Russia, where monasticism was widespread, to the phenomena of prophetic messianism and of the holy fool.[38] Although, on one reading, such a verbal image may unintentionally serve to celebrate the authorities in these "king-ridden, noble-ridden, priest-ridden" countries, it also recalls the vision of monastic communism from early Christianity.[39] Implicitly, Balashov alludes to the book of Revelation, likening the Russians and Spaniards to the forces of Christ, who resist the beast symbolizing unjust authority: "In amazement the whole earth followed the beast [and] worshipped [it], saying, 'Who is like the beast, and who can fight against it?'"[40]

As though to respond, Tolstoy depicts Kutuzov and his fellow generals rallying to discuss how the Spanish reserve army and inexperienced civilian population of Zaragoza, an unfortified city lacking adequate munitions and food, jointly shocked the world by repelling Napoleon's siege for several months in 1808–1809. Ultimately, to rip up the "waving flag of resistance, which animated the rest of Spain and Europe to continue the fight against the designs of the Empire," Bonaparte ordered the city reduced to rubble, and its 60,000 defenders executed.[41] In addition, the Russian high command is shown studying how the allied British forces led by Duke Arthur Wellington laid waste to the French army commanded by Marshal Marmont at the battle of Salamanca (July 22, 1812), provoking the notorious "King Joseph" to flee Spain altogether.[42]

Queer Anarchism and Anti-Militarism

Meanwhile, as Andrei Bolkonsky departs from his family for the last time to rejoin the army, Princess Marya endorses the Tolstoyan ideals of non-resistance and forgiveness to her brother, who in turn decries these as "woman's virtue[s]."[43] As Andrei Nikolaevich leaves his family behind at Bald Hills in the *poema*, he admits to himself that he still doesn't know *why* he is going to the army—thus conceding Peter Kirillich's point from the salon years earlier. Be that as it may, when he arrives at the army's general headquarters, rather than continue to serve in the high command, Bolkonsky requests that the Tsar permit him to fight directly among the troops. Given that this move causes Andrei to "los[e] his standing in court circles forever," it can be viewed as another expression of his queer-anarchist desire for social leveling, class suicide, and homoerotic mingling with the rank-and-file.[44] At the same time, considering the far greater risk Bolkonsky runs serving in the ranks than in command, it can also be seen as a death-wish.

Knowingly, during his inner monologue before requesting this transfer, Bolkonsky reformulates Tolstoy's humanistic critique of hierarchy. Tolstoy/Bolkonsky assert that the theory of "military genius" is an ideology that reflects society's disordered state: "It is only because military men are invested with pomp and power, and crowds of sycophants flatter power," that the idea of one's so-called genius even arises. The mere concept reflects and reinforces the hegemony of power elites over society. In this light, "[i]t is understandable that a theory of their 'genius' was invented for them long ago *because they have the power!*"[45] Tolstoy/Bolkonsky sardonically observe that effective army commanders "need [not have] any special qualities," but instead

> nee[d] the absence of the highest and best human attributes—love, poetry, tenderness, and philosophic inquiring doubt [...]. God forbid that [t]he [commander] should be humane, should love, or pity, or think of what is just and unjust.[46]

Such defamiliarizing comments should be taken as satirical and implicitly critical and utopian, calling into question military hierarchies and the need for war in the first place. That being said, as long as warfare should exist, Prince Andrei and the author conclude that the success of any given military action depends not on the commanding officers but on the "m[e]n in the ranks." This is a striking expression of Tolstoyan anarcho-Populism, as well as a possible echo of Joseph de Maistre's and Clausewitz's stress on the centrality of morale in combat.[47] Likely alluding to Tennyson's bleak poem, the author points out the chaos of such class and power stratification by establishing a psychical contrast between the "depression, uneasiness, and intrigu[e]" regnant at the army headquarters and the purposive, though sometimes oblivious, common soldier: "in the body of the army they did not ask themselves where they were going or why" but simply fought, suffered, and died.[48]

The War of 1812: Lev Nikolaevich's Humanist and Populist Perspectives

With some exceptions—due to lapses into Slavophilism, communitarianism, and nationalism—Tolstoy presents remarkably humanist cosmopolitan-internationalist perspectives on the war between Napoleon's forces and the Russian military. For instance, while describing preparations for the defense of Moscow against Napoleon, Tolstoy portrays Kutuzov as despising "cleverness and learning and *even the patriotic feeling* [...]."[49] In this, he combines the classical martial distrust of intellectuals with an internationalist rejection of patriotism that far surpasses the provincialism of ancient Sparta in terms of inclusivity.[50]

Prior to this moment in the plot, during an initial engagement between the two armies at the battle of Ostrovno (July 13–15, 1812), Count Rostov charges a group of French dragoons and strikes an opposing cavalry officer with his saber in the arm—rather like Prince Andrei, "without knowing why." Upon approach to his "vanquished foe," who has dismounted, Rostov finds "not an enemy's face at all suited to a battlefield, but a most ordinary, homelike face."[51] "[A]ll [of Rostov's] animation vanished" the moment he wounded the French officer, so he did not proceed to kill him. Although the cavalry officer is not seriously injured, Rostov nonetheless receives a St. George's Cross award as well as a promotion for his "gallant deed." In reality, the hussar finds the experience unsettling and traumatizing. In the following days, he will—in an implicit intertextual allusion—revisit Olenin's experience in *The Cossacks* and withdraw from the company of his friends to brood:

> So that's all there is in what is called heroism! And did I do it for my country's sake? And how was he to blame [...]? And how frightened he was! He thought I would kill him. Why should I kill him?[52]

In parallel, within the realm of "always the same life that is no life" in Moscow, Natasha Rostova and her younger brother Petya are viewed as a "nuisance and a hindrance to everyone" due to their energetic play, reflecting their autonomy from the realm of necessity.[53] At a mass held at a private chapel—an exclusive practice observed by the Russian aristocracy—the young countess engages with the service in a very different way than the presiding priest. She prays for "*one community, without distinction of class, without enmity, united by brotherly love*," and equally requests forgiveness for her wrongs against Andrei and her own family. She prays, too, for Anatole Kuragin, despite his abuse of her.[54] In contrast, the priest presiding over the mass in question sacrilegiously likens Moscow to Jerusalem and Napoleon's invaders to heathens, and prays for the blessing of the Tsar and his military victory.[55] However, in favoring human relatedness, Natasha cannot permit prayer "that her enemies might be trampled under foot."[56] Rostova's dignified resistance in this scene illuminates the Orthodox Church's hypocritical claim to represent the teachings of Jesus the Nazarene.

Along similar lines, in 1942, the metropolitan of Moscow blessed Stalin as the "divinely appointed leader" in the face of Nazi invasion, just as the Russian Orthodox Church's patriarch Kirill has blessed the Russian military's October 2015 and February 2022 attacks on Syria and Ukraine, which have involved genocidal crimes.[57] In contrast, in March 2022, the Eastern Orthodox patriarch Theodore II of Alexandria and All Africa knowingly remarked that "[t]he great authoritarian power blinds the eyes and you forget that you are human. It is not possible to cross yourself, pray to God, and at the same time kill children and people in general."[58]

In parallel, Pierre Bezukhov is prohibited from joining the armed struggle against the *Grand Armée* due to his membership in the Masonic Order, which "preached perpetual peace and the abolition of war."[59] Still, due to his blossoming (though platonic and unexpressed) love for Natasha, Bezukhov is aroused: through ideas of reference, he convinces himself that history has chosen him to be Napoleon's assassin. During a spectacular mass-rally in Moscow dedicated to Romanov majesty, Petya Rostov, Natasha's adolescent brother, cyclically finds himself lured to Tsar Alexander's power, much as his elder brother had been at Olmütz. Rather than present this intoxicating same-sex attachment as a necessary expression of in-group sentiment in the face of foreign invasion and occupation, Tolstoy probably means to satirize it as a restatement of *naïve monarchism*—as in the case of the troop-review before Austerlitz. That Petya is nearly trampled to death by the crowd, as thousands would be at the coronation of Nicholas II in 1896, only supports such a critical view.[60]

Furthermore, Lev Nikolaevich would appear to be mocking Pierre's naïvete in imagining that the Tsar's ritualistic summoning of the nobility and merchants on the occasion of the *Grand Armée*'s approach would amount to a consultation akin to Louis XVI's fateful summoning of the *États Généraux*, within the revolutionary turmoil of 1789. Instead, this audience was meant to transmit Alexander's orders that the nobles conscript feudal slaves for the defensive campaign against Napoleon, and that the merchants financially subsidize the feeding of the war-machine.[61]

In the meantime, at the Bald Hills manor, the elder Bolkonsky denies the news about Russia's invasion by the *Grand Armée*, and "tak[es] no steps to secure his safety," even as the French, Poles, and other allies approach Smolensk, just 60 kilometers west of his estate. This episode can be considered a critique in microcosm of the irrationality of patriarchal authority and aristocratic domination, for the evacuation of Bald Hills is delayed during all this time that Prince Nikolai's consciousness is affected by what appears to be an acute case of delirium. Such madness possibly signifies an unconscious reaction to the gravity of the situation. The elder prince sends his serf Alpatych to consult with the local governor, who falsely reports, as a typical bureaucrat enthralled not only to the lure and slavery of sovereignty but also to toxic corporate positivity, that Smolensk is at no risk, and that his troops are about to engage Napoleon's—as they will not.[62]

Just as Alpatych receives this report, though, 130 French artillery guns begin bombarding Smolensk, and a brutish Russian innkeeper kills his mistress for demanding that he arrange her evacuation. Then, Russian soldiers coordinate to set fire to the city, anticipating the fate of a captured Moscow, and Alpatych by chance encounters Prince Andrei, who orders his family to abandon Bald Hills by handwritten note. In the meantime, Smolensk is the scene of wailing, forced displacement, and other misfortunes, such that the hopes of the *Narod* come to rest with the vastly outnumbered Russian military, which is in turn divided into three retreating armies whose commanders compete among each other.[63]

Prince Andrei briefly abandons the regiment he had been given command over—whose rank-and-file troops Tolstoy depicts as idealizing "our Prince" Bolkonsky in a homoerotic way—to visit the newly abandoned Bald Hills estate.[64] Besides conveying an idealization of desertion and/or dereliction of military duties and a reaction formation (or escapism) that would do away with the war, this scene may be interpreted as the encounter of an aristocrat with the menaced dying-away of his world of privilege, secondary to the modernizing march of history typified by the ideals of the French Revolution. Paradoxically, as a queer fifth columnist, the prince sympathizes with these same ideals, just as Napoleon radically violates them. Even so, on an emotional level, it is perhaps when applied to this sequence above all others that the positivist critique of *War and Peace* as "nostalgia for serfdom" resonates most.[65] The centrality of loss in Bald Hills transmits the traumatic significance of the writer's orphanhood, and his perhaps unconscious anxiety over the supersession of feudal relations, despite his anarchist politics.[66]

When Andrei arrives to his childhood home—which he misrepresents as having been "built" by his father *rather than* the serfs—Bolkonsky is disturbed at the marked absence of the numerous domestic servants, the exploitation of whose labor had maintained the manor. "He called for Taras the gardener, but no one replied."[67] Meeting Alpatych, the sole peasant who stayed behind in the ruins of Bald Hills, Andrei cannot desist from ordering *him* to leave, or from commanding that the other serfs he might encounter transfer themselves to one of the Bolkonskys' two other manors. With these orders, Tolstoy conceivably means to point to the illusory nature of Andrei's supposed "emancipation" of his serfs, which mimics the "lip service" Tsar Alexander I paid to the cause of abolishing feudal slavery during his rule. Possibly, he means to express the landowning aristocracy's *Angst* over Napoleon potentially "liberating" the serfs to use for his own purposes, rather than theirs. Otherwise, the positivists may be right, that Lev Nikolaevich is lamenting the twilight of manorial culture.[68]

In the run-up to the approach of the French army to Bald Hills, as Count Tolstoy describes, Prince Nikolai Bolkonsky suddenly regains lucidity of mind, after he reads his son's note to Alpatych. The retired general hastily orders the organization of the defense of the estate, where he intends to fight Napoleon to the death. For all that, amid the erotic and political excitement of reviewing the small army of "peasants and domestic serfs" he has drafted, the old prince suffers a stroke. Soon thereafter, he succumbs to a second cerebrovascular accident, after having been transferred by the peasants to the Bogucharovo estate. Among his last words to Princess Marya are his lament that "Russia has perished. They've destroyed her." The profound love Marya feels for her dying father rapidly yields to horror and depression at the mystery of his passing.[69]

Marya is roused from the existential malaise induced by this encounter with death by occupying herself with the pressing need to evacuate Bogucharovo, in the process of which she commands that the reserve known as the "landlord's grain" be distributed among the starving peasants. In this way, Prince Nikolai's death will dialectically plunge his daughter into existential time, where identity and vocation are clarified. As though awakening from the nightmare of agromanagerial despotism, and echoing the historical experiences of the Buddha, Marya comments on how "strange" it is that "there could be rich people and poor, and [that] the rich could refrain from helping the poor." Before deciding to abandon the manor, Marya expresses her willingness to do "anything [...] for the peasants."[70]

In reality, Princess Marya's unforeseen generosity ironically backfires, for the peasants distrust her supposed magnanimity as masking further exploitation. Like the convicts of *Don Quixote* who repay the knight-errant's amazing intervention to free them by stoning him, the peasants refuse Marya's offer and even imprison her on the estate, in an inversion of the historical relationship of landlordism.[71] This scene appears closely to echo Tolstoy's own unexpected experiences with the serfs at Yasnaya Polyana, who rejected the count's proposal in May 1856 for localized emancipation in favor of waiting on a future decree from the Tsar.[72] As well, it mirrors the fate of the Fourierist *phalanstery* which the utopian socialist landowner Mikhail Petrashevksy (1821–1866) ordered constructed for his peasants, who are reported to have promptly burned it down.[73] Furthermore, it recalls the bathos of *Frankenstein*'s Creature, who is violently punished for having saved a drowning girl.[74]

In a Clausewitzian flourish, Princess Bolkonskaya's distress is alleviated only when Count Rostov and his comrades happen to visit the Bogucharovo estate in search of hay for their horses. They learn of the situation and promptly rescue a fellow noble from the "rough," riotous, and seemingly murderous peasants. Princess Marya's gratitude toward Count Rostov will develop into an erotic attachment and, ultimately, a marital union that, on Gary Morson's account, symbolizes the *poema*'s happy ending, following the great losses of the war.[75]

The Battle of Borodino

The main action of book three—by all means, the very climax of *War and Peace*—comes in its portrayal of the battle of Borodino, which took place on August 26, 1812, over 100 kilometers southwest of Moscow (see Figure 8.1). This cataclysmic battle was one of history's bloodiest battles up until that point.[76] Paradoxically, it took place in an open, pastoral, and otherwise "idyllic" setting, wherein the Russians lacked trenches or other defenses. On the eve of the battle, the Russians lost their Shevardino Redoubt and the high ground surrounding it, together with the 6,000 soldiers who had been ordered to defend it.[77] Accordingly, Kutuzov's hope to have used Shevardino to cover the army's left flank was crushed even before the battle began. Napoleon would immediately exploit this weakness by ordering 40 artillery pieces to fire on this flank, leading to the destruction of an estimated nine-tenths of the Russians on the southwestern front lines.[78] The defending army's center and right flank were better-protected by fortifications, especially the Raevsky Redoubt.[79]

On the eve of the battle, Andrei experiences acute death-anxiety, as he did the night before Austerlitz. This time, Bolkonsky anticipates his mortal injury and thinks of the "three great sorrows of his life": "his love for a woman, his father's death, and the French invasion which had overrun half Russia [...]."[80] Bolkonsky reflects on how Napoleon, previously his hero, unknowingly had "swept" his father "aside," destroyed Bald Hills, and torn Prince Nikolai's "life [...] to pieces."[81] Now, the French Emperor likewise threatened the Russian army, Tsar, and Moscow itself, and to slaughter its inhabitants, including Prince Andrei's person: "To die... to be killed tomorrow... That I should not exist... That all this should still be, but not me..."[82]

Later that same night, Pierre arrives to consult with Andrei in the village of Kniaz'kovo (meaning "princely").[83] Together, they will develop the Clausewitzian thoughts Bolkonsky had begun to formulate at the beginning of the French and allied invasion: that blueprints and outlined war-plans matter less than chance, the moment, and above all, the collective morale, "feeling" (**чувство**), or "spirit of the army."[84] By the same token, General Kutuzov will echo de Maistre's stress on morale on the day of the battle. Speaking with Pierre, Andrei impulsively calls for the summary execution of all French and allied prisoners of war for their atrocities, before denouncing war as "the most horrible thing in life," the "favourite pastime of the idle and frivolous," and a mere game in which life is objectified and subordinated to murder, spying, ruin, and looting.[85] With such an intervention, Bolkonsky is paradoxically channeling Clausewitz's "realist" dismissal of mercy in warfare in response to foreign occupation, while also critiquing the instrumentalism advanced by this very same theorist and the resort to force altogether.[86] Such discordant impulses reflect Tolstoy's fragmented sense of identity, the double-consciousness of dreamers, and the internalized aggression expected of those subjected to military hierarchies.

Along these lines, once the battle begins, the audience confronts the class struggle involving commanders and troops, which is akin to the contradiction between master and slave: "At the battle of Borodino, Napoleon shot at no one and killed no one. That was all done by the soldiers."[87] Further illustrating this estrangement between emperor and subordinates which results from the projection of vertical power, Bonaparte is emblematically blinded by the sun at midday, such that he cannot either follow the battle from afar, or give orders based on the shifting reality.[88] In effect, Tolstoy seeks to demonstrate how utterly ineffectual Bonaparte truly was.[89] In like fashion, in 2022, the top-heavy structure of the Russian military has contributed to its heavy losses not only of rank-and-file soldiers but also of senior generals in Ukraine.[90]

Pierre is our Virgil, or "red [and black] detective," in Tolstoy's depiction of Borodino. The author ahistorically terms this battle to have been both Napoleon's first loss—thus forgetting the Austrians' defeat of the *Grand Armée* at the battle of Aspern in 1809—*and* the ostensible beginning of the end of Napoleonic France. This latter claim would ignore the Empire's temporary recovery after the reversals of 1812, before its final defeat three years later.[91] As in the "Sevastopol Sketches," on which the writer's retelling of the battle is partly based, Lev Nikolaevich uses perceptual (factical), categorical (emotional-iconic), ideological (abstract), and psychological forms of realism, together with agoric denunciation and dramaturgical empathy, to humanize officers and soldiers by depicting their *conditional* agency, which is constrained by the grim chronotope (space-time) of combat imposed by Napoleon's imperialist strategy.[92]

As a Freemason, Pierre participates in the battle only to bear witness to the toil and suffering of the soldiers. He "sees the actions and sufferings of other people pass before him like a spectator."[93] In Bondarchuk's film adaptation, Bezukhov, looking so out-of-place in his upper-class clothes and his "white hat of innocence," is asked several times by the soldiers if he is a physician—in a presumable reflection of the vast needs of the wounded and dying for care.[94] According to Hugh McLean, Pierre's presence "defamiliarizes" the battlefield, helping to convey Tolstoy's critical message.[95] Though presented in a highly dystopian manner, such quixotic defamiliarization of the scene at Borodino constitutes a *deprovincialization* of militarist apologism. Both literary techniques here thus function to link Tolstoy's portrayal of the battle with the radical utopian tradition, propelling his Christian-anarchist alternative through the "religious systole" of outward movement, from self to Other.[96]

Arriving at the Raevsky Redoubt, the central defensive position of the Russian army, Pierre initially feels out of place. Then, the Stranger approaches and befriends a group of soldiers under fire, who welcome him as a newfound comrade. Inspired by this homoerotic love, he will rush to resupply the battery with ammunition, only to be rendered unconscious by allied bombardment of the fort in the process.[97] Fortunately, the count walks away unharmed, but a horse who was injured by the same barrage does not survive. Returning to his previous position, Bezukhov encounters the sudden death of everyone in "that family circle which had received him as a member" moments prior, and shown him the "fire" of patriotism's fury.[98] Though he survives, the Resident cycles out to become estranged again.

As our errant Virgilian-Masonic guide, Peter Kirillich bears witness to the despair experienced on the killing fields. The author likens the ceaseless firing and artillery barrages to individual and collective death-rattles.[99] As at Sevastopol during the Crimean War, Lev Nikolaevich clarifies that the majority of killing and disability on the battlefield of Borodino resulted not from infantry or cavalry charges or movements but rather, from artillery shells and bullets.[100] In keeping with the chronotope's iconic pastoral imagery and the idea of harmonic reason, Tolstoy implicitly contrasts to Borodino's battlefield the peaceful use of its fields for agriculture, and emblematically juxtaposes mass-murder and chaos with the production of art and the tranquil reproduction of life.[101]

At the same time, in keeping with his critique of dehumanization, Lev Nikolaevich compares the soldiers who are killed in these same fields to harvested grain or oats.[102] Indeed, Prince Andrei is fatally wounded at the "edge of a meadow beside an oat-field," and even outside the field-hospital where he will receive emergency treatment, horses are seen "eating oats." Alongside the stacks of oats are visible "a row of thirty-year-old birches with their lower branches lopped off."[103] Such imagery is suggestive at once of war casualties, and of castration anxiety. The author's inversion of safety-danger chronotopes in this sense serves his tragically satirical purpose of denouncing combat and social hierarchy in one stroke.[104]

In reality, the Russians succeeded in repelling seven waves of French assault that day, bolstered doubtlessly by a patriotic "spirit" (дух), but they were ultimately overwhelmed by the eighth such wave.[105] Tolstoy's narrator remarks that, upon approaching the battlegrounds after learning that the Russian defenses had still been holding, Napoleon and his generals were shocked, for they "had [n]ever before seen such horrors or so many slain in such a small area." Rather than a battle, at this point, Borodino had become a "continuous slaughter which could be of no avail either to the French or the Russians." In other words, the sanguinary siege of Sevastopol, with its vast sense of *mortido*, repeated the killing fields of Borodino.[106]

Verily, as the day progresses and the sun begins to set, the scene becomes evermore infernal, as mass-casualties mount, and ultraviolence burgeons, with each successive French wave of attack.[107] The gunfire and shelling is so intense that the conscripted serfs acting as stretcher-bearers "cannot remove all the wounded and dead."[108] Even Prince Andrei's reserve regiment (located in the center of Figure 8.1) is uselessly devastated by artillery fire while awaiting orders, with more than a third of its unit—hundreds of men—injured or killed in this way.[109] Bolkonsky himself is struck in the right flank by a delayed-impact shell during allied bombardment of his troops' position, just as he had been meditating: "I cannot, I do not wish to die. I love life—I love this grass, this earth, this air…"[110]

Donna Tussing-Orwin praises Andrei's observance of his duties as an officer in refusing to take cover as the spinning of the "smoking shell" threatens to take his life, while dialectically modeling "courage and resolve to his men and fellow officers."[111] In contrast, the Slavist Robert Louis Jackson finds Bolkonsky's maintenance of an upright posture in the face of a whirling shell highly unnatural, and reflective of both "his [ostensible] contempt for the ordinary soldier," and of his "adherence to [self-destructive] aristocratic notions of duty and honour." We might add that it combines Andrei's phallic personality with Tolstoy's psychical masochism. Jackson compares the image of the errant, spinning shell to the little bittern (волчок), a wading bird that, when threatened, stands erect and either revolves slowly or whirls rapidly. Such a connotation might further link the scene of Borodino to the prophesied apocalypse, considering the centrality of imagery of birds of prey in the book of Revelation.[112] Peasants will carry Bolkonsky to a field hospital, where the officer is attended to more quickly than the rest, reflecting in part the severity of his wound, but also the inverse care law theorized by Julian Tudor Hart in *The Lancet* a century later, whereby privileged populations receive care more readily in accordance with their needs, compared to more disadvantaged groups.[113]

In the ward, the prince's "general impression" is one of "naked bleeding human bodies that seemed to fill the whole of the low tent." Delirious in his confrontation with death, Andrei Nikolaevich will have the shell removed from his side, but lose consciousness in the process. He will be resuscitated by one of the attending doctors, who kisses him "silently on the lips, and hurr[ies] away." Such an expression of gay love provokes in Bolkonsky "a blissful feeling such as he had not experienced for a long time," as he temporarily conquers finitude with this kiss of life.[114] Then, he will encounter none other than his former nemesis Anatole Kuragin, just after the latter has undergone a possibly karmic amputation of an injured leg, presumably to stave off gangrene.[115] In this cathartic moment illuminated by feelings of Eros, survival, and interrelatedness, Tolstoy's narrator has Andrei emotively recognize the truth of Marya's supposedly "feminine" doctrine of forgiveness and love for one's enemies, based on the teachings of Jesus the Galilean, as an "antidote" to the myriad "atrocities on the battlefield."[116]

Tolstoy's Triumphalist View of the Meaning of Borodino

Although by the time dusk falls, Napoleon's forces appear to have formally defeated the Russian army at Borodino, by having killed half of its soldiers and leaving at least

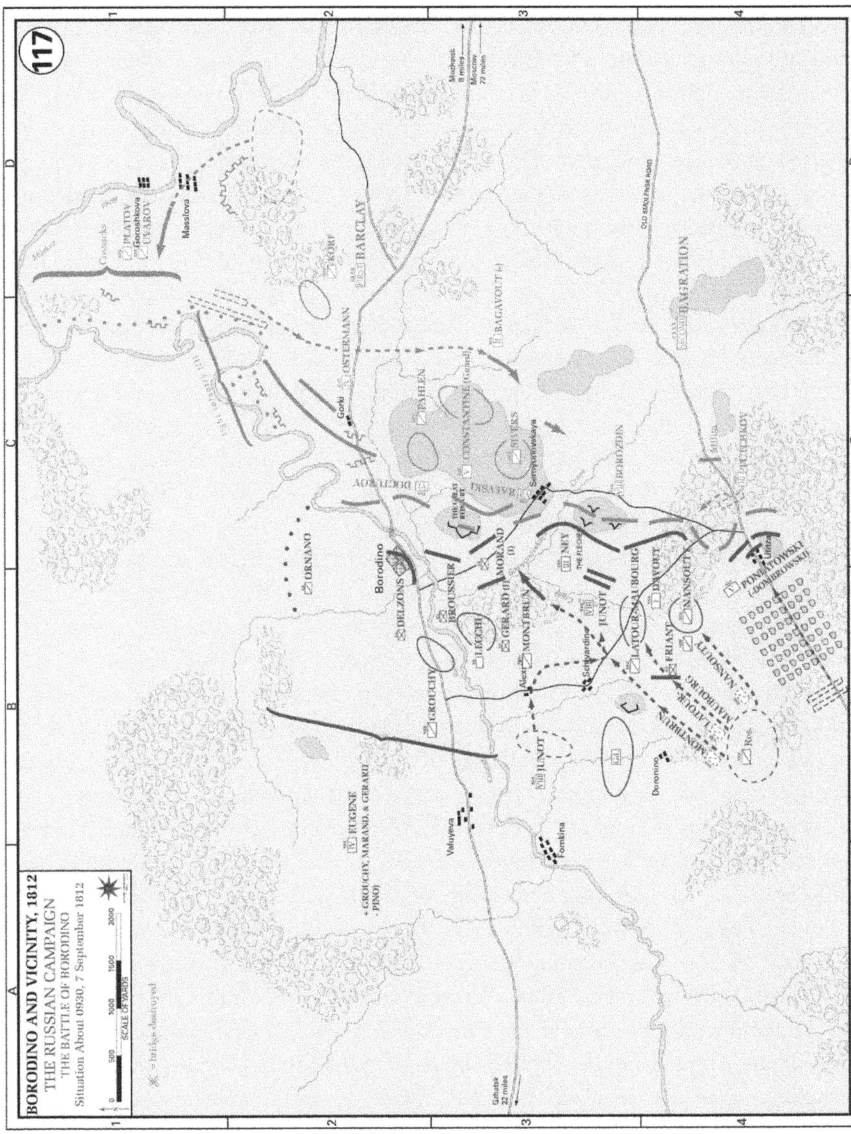

FIGURE 8.1 Map of the battle of Borodino (August 26, 1812).
Credit: Map courtesy of the United States Military Academy Department of History.

10,000 others grievously wounded, Tolstoy presents a patriotic and even chauvinistic framing of the battle. He claims that the morale of the surviving Russian military remained intact at the end of combat, whereas that of the invaders had been exhausted by the false victory they had secured over the Russians. The count asserts that the *Narod*, in its steadfastness, has expressed its putative "moral superiority" over the French and their allies. This "collision" Tolstoy believes to have "deprived [the invading army] of all its force."[117] It is hard to say whether such a triumphalist, quasi-Hegelian interpretation of the devastation at Borodino is Tolstoy's actual view, or whether the author is not satirizing anyone who would make such propagandistic or Panglossian comments, considering Hegel's attraction to Bonaparte.[118]

In certain ways, the pride evinced by Tolstoy's narrator marks the battle of Borodino as a historical moment of equal if not greater importance to the Great-Russian imperial project as the Muscovite State's final defeat of the Tatar khanate of Kazan in 1552. It was for this occasion that Tsar Ivan IV ordered the construction of St. Basil's cathedral in Moscow's Red Square, thus marking the final defeat of the Golden Horde, after a century and a half of war.[119] Tolstoy's pride here regarding the "victory" through defeat at Borodino may also signify an emotional transference linking his political self-concept with the "living past" significance of the *zaseka* and apiary located near Yasnaya Polyana, given that the former wooded area surrounding the Volkona River—source of the surname Volkonsky—had served as a defensive barrier against the Tatars.[120]

If Tolstoy's euphoric "declaration of collective belonging" here is not satirical, it is both uncharacteristically insensitive to human suffering, as well as arguably the loudest of the "chauvinist overtones" Emerson perceives in *War and Peace*. In her view, romantic Eros yields to national-populist Eros, or "common life" (общая жизнь).[121] Certainly, the author's historical narrative situates the Russians as sufferers *and* benefactors of Borodino. Such duality suggests that the writer employs the presentation of emergency *and* ecstatic news in his coverage of the battle, in an attempt to involve and activate the reader, via the politics of pity, to approximate oneself to, and identify with, the *Narod*. Yet, as Chouliaraki observes, the greatest risk of ecstatic news framings is that they serve to arbitrarily privilege certain sufferers "while blocking this same capacity for the largest majority of world sufferings," thus entrenching communitarianism rather than moving audiences toward cosmopolitanism.[122]

According to the war historian Christopher Bellamy, the battle of Borodino resulted in 44,000 Russian and 50,000 French casualties.[123] In this light, rather than advancing the liberatory legacy of the French Revolution, Napoleon's catastrophic invasion of the Tsarist Empire revealed once and for all the general's "gloomy role [as] executioner of the peoples," however much he would prefer to tell himself that his aim—no matter the facts—had always been the common good.[124] This is an exercise in self-rationalization often taken up by sadists, statists, despots, and authoritarians, then as now. Whereas at Austerlitz, Bonaparte had "stood on top of the world like a god commanding its actions," at Borodino, this "heroic fantasy" of domination has yielded to "a nightmare."[125]

To be sure, there are close parallels between Bonaparte's malignant narcissism and Nietzsche's philosophical support for the idea of aristocrats sacrificing countless underlings to maintain power. Such an approach is in turn consistent with the Nietzschean rejection of "a realm of justice and concord [being] established on earth," and the attendant pronouncement that "war is what teaches people to be free."[126]

Historical Flow and the Abandonment and Occupation of Moscow

Tolstoy starkly contrasts Napoleon's self-serving delusions to his own anti-militarist and anarcho-Populist views. He emphasizes that, if we wish to discover the "laws of history," we must "completely change the subject of our observation, must leave aside kings, ministers, and generals, and study the common, infinitesimally small elements by which the masses are moved."[127] In so doing, Tolstoy elucidates the post-colonial goal of decolonizing war.[128] The writer explains his perspective on existence in history as being part of a *flow*, just as "life is movement."[129]

> The commander-in-chief is always in the midst of a series of shifting events and so [s/]he never can at any moment consider the whole import of an event that is occurring. Moment by moment the event imperceptibly shapes itself, and at every moment of this continuous, uninterrupted shaping of events the commander-in-chief is in the midst of a most complex play of intrigues, worries, contingencies, authorities, projects, counsels, threats, and deceptions [...].[130]

Although commanders or leaders may believe themselves to be in control of the situation when the "sea of history" is calm, they still live in constant fear. They know that the arrival of a popular storm will belie this fallacy and uncover the uselessness of authority—just as the periodical flooding of the low-lying St. Petersburg reveals the city's artificial nature.[131] Once the People's allegorical tempest has come and gone, the "flood of nations begins to subside into its normal channels," and sadistic authorities welcome such change, falsely believing themselves responsible for it.[132] The emblematic metaphor of flowing water symbolizes the creative destructiveness of humanity's steadfast collective strength (сила) against constituted power, or власть.[133] After all, rivers provide silt for the cultivation of crops and waterways for exploration; the movement of water also calms the nervous system.[134] In this sense, Tolstoy's concept of flow may resemble social-movement theory. By definition, systems of centralized water management function on the basis of the channeling of hydraulic flows to control dynamism and turbulence.[135] Whereas any single individual may represent but a drop in the proverbial ocean, masses of humanity can act in concert like waves.[136]

In a sense appreciated by Buddha, Lao-Tzu, Aristotle, Proudhon, and Le Guin alike, time and motion are continuous, and all phenomena impermanent.[137] Likewise, in Eastern Christianity, life is considered "eternal movement, eternal resurrection, eternal growth," and God, who is considered immanent, is symbolized by energy, movement, and light.[138] Consequently, that the writer in his *poema* mindfully centers *anitya* (impermanence), the first of three marks of existence identified in Buddhism, may conceivably link the novel's theme of acknowledging harmonic or circular reason (*samsara*) with its Christian-anarchist and anarcho-Populist messages, aimed at relieving *dukkha* and achieving political Nirvana by going beyond the given "order of domination."[139]

Shifting from theoretical inquiry back to narrative form, Tolstoy differentiates between the responses of the divergent social classes comprising the *Narod* to the approach of the *Grand Armée* to Moscow: while the wealthy flee, the poor majority of serfs, who comprised an estimated 61 percent of Moscow's inhabitants in 1811, remain to burn the property of the rich.[140] These inequalities in labor and safety notwithstanding, privileged and working classes alike are depicted as commonly supporting the struggle for national liberation, and rejecting subjugation to the French as "the worst thing that could happen" to them.[141] Curiously indeed, in Tolstoy's Moscow of 1812, the middle classes are more or less absent, with the exception of Napoleon himself, whom the prose poet resents from his aristocratic vantage point as an opportunistic social climber.[142]

Remarkably, in a "salvific act of life and love," as the Rostovs order several dozen carts to be packed with their wealth and possessions to prepare for evacuation, Natasha and Petya rebel, demanding that the carts be used instead to transport the war-wounded from Borodino.[143] Although Natasha's noble gesture is consistent with Tolstoy's anti-militarist avowal of non-cooperation with evil, it likewise reproduces authority, in that "the servants [now] gathered around Natasha" to carry out her different, more compassionate orders—instead of autonomously organizing to carry out this humane project themselves.[144] Rather than disassembling the estate on behalf of the Rostovs as they previously had been, the workers are portrayed as laboring "at this new task with pleasure and zeal," in light of the more righteous content of the order governing it—as they exchange the movement of cases of "china, bronzes, pictures and mirrors" for that of their injured compatriots.[145] This verbal image recalls Pierre and Andrei's paternalistic assistance to the serfs: like Tolstoy's Aunt Ergolskaya, whom the novelist idealizes as having used her privilege only to serve the Other, they will "help" them, and consider their lot their charge, according to the doctrine of *noblesse oblige*. Still, they stop short of contemplating manumission or emancipation.[146]

As with the troop-review at Olmütz and Petya's witnessing of the crowd hailing Tsar Alexander in Moscow, it is ambiguous whether Lev Nikolaevich means to satirize such vertical forms of communication and social organization during the exigent circumstances of war that lead to the progressive reorientation of privilege in service of the *Narod*, or to endorse them. There is no doubt that, all of Tolstoy's sympathy for anarcho-Populism notwithstanding, *War and Peace* centers aristocratic characters, and effectively reduces the peasant base of the *Narod*—comprising 84 percent of the Russian population in 1850—to mere cameos or bit players.[147] Like Dostoevsky's *Crime and Punishment* (1866), wherein the murderous protagonist Rodion Raskolnikov's elderly female victims serve as mere objects for the plot's progression, the text of *War and Peace* remains "too focused [...] on the life of the rich and learned."[148]

Tolstoy's, then, is a "Paternal Populism" that may serve the cause of national liberation, but which can never deliver the self-emancipation of the working classes and peasantry.[149] Princess Marya declares to the Bogucharovo serfs that "[o]urs is a common misfortune and we will share it together. All that is mine is yours."[150] Although such egalitarian affect may impart an anarchism of love that would level social hierarchy, according to the idea that tenderness and affection undermine authority, her statement nevertheless appears misleading, considering that her family owns her audience's land and labor.[151]

Count Rostopchin Incites Vereshchagin's Lynching and Confronts his Guilt

The remarkable mass-abandonment of Moscow before its occupation by the *Grand Armée* represents a striking example of mass non-cooperation with evil. If the *Narod* rejects Bonaparte, over whom will he legislate, and precisely whom will he exploit? The Muscovites will self-estrange in the hopes of returning later in residence.[152]

In covering the fall of the city as an anachronous war correspondent, Tolstoy draws a stark contrast between the fate of Moscow and that of Berlin and Vienna following their occupation by the *Grand Armée*. Specifically, the French Emperor's war-drive would press on rather than be stopped in its tracks in these Central European cities, because their populaces had not done as the Russians had, by refusing to "welcome the French with bread and salt" or to "bring them the keys of the city."[153] With this foil, the author accentuates his Slavophilic differences with many contemporary Russian writers, who from the 1830s on commonly portrayed Russian urban life as being tantamount to the ostensible seediness of existence in London or Paris. Such a contrast helps to transmit his anarcho-Populist critique emblematically.[154]

Naturally, the decision to abandon Moscow could not be made lightly, considering the great suffering and death such displacement would imply, particularly for the masses of "factory hands, house-serfs and peasants," who faced the dilemma of risking death by exposure or remaining to be abused and potentially massacred by Napoleon's forces.[155] By the same token, to flee Moscow implied risking its mass-looting and utter destruction. In reality, the *Narod*'s decision to overwhelmingly abandon the city constituted a repudiation not only of Napoleon *but also* of Count Fëdor Rostopchin, the city's governor-general, who deluded himself into thinking he could control Moscow's inhabitants, according to Tolstoy. As a self-interested Tsarist bureaucrat, Rostopchin mirrors Bonaparte.[156] In effect, the *Narod*'s mass-expression of their "national feeling" illuminates the uselessness of Rostopchin as their administrator, and potentially, of all administrators.[157] However, whether this confrontation between *Narod* and governor-general is historically accurate is another story.

In an illustration of the irrationality of State power, Rostopchin will project his feelings of frustration, isolation, and superfluity over Russian losses and Muscovite disobedience onto the youth Vereshchagin. He uses his power to sadistically accuse this young man of spying for the French, without any sort of evidence or process. In effect, Rostopchin incites the bewildered Muscovites to lynch this son of the *Narod* in the streets as the bureaucrat escapes the city by coach through a rear gate. The count hence manages his anxieties in the face of defeat and capture by seeking to reassert his power and ensure compliance through the punishment of an illusory deviance.[158] With Vereshchagin freshly murdered, Rostopchin will suddenly repent, hypocritically remark on how "terrible" and "disgusting" the "mob" is, and conveniently overlook his own complicity in inciting the crime against the scapegoat in question by incredulously pinning the loss of Moscow on the young man—rather like a Pontius Pilate, or a Donald Trump.[159]

Though he quickly represses memory of this atrocity, having retreated to his *dacha*, Rostopchin will have to soon confront his guilt once again. This comes at the apocalyptical suggestion of an anonymous ex-inmate of a psychiatric institution who, as a "holy fool," challenges the carriage-riding count's effective usurpation of divine authority through his summary execution of Vereshchagin.[160] Swarmed by escapees from the mental ward dressed in white—thus, connotative of the martyred souls demanding judgment, as delineated in the biblical story of Revelation, as of the "emissaries of anarchic revolt from the French Revolution," *and* of the apparitions of those killed in the war against Napoleon—Rostopchin, gripped by death-anxiety, tremulously orders his coach-driver to go "fas... faster!"[161]

These truth-telling inmate-escapees thus embody the hope that there might be a "price to pay for violence, oppression, war. It is the messianic King, the Lion of Judah, Christ himself who opens the seven seals and releases a hail of destruction upon the world of wickedness."[162] Resurrected by this voice of conscience, the governor-general will change his mind, and come to support the evacuation effort.[163] Despite Rostopchin's conversion, Tolstoy in this sequence fashions a verbal icon lamenting chaotic impersonalization as perpetrated not only on the front lines, between the advancing French and retreating Russian forces, but also by despotic Russian authorities on the home front.

Tolstoyan Anarchism, Appropriated by Stalinism

Considering the implicitly internationalist and anarchic verbal images from this part of the *poema*, it is no surprise that, beginning in 1946, the entire "Moscow in Flames" sequence was excluded from Prokofiev's adaptation of *War and Peace* at the Kirov Opera House. Workers at the Opera House feared retaliation from Stalin's ultra-nationalist cultural minister, Andrei Zhdanov (1896–1948), had they included it.[164] That the *poema*'s finale endorsing the Decembrist revolutionaries was not reproduced either in Bondarchuk's film version—released under the hardliner Leonid Brezhnev's regime, though mostly filmed during the revisionist Nikita Khrushchëv's rule—presumably follows a similar logic. In an affirmation of Soviet patriarchal norms, in Bondarchuk's adaptation, it is Count Ilya Rostov *rather than Natasha* who magnanimously proposes redirecting the labor dedicated to the evacuation of his manor to the evacuation of the wounded and dying at Borodino.[165]

Likewise, in 1928, Stalin observed a "false jubilee" for the centenary of Tolstoy's birth. In parallel, the Russo-Soviet philologist Leonid P. Grossman (1888–1965) and writer V. Rozenblat concurred in their assessment of Dostoevsky's novel *Demons* (1871–1872) as being anti-anarchist in orientation—hence, of use to the Soviet State, despite the art-work's reactionary politics.[166] Then as now, Stalinist self-promoters ignore that Marxist-Leninist statist despotism is fundamentally incompatible with the Tolstoyan centering of разумение, or self-determination, in both theory and practice.[167]

Despite Lev Nikolaevich's unambiguous condemnation of the "forcible construction of other people's lives," whether perpetrated by a reactionary-authoritarian State or its "revolutionary" opposition, Stalin's regime opportunistically profited from using the *poema* during World War II. It did so by enshrining the work's triumphal portrayal of a national struggle against an invading force led by a megalomaniacal dictator, in an attempt to rouse the titanic popular effort to repel Hitler's war-machine.[168] During the siege of Stalingrad, in fact, a million copies of *War and Peace* were sold, and sections of the "Sevastopol Sketches" were broadcast via loudspeaker in Leningrad's Palace Square to boost morale during the Nazi siege. Even as the authorities had shuttered the Tolstoy Moscow Vegetarian Society in 1929; persecuted, banished, and murdered peasant-intellectual followers of Tolstoy for establishing autonomous communes; and permanently closed the Kropotkin Museum in 1939, Stalin's regime brazenly evacuated the contents of the Tolstoy Museum in Moscow to Tomsk and Tashkent.[169]

The Great Fire of Moscow

Tolstoy views the infamous Great Fire of Moscow as the turning point that would result ultimately in Napoleon's defeat. He believes that this conflagration was the outcome not of any conscious arson on the part of the city's displaced inhabitants or their leaders, but rather, the plausible consequence of blazes set by the occupying army in an otherwise abandoned city built of wood that lacked fire-suppression services of any sort.[170] In contrast, according to historian Catherine Evtuhov and her colleagues, "fires were intentionally started throughout the city" on the orders of the Russian authorities, a conclusion with which Orlando Figes agrees. In contrast, the war historian David Gates asserts that it was Napoleon who mandated the city's arson upon its capture.[171] Some memoirs of French eyewitnesses blame the arson on convicts who were released during the chaos.[172] Clausewitz, for his part, claims the fires were either the outcome of an intentional order on the part of the Muscovite government, or unintentional acts for which Cossacks supposedly were to blame.[173] In a similar vein, according to Herzen, whose own father was summoned to Bonaparte as an *ad hoc* representative of the Tsar, Napoleon "blamed Rostopchin for the fire, sa[ying] that it was vandalism."[174]

Whatever its true cause, the Great Fire that raged for nearly two weeks after the battle of Borodino consumed some 80 percent of the metropolis.[175] In this light, Tolstoy appears not to have fully appreciated the degree of despair and social collapse evident among the populace of Moscow after its occupation, especially considering the ruination of the municipal sanitation system, which he does not integrate into his portrait. Such a lacuna notwithstanding, the writer's depiction of Vereshchagin's plight may be taken as standing in for the ruthless mob violence that surged in the city against those who appeared foreign. Still, considering that Count Rostopchin himself came from mixed Slav and Tatar background, the prose writer's choice to weave in a parable about the governor's incitement of mob violence against the scapegoat Vereshchagin may simultaneously betray his Christian anarchism, Orientalism, *and* Great-Russian chauvinism.[176]

In like fashion, whereas the novelist illustrates the serfs' looting of Moscow following Napoleon's withdrawal as regenerative, contemporary accounts by a number of priests and their relatives liken these same peasants to locusts, and decry their anarchic reappropriation of private property and associated proclamation of a society without masters.[177] In keeping with Shklovsky's critique, in fact, Tolstoy fails to render either of these latter realities visible in his narrative. The author nevertheless implicitly contrasts the cowardice of the fleeing gentry with the authentic courage and steadfastness of the serfs and peasant conscripts, following the juxtaposition noted by the poet Fëdor Glinka (1786–1880), who fought alongside Sergei Volkonsky as a partisan.[178]

Pierre stays behind in Moscow, dressed in peasant's clothes, with an idea to sacrifice himself by assassinating Bonaparte. Bezukhov bears witness to how the occupying French desecrate the city in their drunken revelry, abuse the remaining Muscovites, and loot *en masse*. The occupiers would use churches as "barracks, stables, and slaughterhouses," defile mansions, attempt to bomb the Kremlin, and turn Moscow's new boulevard into a mass-execution site.[179] As the infantile Herzen's family and servants flee their wooden Muscovite family home for their uncle's stone dwelling, they are beset by French soldiers who tear Alexander's baby-clothes to shreds in search of concealed riches.[180] Marching bands of the occupiers play artificially celebratory pomp, as the *Grand Armée* utterly ruins the city, illustrating the horrors of imperialism, necropolitics, accumulation by dispossession, and the specifically Napoleonic pretension to resurrect the Roman Empire. This is not to mention the historical echoes of Bonapartism in Mussolini's Fascism—as laid bare in the Spanish Civil War and World War II.[181]

A French soldier's victimization of a "Georgian or Armenian" woman will provoke Pierre to lash out with incredible strength, as though channeling the *Narod*'s сила (force), before he has a chance to confront Bonaparte, leading to his arrest.[182] During his incarceration, Bezukhov is initially rejected by the other detainees due to his class privilege, though later on, he will become their leader—thus exemplifying the anarcho-Populist ideal of class fusion.[183]

During his captivity, Peter Kirillich witnesses summary executions of Muscovites by the occupying army carried out ostensibly to punish and deter arson.[184] In Bondarchuk's film, these atrocities unmistakably take after Francisco de Goya's 1814 painting, *El tres de mayo 1808* ("The third of May, 1808"). Goya's work condemns the mass-executions carried out by Napoleon's troops as retaliation against the People of

Madrid for rising up against the invaders the previous day, as the transfer of power from the Bourbon monarchy to King Joseph Bonaparte was being finalized.[185] This prior revolt is memorialized in another Goya painting, *El dos de mayo 1808.*

As the French serially execute Russian prisoners accused of arson, an adolescent male factory worker who is about to be murdered bonds ephemerally with his neighbor Pierre, seeking intimate solace through a "precarious commune" with a would-be *erastes*, or elder male partner, as he confronts the absurdity of premature death at the hands of occupiers.[186] Though this boy is killed, Pierre's life is spared at the last moment, quite like Dostoevsky's—hence, allowing Bezukhov to discover his life's meaning through revolutionary suicide, as we shall see in the next chapter.[187]

These summary executions of ostensible arsonists have echoes in the massacres which followed the occupation of Rome by Napoleon's forces in 1797 and the *Armée*'s destruction of Zaragoza in 1809, as well as in the Versaillais troops' brutal suppression of the Paris Commune in 1871, two years after *War and Peace*'s release. In a chilling parallel to the rationale later used by the Versaillais commanders to massacre up to 30,000 Communards, the French General de Ségur lays bare the fundamental barbarism of Bonapartism in his memoirs. He comments that the Muscovite arsonists, in representing the internal enemy, required extermination in the interest of "civilization," in keeping with the Napoleonic doctrine of total war (see Figure 8.2).[188] Now, in 2022, Putin's regime commits genocidal crimes against Ukrainians, such as the mass-deportations of survivors of the siege of Mariupol and the massacre of a thousand civilians in the town of Bucha, to the approbation of many fascistic Russians.[189]

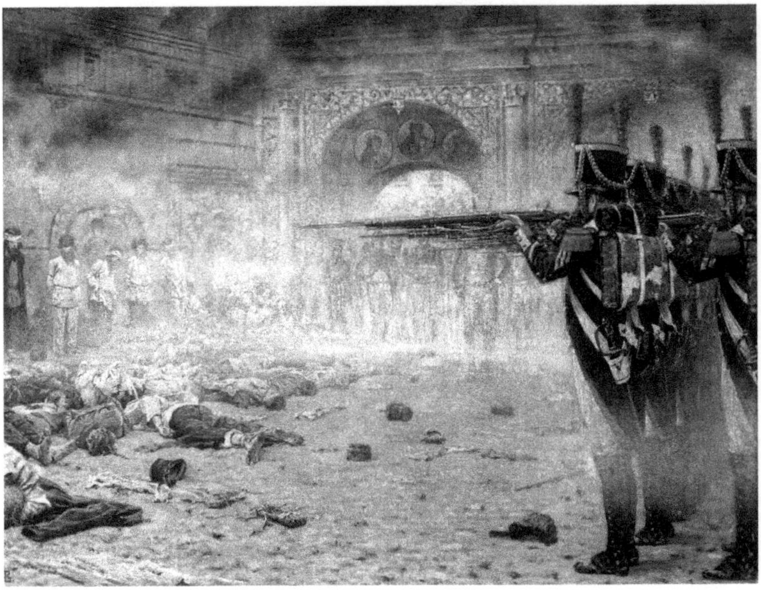

FIGURE 8.2 Vasili Vereshchagin, *In Defeated Moscow* (1898)

Notes

1 Tolstoy 2010: 647.
2 *Ibid* 668; Evtuhov et al. 326.
3 Tolstoy 2010: 877–8.
4 Gerth and Mills 224. Hopefully, with the continued support of Western allies, the Ukrainian resistance to the "special military operation" that Putin launched on his neighboring country in February 2022 will have a similar outcome, helping to put an end to Putin's rule, democratize Russia, rebuild Ukraine, and accelerate a global transition to renewable energy.
5 Tolstoy 2010: 1153–6; Evtuhov et al. 311–13; Ludwig; Gerth and Mills 212.
6 Tolstoy 2010: 1147; Foster J 112, 152; Bondarchuk 1966–1967; Gerth and Mills 217; Du Bois 935.
7 Du Bois 929 (emphasis in original).
8 Medzhibovskaya 2005: 49; 2004: 22.
9 Tolstoy 2010: 649.
10 Gerth and Mills 199; Bronowski.
11 Tolstoy 2012: 224.
12 Knapp 1991: 35–8.
13 Tolstoy 2010: 649.
14 Love 2012: 86.
15 Medzhibovskaya 2005: 47.
16 Freire.
17 Tolstoy 2010: 650, 841, 881 (emphasis added).
18 Orwin 1993: 26, 102; Zorin 46–7.
19 Tolstoy 2010: 652, 974.
20 Forrest 64.
21 Figes 2002: 154–5, 361.
22 Tolstoy 2010: 762 (emphasis in original).
23 Mbembe 2003: 23–4; Forrest 68–71.
24 Tolstoy 2010: 935–6.
25 Bulgakov 29; Gerth and Mills 225.
26 Tolstoy 2010: 654; Love 2012: 91; Becker 265; Medzhibovskaya 2004; Browne; Fuchs 13; Fromm 1969: 165; Gustafson 1986: 409; Benjamin 60; Fischer et al.
27 Tillich 49, 130; Tolstoy 2010: 842. Compare the Roman address, "*Ave* [hail] Caesar!"
28 Tolstoy 2010: 654–5; Evtuhov et al. 326.
29 Orwin 1993: 123; Tolstoy 2010: 661–3.
30 Herzen 678; Bondarchuk.
31 Evtuhov et al. 379; Currie.
32 La Botz 138.
33 Tolstoy 2010: 668.
34 Herzen 346.
35 Figes and Kolonitskii 69.
36 Tolstoy 2010: 669.
37 *Ibid* 670, 1336n670; Evtuhov et al. 323–6. Alexander would similarly take advantage of this "peace" to wage war for territory with Sweden, Turkey, and Georgia.
38 King Philip II (r. 1556–1598) ordered the construction of the vast Escorial monastery to commemorate the Spanish victory over the French at the battle of St. Quentin in 1557 (Abellán; Hall 134).
39 Bergamini 152; Kautsky.
40 Revelation 13: 3–4.
41 Tolstoy 2010: 887; Olaya.
42 Gates 626–7; Holmes 802.
43 Tolstoy 2010: 677. Besides through Eastern Christianity, it was likely from his Aunt Toinette Ergolskaya that Tolstoy confronted this lesson most vividly, when he

discussed with her a real-life instance of infidelity. In this case, she advised compassion instead of vindictiveness or resentment (Bartlett 2011: 221–2).

44 Tolstoy 2010: 691.
45 *Ibid* 691 (emphasis added).
46 *Ibid* 690.
47 Berlin 1978: 59.
48 Tolstoy 2010: 692.
49 *Ibid* 796–7 (emphasis added).
50 Gerth and Mills 344–9.
51 Tolstoy 2010: 701.
52 *Ibid* 702.
53 *Ibid* 709, 914.
54 Martin 46; Tolstoy 2010: 710 (emphasis added).
55 Tolstoy 2010: 711.
56 *Ibid* 712; Gustafson 1986: 40.
57 Evtuhov et al. 712; Aubin; Borshchevskaya; Schneider and Lütkefend; *Guardian*.
58 The New Arab.
59 Tolstoy 2010: 715.
60 *Ibid* 713–15, 723–5; Bartlett 2011: 365.
61 Tolstoy 2010: 725–31.
62 *Ibid* 730–42; Klikauer. This letter from the governor to the General Prince satirizes General Barclay's own assurance to the governor of Smolensk that the city was in no danger—precisely as it was being captured and destroyed. Compare the haughtiness of an Afghan provincial governor in August 2021, who announced that the city of Herat was at no risk from the Taliban, just hours before he and his forces left Herat, precipitating its downfall (Ungurianu 32; Makoii).
63 Tolstoy 2010: 654–68, 746–57.
64 Colonel P. N. Glebov observed that, during the Crimean War, "Count Tolstoy, a Sub-Lieutenant of artillery, is in command of two mountain batteries, but he himself roams anywhere he pleases" (Maude 1987a: 126).
65 Sloane 2005: 104.
66 Figes 2002: 129; Bartlett 2011: 55–60; Foster R.
67 Tolstoy 2010: 753.
68 *Ibid* 754; Evtuhov et al. 321, 371.
69 Tolstoy 2010: 764, 769–71.
70 *Ibid* 779–80. Compare Tolstoy's "strange feeling of consternation" as a child encountering his half-brother Mishenka, whose class status was very different than that of Lev or his "legitimate" brothers (Maude 1987a: 5).
71 Cervantes 176–86.
72 Zorin 36–7.
73 Berdyaev 1966: 32.
74 Shelley 142–3.
75 Tolstoy 2010: 784–90; Morson 2002: 76.
76 Evtuhov et al. 327.
77 Tolstoy 2010: 810; Orwin 2012c: 135. For the Shevardino Redoubt, see the lower-left quadrant of Figure 8.1.
78 Tolstoy 2010: 1099.
79 *Ibid* 817, 837–9. See center of Figure 8.1.
80 *Ibid* 824–5. Does Andrei mean Lise, Natasha, or possibly Tushin? Tolstoy leaves this up to the reader's imagination.
81 Compare Hegel's treatment of Bonaparte as the "World-Spirit on horseback" in an 1806 letter to Friedrich Immanuel Niethammer (Hegel).
82 Tolstoy 2010: 826.
83 Orwin 2012c: 130.
84 Tolstoy 2010: 678, 829, 864.

85 *Ibid* 831–2, 864. Ironically, Napoleon himself believed that, "in the last analysis, the sword is always vanquished by the spirit" (Ludwig).
86 McPeak 121.
87 Tolstoy 2010: 841.
88 Orwin 2012c: 133; Mbembe 2003.
89 Welch 178.
90 Barnes et al.
91 Stites 1989: 174; Tolstoy 2010: 880; Lieven 2012: 14–15.
92 Chouliaraki 79–93, 119–33.
93 Freud 1953: 426.
94 Bondarchuk; Gustafson 1986: 211.
95 McLean 2008: 84.
96 Reitz 84–5; Bounds; Feuerbach 31.
97 Gustafson 1986: 245; Orwin 1993: 114.
98 Tolstoy 2010: 850–6; Orwin 2012c: 126.
99 Orwin 2012c: 127.
100 Tolstoy 2010: 859.
101 Eisler 13.
102 Orwin 2012c: 136–9.
103 Tolstoy 2010: 825, 869–71.
104 Chouliaraki 177; Cervantes.
105 Orwin 2012c: 124; Bellamy 2001a: 142.
106 Tolstoy 2010: 863–4; Tolstoy 2006a: 326–32.
107 Bellamy 2001a: 142; Kaur.
108 Orwin 1993: 113.
109 Tolstoy 2010: 868; Orwin 2012c: 127.
110 Tolstoy 2010: 870.
111 Orwin 2012c: 125; Tolstoy 2010: 870.
112 Jackson 29–30.
113 Cookson et al. As though Tolstoy were anticipating his own death when composing this scene, in much the same way, peasants will carry his coffin to its burial site in the woods of Yasnaya Polyana in November 1910 (Bartlett 2011: 413).
114 Tolstoy 2010: 872–3; Berdyaev 2009: 251–2.
115 Tolstoy 2010: 868–74; Orwin 1993: 129.
116 McPeak 122.
117 Tolstoy 2010: 880, 884, 906.
118 Ewing; Herberg-Rothe. An allusion to Professor Pangloss, the ever-optimistic foil to Voltaire's *Candide* (1759).
119 Figes 2002: 151–2, 376.
120 Newlin 366; Bartlett 2011: 21–22; Chodorow 1999.
121 Chouliaraki 33; Emerson 2002: 3, 10; Orwin 1993: 123.
122 Chouliaraki 165–81, 179–90.
123 Bellamy 2001a: 142.
124 Tolstoy 2010: 877.
125 Orwin 2012c: 124.
126 Fromm 1947: 124; Beiner; Nietzsche 1974: 338–9; Nietzsche 2002: 213.
127 Tolstoy 2010: 883.
128 Mälksoo.
129 Denner 2011: 95.
130 Tolstoy 2010: 885.
131 *Ibid* 952; Figes 2002: 158; Berdyaev 2009: 193.
132 Tolstoy 2010: 1223.
133 Banister; Orwin 1993: 138; Orwin 2002c: 223.
134 Cocker.
135 Banister.

136 Stites 1990: 79.
137 Love 2012: 90; Clark 2019: 184–5; Kinna and Harper; Capra; Le Guin.
138 Gustafson 1986: 108, 450.
139 Clark 2019: 201.
140 Tolstoy 2010: 892; Martin 46.
141 Tolstoy 2010: 893.
142 Martin 43–7; Gerth and Mills 211.
143 Tolstoy 2010: 922–6; Gustafson 1986: 289.
144 Tolstoy 2010: 926; Shantz and Williams 123.
145 Tolstoy 2010: 926.
146 Bartlett 2011: 42; Maude 1987a: 50, 197.
147 Martin 42–5, 57; Evtuhov et al. 371; Abromeit.
148 Shestov; Gustafson 1986: 162.
149 Figes 2002: 226.
150 Tolstoy 2010: 781.
151 Gilman-Opalsky; Stites 1989.
152 Gustafson 1986: 39.
153 Tolstoy 2010: 964.
154 Martin 43.
155 Tolstoy 2010: 920, 942–9.
156 Gustafson 1986: 233.
157 Tolstoy 2010: 949–51.
158 *Ibid* 953–9; Gustafson 1986: 287; Solomon et al. 14; Hall 164.
159 Tolstoy 2010: 954–7.
160 Jackson 25–7.
161 *Ibid* 26–7; Tolstoy 2010: 959.
162 Jackson 32.
163 Gustafson 1986: 287–8.
164 Emerson 2002: 5.
165 Bondarchuk.
166 Goodwin.
167 Medzhibovskaya 2005: 49.
168 Tolstoy 1987: 218–19; Emerson 2002: 9.
169 Clay 217; Bartlett 2011: 444–8; Goodwin 176; Christoyannopoulos 2010.
170 Tolstoy 2010: 964.
171 Evtuhov et al. 327; Figes 2002: 150; Gates 626.
172 Martin 51.
173 Herberg-Rothe 148.
174 Herzen 6–8.
175 Figes 2002: 150.
176 Martin 50–3; Said; Figes 2002: 363.
177 Martin 56.
178 Figes 2002: 74–6.
179 Martin 50–3.
180 Herzen 4.
181 Ludwig.
182 Tolstoy 2010: 995–1001; McPeak 117.
183 Tolstoy 2010: 1032; Orwin 1993: 135.
184 Tolstoy 2010: 1040.
185 Gates 702.
186 Tolstoy 2010: 1038–40; Gilman-Opalsky 262.
187 Yalom 33.
188 Shafer 93–5; Martin 52–4; Gerth and Mills 224–5.
189 Garner; Chulov; Kirby.

9

WAR AND PEACE, BOOK FOUR

"Pierre Bezukhov"

Imprisoned as the French occupy and despoil Moscow, Pierre feels deep existential despair. In fact, the violence and destruction surrounding him shatter his belief in progress and meaning.[1] Then, as if in response to such distress, "God's messenger to Pierre" appears: Platon Karataev, the epitome of a "natural man," who tells Bezukhov immediately upon their meeting, in anarchist fashion, that "[w]here there's law there's injustice."[2] As a simple Christian (христианин) and peasant (крестьянин) without a master, Karataev is a uniquely tender character, for he expresses grief that Bezukhov's parents have passed away, laughs and smiles heartily and often, shows generosity, and endorses prayer and pity for animals.[3] Resembling a wandering *Strannik* in his apparent lack of concrete attachments—besides that to his adorable dog, whom he calls Grey or Flop-ear—Karataev observes both the Christian law of love and the Schopenhauerian stress on compassion in a remarkable way.[4] He does not view himself as distinct from others, but rather as an integrally fluid component of the human whole.[5]

Platon symbolizes the humanistic character of the commoner, the democrat, and the friend, in stark contrast to the exploiters, dictators, and demagogues who fill the pages of *War and Peace*.[6] Likewise, he embodies the Rousseauvist rejection of social artifice, living out Buddhist ideals of hospitality, non-attachment, non-egoism, and an ethics of care, thus exemplifying the traditional Russian peasant values of *pravda* (truth) and *volya* (freedom). In parallel, Karataev resembles the itinerant *bhiksu*, or monk, as well as the neo-Hinduists and *bhakti* followers such as Vivekananda (1863–1902), who criticized the ascetic and egotistical ideal of Hindu sainthood in favor of an engaged, loving approximation with other human beings.[7] In short, he is the archetypal holy fool.

Equally important, in light of the observed normalization of same-sex relations between Buddhist priests and their novices in China, Burma/Myanmar, and Japan, and of the general affinities postulated by Carpenter among religion, free love, and

DOI: 10.4324/9781003328964-9

homosexuality, there is a distinctly queer element to the spontaneously forged bond between Platon and Pierre. Through transference, this relationship builds on Bazdeev's prior mentorship of Bezukhov, Bolkonsky's encounter with Tushin, and Tolstoy's infantile symbiosis with his mother.[8] Indeed, Karataev treats Pierre with a "kindness and consideration" that is reminiscent of maternal love.[9]

In Bondarchuk's portrayal, Karataev first greets Pierre within their shared context of the "terrible time" (ужасный время) of defeat and captivity by the French by referring to Bezukhov as "guy" (парень) and "love" (дружок). As a motherly figure, this *muzhik* attends first to Peter Kirillich's needs for food, warmth, and rest, such that they jointly found a precarious interpersonal commune.[10] The strength, simplicity, kindness, and dignity symbolized in Karataev's person eases Pierre's demoralization and fear within the darkness of their prison, leading him to feel that "the world that had been shattered was once more stirring in his soul with a new beauty and on new and unshakeable foundations."[11] Platonically reinvigorated by Eros, as revealed to him by Karataev, Bezukhov perceives in the striking Moscow landscape and river the next morning a reflection of the "new joy and strength in life such as he had never before known."[12] This revitalization will then allow Pierre to respond to his captivity by laughing heartily at its absurdity, in a resounding affirmation of human autonomy.[13]

On another difficult front—in this case, the Rostovs' Yaroslavl estate—the fatally wounded Prince Andrei grieves his fate. Natasha and Marya care for him, expressing their erotic and filial love for him, respectively.[14] Still, the moribund Bolkonsky increasingly detaches from life. Once Princess Marya passes through the door into the darkness to visit her brother, whom Natasha is nursing, she struggles to communicate with him; their conversation is "cold and disconnected."[15] When Andrei's young son Nikolushka is brought to see his father, the estranged prince kisses him but "evidently did not know what to say."[16] As he lies suffering at life's end, this "all too cerebral hero" remains incapable of "unlock[ing] the mystery of divine love."[17] His prognosis worsens, due to a lack of proper medical treatment from his doctor. In a letter to the journalist A. S. Suvorin in 1891, the physician Anton Chekhov declares that, had the prince been under his care, he could have saved Bolkonsky's life.[18]

In Bondarchuk's film, the dying prince is transferred into an aesthetically pleasing room, full of light. Even so, Andrei Nikolaevich feels an "estrangement from everything belonging to this world." He reflects on how that errant shell had brought him to this "last spiritual struggle between life and death, in which death gained the victory."[19] How equally cruel *and* lovely it is for the love-bond between Natasha and Andrei to be reconstituted just before his death! The couple will discuss their hopes, illusions, and delusions regarding his recovery and their future life together on his death bed.[20] "How good it would be!" (Как хорошо бы!), cries Andrei, as he recognizes the pervasiveness of love and the plenitude of Eros—despite the immediacy of Thanatos and the grip of *mortido*—within him:

> Love? What is love? [...] Love hinders death. Love is life. All, everything that I understand, I understand only because I love. Everything is, everything exists, only because I love. Everything is united by it alone.[21]

Just as he comes to this realization, that love is an "active force reaching out to receive the other," Andrei succumbs in the final struggle against death at his door.[22] Only by perishing does he come to understand love as a simultaneous self-expression, identification with the Other, and manifestation of God, and so paradoxically achieve a love of everything.[23] Given that, ideally, this insight should be gained in life, Prince Andrei in reality achieves a masochistic "victory through defeat."[24] Lamenting the tragedy of death as the basic tragedy of eternal separation, Marya asks, "Where has he gone? Where is he now?..."[25]

Forward: The *Narod* Avenges Russia

Following his depiction of Prince Andrei's passing, Lev Nikolaevich returns to theoretical inquiry. He reiterates his stress that the "essence of any historical event [...] lies in the activity of the general mass of the people who take part in it." For this reason, history should not be viewed as the outcome of the supposed work of "those who stood in the most prominent position[s]" at any given time. Then again, Tolstoy celebrates the *poema*'s spiritual aristocrats as productive expressions of the *Narod*, as in the concept of *sobornost'*: for example, Captain Tushin, General Kutuzov, Prince Andrei, Natasha Rostova, Pierre Bezukhov, and Platon Karataev, among others.[26] On one front, these heroes defy the *ancien régime* upheld by the Kuragins and Tsarist autocracy, while on another, they resist the foreign onslaught of bureaucratic centralists.

Returning to narrative form, we see that Kutuzov's brief response to Napoleon's call for negotiations refers to his historical purpose, as an (unelected) representative

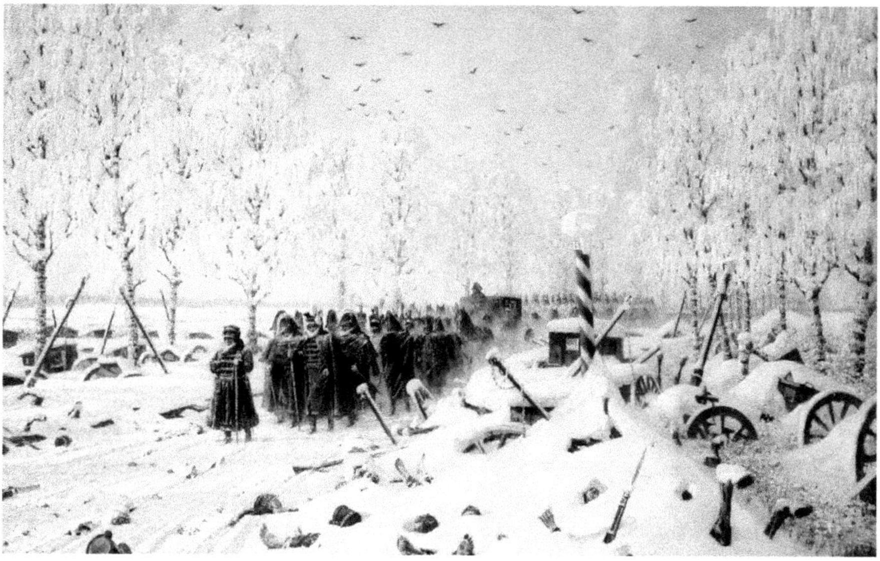

FIGURE 9.1 Vasili Vereshchagin, *On the Road. Retreat and Escape* (1895)

of the *Narod*. Replying that he would be damned by posterity if he were to come to any agreement whatsoever with the invaders, the commander-in-chief exclaims that he represents the "spirit of my nation" in rejecting his counterpart's entreaty. In turn, the Russian troops' morale improves upon hearing reports of the "easy successes gained by peasants and guerrilla troops over the French," and their desire to avenge the capture and arson of Moscow is inflamed—resulting in a newfound sense of optimism in the struggle against the French Emperor and his allies. This strengthening of the "national feeling" is bolstered by the Russians' victory at Tarutino a month after the French take Moscow. In point of fact, suffering such a loss will contribute to the occupiers' decision to abandon the city altogether.[27]

Napoleon's Expulsion as National Liberation and Anarcho-Populist Victory

Tolstoy continues to feature his classic humanistic critique of hierarchy and militarism in this penultimate book of *War and Peace*, wherein the *Narod* is revitalized through its expulsion of the occupying forces.[28] This resolution of the plot recalls the prophet Isaiah's vision of punishing the wicked and "lay[ing] low the insolence of tyrants."[29] Indeed, the supposed military genius Bonaparte will fail to provision his army with either adequate winter clothes or supplies before ordering them to withdraw from Moscow in October 1812. The French soldiers' distress will lead to stampedes and mass-desertions upon the *Grande Armée*'s exit from the ruined city, and Napoleon will order a general retreat along the Smolensk road following a close personal encounter with a Cossack unit (see Figure 9.1). Anticipating the Ukrainian peasantry's resistance to Stalin's forcible collectivization in the twentieth century, the serfs will refuse to cooperate with the retreating French and allied forces.[30] Rather, they burn the available stocks of hay to systematically starve Napoleon's draft animals and impede the movement of foraging parties.[31] In this brutal war of attrition—which Tolstoy, Evtuhov, and Goldfrank agree as having constituted a significant "departure" from the norms which had informally governed established European warfare up until that time—the *Narod* supported and resorted to informal tactics such as guerrilla warfare to avenge the scorched-earth tactics used by the *Grand Armée*. Hundreds of irregular military formations were formed to repel the invaders.[32]

Hence did the People in 1812 repudiate Napoleonic imperialism, reproducing the tactics of asymmetrical warfare which the Spanish national-liberation forces would use against Bonaparte's occupation, and which the indigenous peoples of Transcaucasia would similarly employ against Great-Russian expansionism itself.[33] In parallel, the Haitian people defeated Napoleon's 1802 invasion, which had sought to suppress the first Black republic—itself inspired by the ideals of the French Revolution—and reinstitute slavery.[34] In the end, just as yellow fever helped decimate the Napoleonic forces in Haiti, the combination of desertion, disease, hunger, bitter winter cold, "General Mud," and resistance from partisans *plus* the army led by Kutuzov devastated the French and allied forces in Russia, leaving their corpses to the wolves by the thousands.[35] Then, in World War II, history repeated itself, as the Red Army, partisans, and People jointly defeated the German invasion of the Soviet Union.[36] After all, as at Borodino in 1812, the 1941 battle of Moscow amounted to the *Wehrmacht*'s first loss, foreshadowing Nazism's ultimate downfall.[37]

The Deaths of Platon and Petya, and the Globe of Life

Toward the end of *War and Peace*, Tolstoy critically examines the psychosocial dimensions of authoritarianism through his illustration of the plight of Russian prisoners of war captured in Moscow. Complying with orders from above, the retreating French will subject even their mortally ill prisoners to forced marches. Pierre notices a violent change in the personality of the guards at this time. Namely, their "former friendly relations" shift to an outright denial of the humanity of their neighbors and would-be victims. To conform with the orders passed down through the military hierarchy, these soldiers will "blind" themselves willfully through a malice that simultaneously prepares the stage for, while also perpetuating, the dehumanization of the Other. Though over two-thirds of these prisoners of war will die, mostly from starvation, disease, exposure, and summary execution, the rest will be liberated by a Cossack unit which the boldly passionate teenager Petya Rostov has joined. Young Petya, who attaches homoerotically to the brave Dolokhov and collaborates courageously with him to free these prisoners, is himself killed leading the charge.[38]

Upon his visit to the Rostovs' after his liberation and the death of Petya, Peter Kirillich foreshadows Fëdor Dostoevsky's character Ivan Karamazov in *The Brothers Karamazov* (1880). Ivan, possibly having been based on the philosopher Vissarion Belinsky, famously tells his brother Alësha that the concept of the all-loving and omnipotent God stipulated by Christianity is called into question by the very existence of suffering and abuse of children. Along these lines, Pierre declares before Petya's family that there is *nothing* he can "say or think of as a consolation [...]. Why did such a splendid boy, so full of life, have to die?"[39]

Furthermore, Lev Nikolaevich examines the coldness with which Pierre manages the mortality salience of which Platon Karataev reminds him, as the latter's constitution weakens over the course of their joint captivity. Toward the end, Pierre avoids Platon altogether, and even looks away from his authentic, tender human gaze requesting friendliness as a last summons before the French kill him for straggling behind.[40] At the same time, while this scene may affirm "amoral vitality" and the "necessity of natural selfishness" in the face of summary execution at the hands of sadistic captors, Tolstoy appears to suggest that Bezukhov's refusal of compassion to Karataev at life's end was not entirely his fault. Rather, it was due to a state of delirium akin to the one suffered by Prince Nikolai Bolkonsky before his arousal and death at Bald Hills, the fog within which Countess Natalia Rostova is lost upon learning that "her beloved boy [Petya] was killed in the bloom of life," and the dissociative dream-state Natasha experiences while caring for Andrei and inuring herself to Moscow's fate.[41] Soon enough, Pierre comes to his senses and realizes lamentably that Platon's life, too, has been destroyed.

On the one hand, this scene exhibits the reification of human feeling through bourgeois coldness, understood as a pathological derogation of the interests of the Other—consistent with the Kantian concept of radical evil. On the other, the homophilic bond between Bezukhov and Karataev is also featured, considering the rush of concerned human passion which returns to Pierre upon his regaining an alert and oriented consciousness.[42] In an inversion of the relationship described in the fleeting comrade-love experienced by Tushin and Bolkonsky at the battle of Schön-Grabern, Pierre *sotto voce* becomes the *eromenos/kleinos* (the beloved junior partner), and Platon the *erastes/philetor* (the lover/befriender), who in turn transmits his teachings to his *protégé*.[43]

Following Karataev's death, together with that of Andrei and Petya, the author avers that Pierre's "sympathy for others shone in his eyes," as he intuitively comes to an understanding of the importance of mutual aid and his connection with all life (**всежизнь**), and accordingly beseeches service to humanity and a caring reconstruction of the life-world.[44] Ultimately, then, in spite of separation and loss, Bezukhov comes to resemble Kutuzov, a fellow war survivor, as he finds residence in the Kingdom of God through communal love and achieves the "true life" through participation in the reorientation of "evil" into "good life."[45]

Nevertheless, this profound understanding is arrived at only through an emblematic dream Pierre experiences after falling asleep shortly following Karataev's execution, which in turn follows soon after Petya's death in combat. Overcome with powerlessness, the personality resorts to fantasy to restore life.[46] In this trance, which "does not follow the laws of space, time, or causality," Peter Kirillich discerns a liquid world wherein existence is fluid and transient.[47] The spirit of his mentors Platon and Bazdeev describes cosmic space to him:

> Life is everything. Life is God. Everything changes and moves and that movement is God. And while there is life there is joy in consciousness of the divine. To love life is to love God. Harder and more blessed than all else is to love this life in one's sufferings, in innocent sufferings.[48]

In this dream-state—a prime example of "'theologiz[ing]' through literature"—Bezukhov encounters his Swiss childhood geography tutor (presumably modeled after Friedrich Rössel, the author's German tutor at Yasnaya Polyana), who shows him a pulsating liquid globe comprised of droplets of water, which move around, compress, and sometimes merge with each other, or divide.[49] Pierre's tutor explains, "God is in the midst, and each drop tries to expand so as to reflect Him to the greatest extent. And it grows, merges, disappears from the surface, sinks to the depths and again emerges."[50] This karmic "globe of life," presumably symbolizing the world and/or the mind, centers the importance of swarming and union in humanity's collective life, accentuating our liquid mass.[51] Each person is but a tiny particle of the species, and death, reversal, and return are necessary parts of life.[52] By all means, in her novella "Whose Fault Is It?" Countess Sofia Tolstaya expresses a similar understanding when citing the Stoic philosopher-slave Epictetus

(50–135 CE), who held that "death is the absorption of the human mind into the universal mind."[53]

In keeping with the motif of flow, "[o]ne must immerse oneself in the river of life [...]," as the existential psychotherapist Irvin Yalom (b. 1931) writes.[54] During our earthly existence, as "atoms of love for all," we "strive outward and toward each other," substantiating the hope that "[a]narchistic community is possible," because we are "not individuals, at war with each" other, but rather, "concerned with the whole." Consequently, meaning and engagement reside not at the individual level, but "in the units linked together into a whole," reflecting the reality that "[l]inkage makes the world coherent."[55]

Upon their reunion at Princess Marya's in Moscow, Pierre and Natasha share their mutual experiences of the war with each other, as the latter recounts her three weeks of journeying with and caring for the dying Andrei. Mirroring such lessons, Peter Kirillich remarks on how much he as a noble learned from the peasant Karataev, portending his own effort to put Platon's teachings into practice, and distinctly imparting Tolstoy's iconoclastic commitment to anarcho-Populism, as well.[56] Here, near the *poema*'s close, and in parallel to his comrade Prince Andrei's epiphany at life's end, Peter Kirillich will finally apprehend "what his nanny told him long ago: that God is here and everywhere." Rather than have "looked over the heads of the men around him," he "should have merely looked in front of him without straining his eyes." Still, a gap exists between theory and practice, at least for the time being, as the footmen attending to the candles illuminating Pierre and Natasha's rapture remind us.[57]

Epilogue

In the first part of the epilogue to *War and Peace*, Lev Nikolaevich denounces Bonaparte for his willingness to rationalize and command all the crimes and atrocities he and his subordinates would commit to invade and occupy Russia. In a complementary manner, he condemns Napoleon's Egyptian and Syrian campaigns in 1799 as outrages that anticipated the ruthless tactics later employed against Russia.[58] The writer then pivots to advance an implicit critique (and self-critique) of the landowning class in his portrait of Count Nikolai Rostov's move to Bald Hills upon his marriage with Princess Marya Bolkonskaya. Rostov hypocritically announces his love for "*'our Russian folk'* and their way of life with his whole soul," just as he extracts "brilliant results" from the serfs he owns, imposes his own stooges as the authorities of the peasant commune, and works assiduously to expel "the lazy, the depraved, and the weak" from the land. That Rostov is approached by numerous serfs who request that he buy them so they might suffer less under his ownership, relative to where they are currently enslaved, does not absolve Rostov of complicity with the violence inherent to landowning, labor, or management.[59]

The conclusion of the narrative counterposes to this predicament an historical *and* allegorical solution, one that previews *The Decembrists*, the incomplete sequel to *War and Peace*, thus constituting an important "signpost" along the journey of the poet's life.[60] Pierre arrives to his reunion at Bald Hills having just visited with a certain "Prince Fëdor," from the secret "Union of Salvation," which seeks to introduce constitutionalism to Russia. Whereas Bezukhov, by the novel's end, has learned to embrace the "ever-changing, always majestic, incomprehensible, and infinite" world of life with joy, he believes that not only "culture and philanthropy" but also "action" is needed to change the world.[61] In this, he signals his cosmopolitan-humanist support for immediate remedial policies, as well as long-term social restructuring, to relieve the plight of proximal and distant sufferers alike.[62] Though the married couple Pierre and Natasha are vague about the meaning of the "action" they intend, the allusion to the Decembrists itself reveals that their strategy aims at revolutionary suicide and the overthrow of Tsarism. In the presence of Nikolenka, Prince Andrei's orphaned son, Pierre tells Count Rostov that his own commitment to the Decembrist cause and radical struggle against the autocracy is consistent with the Christian law of love.[63]

For the author, Marya and Natasha's love for their families and humanity are expressions of this same law. Then again, in Natasha's case especially, Tolstoy's perspective is decidedly misogynist: being "wholly engrossed" by her family, Countess Bezukhova readily accepts her position as "slave to her husband." Lev Nikolaevich furthermore explicitly endorses sexism by having Pierre express agreement with Rousseau's arbitrary opposition to wet-nursing.[64] Indeed, several of the characters' derogatory declarations in the epilogue are consistent with an affirmation of patriarchal despotism. For instance, Natasha calls Sonya a "*sterile flower*" for being unmarried and childless, while her mother ostensibly "realize[s]" that Natasha's "outbursts had been due to her need of children and a husband."[65] In parallel, the matriarchal Marya Dmitrievna Akhrosimova chastises Rostova as a "Cossack" for her ostensibly "unladylike behavior"—signaling possible lesbian tendencies.[66] In reality, the seemingly progressive Tolstoy adhered to the backward belief that single women without children retain value only as "aides to mothers."[67]

Beyond this lapse into misogyny, the *poema*'s finale conveys the author's view that the world is governed by harmonic or circular reason, as suggested in the two concepts of the work's title: the "alternation of peace and war."[68] Life succumbs to death, which through decomposition in turn yields life. This theme resurges in the deaths of Andrei, Petya, and Platon preceding the marriages of Nikolai Rostov and Princess Marya, and of Pierre and Natasha. In book two, Prince Andrei's heterosexual desires, shattered by his wife Lise's death, are revitalized after his meeting Natasha—as symbolized in the motif of the barren oak tree, which is suddenly reborn in spring.[69]

In turn, Bolkonsky's queerness is stimulated at the battle of Schön-Grabern by his spontaneous attraction to Captain Tushin, and especially during his surreal, near-death experience at Austerlitz. He will come ever-closer to the queer-anarchist understanding of kenotic, ubiquitous love after suffering a mortal injury at Borodino. Likewise, as the cycle of *samsara* turns, Petya's passing leads paradoxically to Natasha's revitalization, as she attends to her grieving mother.[70] Significantly, Natasha and Pierre will name their first-born son after the martyred Rostov youth.[71] In this way, "[e]ach death [...] leads to a rebirth bearing seeds of the next death, which in turn is transformed into another regeneration."[72]

Collective Strength (Сила) against Despotic Authority (Власть)

In the second part of the epilogue to *War and Peace*, Tolstoy switches from the previous narrative format back into essay form. Here, he restates two significant concerns from the *poema* which lie in tension with each other:

1. An anarcho-Populist interpretation of history emphasizing the movement of nations and peoples rather than leaders, States, or empires.
2. A puzzling determinism that denies human freedom.

Both points constitute recurring themes of the novel itself, but it is the latter which is more roundly contradicted, both internally in the plot of *War and Peace*, as well as generally in Lev Nikolaevich's later works. Readers hence confront conflicts between "the feeling of responsibility" and "the values of private life" on one side, and the stipulated "reality of inexorable historical determinism" on the other.[73] Presumably, this tension results from Tolstoy's basing his argument here, as the Formalist Boris Eikhenbaum elucidates, on Schopenhauer's *The Two Fundamental Problems of Ethics* (1841), wherein the German idealist recognizes the existence of both determined and free wills.[74]

At the outset of the second part of the epilogue to his study of the wars of 1805 and 1812, the writer begins by declaring that "[h]istory is the life of nations and of humanity." He criticizes historians throughout the ages for focusing on rulers, statecraft, and supposed heroes rather than what is "apparently elusive—*the life of a people*."[75] This criticism is embodied within the *poema* in the opposition Tolstoy draws between "the concrete and multi-coloured reality of individual lives," as reflected in the work's effective pantheism, and "the pale abstractions of scientists or historians."[76] In this sense, one may think of the foils Natasha and Bonaparte, Kutuzov and the Tsar, or Platon Karataev and the French guards. According to the dominant fallacy which Tolstoy critiques, historical events "occur solely by the will of a Napoleon, an Alexander, or in general the persons they describe."[77] Similarly, in book three of *War and Peace*, Pierre Bezukhov "wanders about 'lost' on the battlefield of Borodino, and looks for something which he imagines as a kind of set piece; a battle as depicted by the historians or the painters. But he finds only the ordinary confusion of individual human beings haphazardly attending to this or that human want."[78]

On the contrary, Tolstoy suggests that, if we desire to understand history as "the movement of humanity and of the peoples," we should first ask, "What is the power that moves peoples?"[79] In *War and Peace*, we see that Tolstoy answers the question he poses by identifying a "power" (сила) which mainstream historians "apparently do not recognize," and by suggesting that the movement of peoples can be explained only with reference to this conception of force (сила) that corresponds to the "whole [collective] movement" of the Peoples.[80]

Consistent with his anarcho-Populism and affinities for Proudhon and Bakunin, who detested "bourgeois intellectuals," and his contrarian resentment of the very intelligentsia of which he formed a key part, Tolstoy in the *poema*'s epilogue denies that "intellectual activity" contributes to the movement in concert of peoples which constitutes history.[81] Utterly rejecting liberalism and representative government as false expressions of the popular will—which the People never in fact transfer to the State authorities—Tolstoy concludes that the "*force that moves nations lies [...] in the nations themselves*," such that they have no need for rulers or great men.[82] This formulation is remarkably close to the title and basic argument of the artist's 1893 Christian-anarchist classic, *The Kingdom of God Is Within You*. Within the plot of *War and Peace* itself, Prince Andrei comes to this same realization after his queer-anarchist epiphany, when he first encounters Napoleon at the conclusion of the battle of Austerlitz. Restating his Populist position once again, the prophetic humanist writer asserts that it is through "the activity of *all* the people who participate in the events" that the movement of nations and history proceeds.[83]

Illustrating his point with implicit reference to the *poema*, Tolstoy contemplates the pyramidal structure of an army, which can be considered an allegory of feudal-capitalist society as a whole. At the bottom, the soldiers, "of whom there are the most," are the ones who actually "d[o] the stabbing, hacking, burning, and pillaging" on the orders of their commanding officers, each of whom do less labor, and/or are otherwise protected from the risks of combat, as one rises in the ranks of the command hierarchy.[84] This master-slave relationship of privilege between commanders and rank-and-file troops is derived from "power" (власть), and Tolstoy completely rejects its role in advancing the movement of the nations, whether alone and directly—as in classical despotism, including Tsarism—or together with intellectual activity—as is proposed by Jacobinism, Marxism, and Leninism.[85]

Like Proudhon, Lev Nikolaevich seeks the creation of a new popular history filled with a "flow" of events that is not to be "prescribed, decreed, or ordered by monarchs, ministers, parliaments, or newspapers," but rather, one that advances producerist Populism by repudiating "political unity," "patriotism," "balance of power," and so-called "civilization."[86] Here, the circle linking the motif of collective strength through hydrological flows (сила) with the People liberating themselves from despotism (власть) through self-determination (разумение) is completed.

Even so, we must reiterate that Tolstoy's Populist framing of the Russian *Narod* acting in concert to repel the French invaders "deliberately minimizes the tensions among the classes" in the plot.[87] In both focusing on the gentry as protagonists of the popular-defensive war and considering them to be an integral part of the *Narod*, Lev Nikolaevich runs the risk of presenting an anarcho-Populism that becomes a self-parody, due to its programmatic perpetuation of social hierarchy and class privilege—however much that risk is tempered by the author's Christian-anarchist ideal, as reflected throughout the *poema*.

Freedom, Necessity, and Enlightenment

Finally, after sharing these profoundly insightful Populist observations about history, politics, and the future of humanity in the Resident mode, Tolstoy dedicates the remainder of the epilogue of *War and Peace* to outlining an ill-conceived historical determinism as a Stranger. In so doing, he contradicts his underlying anarchist hopes, as expressed both in *War and Peace*, and in the four decades of life that followed its publication.[88] Challenging the idea of humanity as the subject of history, Tolstoy in the final pages of the epilogue fetishizes the Russian ideal of судьба, or destiny, in presenting a depressing, fatalist account of human existence.[89] He goes so far as to claim that freedom is a comforting myth akin to the idea of heaven, and that, "[t]o conceive of a man being free we must imagine him outside space."[90] By making such comments, Lev Nikolaevich may be following his mentor Kant, who believes that the lack of self-determination and perfectibility open to us in this life implies that these struggles must persist on after death, suggesting our immortality.[91]

Without a doubt, Tolstoy means to emphasize the instrumentalization of human life perpetrated by hegemonic institutions, as well as humanity's own vulnerability and fundamental finitude, both in these closing reflections, and in the narrative critique of militarism, exploitation, and hierarchy. At the same time, he momentarily takes these interrelated concerns for social oppression on the one hand and human mortality and contingency on the other to an extreme that anticipates the ahistorical gloominess evinced by Martin Heidegger in *Being and Time* (1927).[92] Whereas suffering, toil, and death reflect human boundedness within natural laws, the social contexts mediating these realities must not be overlooked, as they can greatly affect how these truths are experienced.[93]

As Isaiah Berlin explains, Tolstoy argues here that people, "unable to face this [supposedly] inexorable process [of external determination], seek to represent [life] as a succession of free choices." The critic is right to link such pessimism to Tolstoy's affinities for Schopenhauer, who similarly presents "a gloomy picture of the impotent human will beating desperately against the rigidly determined laws of the universe."[94] Echoing Schopenhauer, Tolstoy fails to show convincing evidence for his deterministic claims. In attributing historical causality to an amorphous "Providence," Tolstoy is being obscurantist, as well as engaging in a performative contradiction. Above all, in the narrative of *War and Peace*, the poet illustrates how the actions of a Captain Tushin, a General Kutuzov, or a Natasha Rostova can change the course of history—yet, he negates just this very possibility in his theoretical conclusion.[95] Hence, the paradox of Tolstoy's having written "a monumental work of fiction replete with choice in which he professes that there is no such thing as choice."[96] Therefore, if Tolstoy is being serious, this is a confused and reductive account that leaves nothing more to human life than allegorical victimization at the hands of reified forces, such as can be seen reflected in the various combat sequences of the *poema*, which constitute dramatizations of our "fundamental expendability in nature," and hence, perhaps, "the real despair of the human condition."[97]

It is evident as well that Tolstoy's argument here may constitute a contrarian *overreaction* to the positivism, physiological materialism, and Darwinism so popular among European intellectuals at the time. Its pessimism may also reflect his enthrallment to the Russian tradition of fate (судьба), whereas its internally self-contradictory nature evinces Tolstoy's fragmented sense of identity, owing perhaps to trauma, and his impulsivity.[98] Like the Romantic-medievalist Slavophiles, Tolstoy rejected British empiricism, liberal reformism, and Marxist socialism. He equally disputed the materialism advanced by Nikolai Chernyshevsky and Dmitrii Pisarev, despite his close affinities with these latter two writers. Tolstoy converged with Pisarev's radical critique of civilization, and agreed with Chernyshevsky in disparaging Hegel, advancing a rationalist and moralist critique, and emphasizing didactic prose.[99] Despite their rivalries, Tolstoy would have agreed with the following declaration Nikolai Gavrilovich made in his diaries:

> The problem is not whether there should be a king or not, or whether there should be a constitution or not. It is, rather, one of social relations, and lies in the fact that one class should not suck the blood of another.[100]

Such radical intransigence echoes the intellectual pride uncovered by Prince Golitsyn's agents within Herzen's letters, following the revolutionary youth's arrest in 1834:

> All constitutional charters lead to nothing: they are contracts between a master and his slaves; the task is not to make things better for the slaves, but that there should be no slaves.[101]

Notwithstanding the pessimism conveyed in the second part of the epilogue, Tolstoy's messianic concept of the Kingdom of God reiterates Chernyshevsky's condemnation of the fatalist idea that "the idyll is inaccessible" as "pure nonsense": in reality, it is "even feasible, very much so [...] for all people."[102] For all that, whereas Tolstoy was an anarchist rooted in the traditions of Eastern Christianity, Chernyshevsky and Herzen were radicals who sympathized more with statism and Westernizing tendencies, respectively, than did Lev Nikolaevich—Chernyshevsky's contempt for Herzen's idealism to the side.[103] Tolstoy also fundamentally disagreed with Chernyshevsky and Herzen on the woman question.

Besides finding Chernyshevsky's lack of aesthetic sense repellent, Tolstoy evidently resented his counterpart's self-confidence, considering his lowly social origin.[104] Their spat would continue until 1862, when, to stifle a myriad of sources critiquing the limitations of emancipation without land, *The Contemporary* was shuttered, Chernyshevsky arrested, and Tolstoy's manor at Yasnaya Polyana raided by the secret police. Such State retaliation would come as the count was taking a *kumys* cure with Bashkirs on the borderland steppe near Samara.[105] Tragically, this police raid would frighten the writer's beloved Aunt Ergolskaya to death.[106]

In a reflection of the emotional intensity of the bond between Tolstoy and Chernyshevsky, in spite of their disagreements, Lev Nikolaevich implicitly pays tribute to the revolutionary political prisoner when he has Kutuzov pose the question of "What is to be done?" no less than four times in his final address to the troops. The field marshal answers with reference to the anarchic Daoist concept of *wu-wei* (non-action, or non-government), implying a disavowal of all will to power.[107]

At the close of the epilogue of *War and Peace*, Tolstoy moderates his deterministic pessimism by conceding that, in each human action—and therefore, in history—there are elements of *both* freedom and necessity, or inevitability. Humanity cannot exist without freedom, and consciousness "gives expression to the essence of freedom."[108] Although he fails to explain to what extent freedom and necessity can interrelate, the poet does appear ultimately to acknowledge the reactionary implications of a predominant determinism in the work's final page. Anticipating Bakunin's anarchist analysis in "God and the State," together with Freud's similar view that "a personal God is [...] nothing other than an exalted father," Tolstoy observes how the "law of inevitability in history [...] strengthens the foundations on which the institutions of State and Church are erected."[109] Such insight nevertheless remains in tension with his ascetic insistence, made in the penultimate paragraph of the text, that we "renounc[e] the direct feeling of the independence of [our] own personality" as a precondition to accepting the external determination of our fate.[110]

Undoubtedly, the ambivalence of this conclusion may prove frustrating and "unsatisfactory" to its readers.[111] Most charitably, Lev Nikolaevich means to contest the atomistic concept of Western individualism with a sense of social interdependence that is cognizant of our equality, uniqueness, and oneness, as Eastern Christianity, Daoism, Buddhism, and Sikhism teach, and as his "globe of life" allegory suggests.[112] Truly, Tolstoy's stature as a Russian *philosophe* who unified Enlightenment and Romanticism while supporting the collective liberation of humanity and history from their domination by the State, capital, and Church is more consistent with the anarchist emphasis on collective struggle for freedom than any sense of historical determinism.[113] After all, Tolstoy's practice of "embod[ying] some type of doctrine, conception, learning, thesis, or idea for the reader" in the struggles of his characters is consistent with the Enlightenment practice of refashioning morality plays for progressive purposes.[114]

To this point, Kant, an icon of German idealism, appears numerous times in the text. This happens through veiled allusions—such as to the works of "Abbé Morio," namely, "Perpetual Peace" (1795)—and via Tolstoy's affirmation of cosmopolitan internationalism, which acknowledges humanity's "universal community" and attendant rights.[115] In avowing the metaphysical reason of *Vernunft*/сознание as an autonomous and productive force, Tolstoy closely follows Kant's formulation of the categorical imperative as a human rather than divine commandment: one to be best observed through global humanist Enlightenment.[116] Beyond Bondarchuk's cinematic depiction of General Prince Nikolai Bolkonsky as a Kantian avatar, the "queer big fellow" (странный большой человек) Pierre begins laughing uncontrollably at his captivity—his reduction by the French to a mere means, in violation of the categorical imperative. Then, he

> glanced up at the sky and the twinkling stars in its far-away depths. "And all that is in me, all that is within me, and it is all I!" thought Pierre. "And they caught all that and put it into a shed boarded up with planks!"[117]

Bezukhov contemplates the stars above, and considers his own internal strength (сила), intuitively sensing the common mineral elements we contain as stellar human beings, or ideal-material emblems of individual and collective resilience and transcendence in the face of death and loss. Following Prince Andrei's discovery of the meaning of love through confronting finitude, Peter Kirillich will experience a profoundly animating sense of union with all (всежизнь) at this most extreme alienation from others.[118] At last, he lies down to rest with his comrades. This meditative thought-image is unambiguously a restatement of the conclusion to Kant's *Critique of Practical Reason*:

> Two things fill the mind with ever new and increasing admiration and awe, the oftener and the more steadily we reflect on them: *the starry heavens above and the moral law within.*[119]

As well, celestial imagery connotative of human dignity and queer sexual union will adorn the night sky to anticipate the end of the war, when the Russians welcome French deserters, in a verbal icon conveying the Christian love of neighbor, "enemy," and Other.[120]

Notes

1 Tolstoy 2010: 1041.
2 *Ibid* 1043; Orwin 1993: 105. In parallel, Feuerbach notes, "[t]he law holds man in bondage; love makes him free" (Feuerbach 48).
3 Zorin 115; Tolstoy 2010: 1044–7.
4 Bartlett 2011: 4, 184; Tolstoy 2010: 1047, 1085.
5 Gustafson 1986: 78.
6 Fuchs 10.
7 Zorin 18; Clark 2019: 184–90; Milivojevic 1991; Stites 1989.
8 Carpenter 1919: 33–56; Chodorow 1999; Rancour-Laferriere 1995.
9 Freud 1961b: 57.
10 Gilman-Opalsky.
11 Tolstoy 2010: 1045.
12 *Ibid* 1090; Orwin 1993: 131–2.
13 Orwin 1993: 137, 204.
14 Tolstoy 2010: 983–91, 1051. Compare the nursing of Tolstoy's dying brother Dmitri by the latter's partner Masha and Aunt Ergolskaya in 1856 (Maude 1987a: 148).
15 Tolstoy 2010: 1053–5; Orwin 1993: 128.
16 Tolstoy 2010: 1055.

17 Gregg 18.
18 Chekhov 2004.
19 Bondarchuk; Bloom 73n9; Tolstoy 2010: 1053–7.
20 Tolstoy 2010: 1057–8.
21 *Ibid* 1058. Similarly, according to Feuerbach: "Love is God himself, and apart from it there is no God. Love makes man [*sic*] God and God man" (Feuerbach 48).
22 Gustafson 1986: 70; Tolstoy 2010: 1059.
23 Gustafson 1986: 71; Orwin 1988: 21.
24 Rancour-Laferriere 1995: 96.
25 Tolstoy 2010: 1060; Berdyaev 2009: 54.
26 Tolstoy 2010: 1062, 1109.
27 *Ibid* 1066, 1077; Evtuhov et al. 327.
28 Clay.
29 Isaiah 13: 11.
30 Tolstoy 2010: 1077, 1104–6; Plokhy 250.
31 Tolstoy 2010: 1110; Lieven 2012: 18.
32 Tolstoy 2010: 1111–14; 2004: 327–8; Lieven 2012: 21; Forrest 67. After all, the Geneva Conventions would not come into effect for more than a century after the Napoleonic Wars.
33 Tolstoy 2010: 732–3, 1111.
34 James; Buck-Morss.
35 James; La Botz 138; Tolstoy 2010: 1177.
36 Plokhy 278–82.
37 Bellamy 2001c.
38 Tolstoy 2010: 1092–6, 1127–47; Orwin 2002c: 227.
39 Berdyaev 1966: 40–2; Evtuhov et al. 511; Dostoevsky 1990; Tolstoy 2010: 1199.
40 Tolstoy 2010: 1140–5; Orwin 1993: 108; Orwin 1988: 20.
41 Orwin 1988: 20–1; Tolstoy 2010; 983–91, 1146, 1162. Countess Natalia's grief almost presages Countess Sofia Tolstaya's own bereavement over the loss of her seven-year-old son Ivan (Vanechka) in 1895 (Zorin 144–7; Bartlett 2011: 357–8).
42 Reitz 146.
43 Fone 14.
44 Tolstoy 2010: 1189; Harris; Lazar.
45 Gustafson 1986: 103–4, 233, 284, 372; Ziarek 135.
46 Benjamin 173.
47 Gustafson 1986: 317; Gilman-Opalsky 251.
48 Tolstoy 2010: 1145.
49 Newlin 381–2; Bartlett 2011: 44.
50 Tolstoy 2010: 1146.
51 Gustafson 1986: 315, 380; Clark 2019: 38; Rule 21; Berdyaev 2009: 21–2.
52 Zorin 131; Gustafson 1986: 102.
53 Tolstaya 2014b: 137.
54 Yalom 483.
55 Gustafson 1986: 176, 291–2, 401; Yalom.
56 Tolstoy 2010: 1199–203; Orwin 1993: 105.
57 Tolstoy 2010: 1189, 1204.
58 Compare how Putin's 2015 intervention in Syria prepared the ground for Russia's 2022 "special military operation" in Ukraine (Borshchevskaya).
59 Tolstoy 2010: 1219–20, 1232–4 (emphasis in original).
60 Orwin 2002a: 49; 1993: 10.
61 Bondarchuk; Tolstoy 2010: 1258.
62 Chouliaraki.
63 Newton; Tolstoy 2010: 1262–3.
64 Tolstoy 2010: 1244–5, 1264.
65 *Ibid* 1236, 1243 (emphasis in original).

66 Cruise 196; Healey 52.
67 Bartlett 2014: 11.
68 Orwin 1993: 107–9.
69 *Ibid* 163.
70 Vinitsky 84; Orwin 2013: 109.
71 Tolstoy 2010: 1247.
72 Clay 212.
73 Berlin 1978: 43.
74 Orwin 1993: 150–1.
75 Tolstoy 2010: 1270 (emphasis added).
76 Berlin 1978: 43; Orwin 1993: 168.
77 Tolstoy 2010: 1274.
78 Berlin 1978: 34–5.
79 Tolstoy 2010: 1273. In *The Decembrists*, the incomplete sequel to *War and Peace*, Lev Nikolaevich describes how during the repulsion of Napoleon's forces in 1812 and following the Russian Empire's loss in the Crimean War in 1856, the *Narod* "found themselves in indescribable enthusiasm" (Tolstoy 2017: 2).
80 Tolstoy 1277–8; Толстой 2012b: 477.
81 Berlin 1978: 55; Tolstoy 2010: 1276–7; Berdyaev 1966: 67.
82 Tolstoy 2010: 1279–85 (emphasis added).
83 *Ibid* 1292 (emphasis in original).
84 *Ibid* 1289; Child J.
85 Tolstoy 2010: 1292; Толстой 2012b: 488; Bakunin 2005.
86 Tolstoy 2010: 1291; Abromeit.
87 Orwin 2002a: 52.
88 Gustafson 1986. After all, in 1895, Tolstoy will write that free will "is God within us" (Gustafson 1986: 10).
89 Rancour-Laferriere 1995: 69–77.
90 Tolstoy 2010: 1293–5, 1302.
91 Poole.
92 Beiner. As though to anticipate Heidegger, one Russian proverb goes, "We are born not for life, but for death" (Rancour-Laferriere 1995: 75).
93 Marcuse 1955.
94 Berlin 1978: 41, 56.
95 Orwin 2012b: 101.
96 Welch 181.
97 Becker 52, 269.
98 Rancour-Lafarriere 1998: 149; Kaufman and Paul.
99 Berlin 1978: 53–6, 63; Orwin 1993: 8–22.
100 Venturi 138.
101 Herzen 155.
102 Chernyshevsky 232–3.
103 Gustafson 1986; Venturi 167–9; Berdyaev 1966: 123.
104 Berlin 1978: 229.
105 Zorin 47–9; Bartlett 2011: 147–8. *Kumys* is soured and fermented mare's milk, believed to have healing properties (Maude 1987a: 280; Zorin 51).
106 Kropotkin 1991: 128.
107 Denner 2001: 16; Berdyaev 2009: 150.
108 Tolstoy 2010: 1297, 1303–4.
109 Tolstoy 2010: 1308; Orwin 2012a: 1; Bakunin 1973: 125; Freud 1961b: 83.
110 Tolstoy 2010: 1308.
111 Welch 184.
112 Rapp; Takhar.
113 Berlin 1978: 239–41; Orwin 2012a: 6.
114 Polosina 55.

115 Kant 1991: 105–8.
116 Reitz 104–5.
117 Tolstoy 2010: 1097–8; Толстой 2012b: 344.
118 Gustafson 1986: 80.
119 Kant 2004: 170 (emphasis in original).
120 Tolstoy 2010: 1178–80; Gustafson 1986: 282–3.

10

CONCLUSION

The Psychodynamics of Hierarchy

To conclude *Queer Tolstoy*, let us summarize some of the enduring themes, lessons, and doctrines presented by Tolstoy in "The Sevastopol Sketches" (1855), *The Cossacks* (1863), *War and Peace* (1869), and *Hadji Murat* (1912).

In the numerous literary works Lev Nikolaevich Tolstoy produced in life, he expresses themes critical of militarism, imperialism, capitalism, heteronormativity, and social hierarchy—with the notable exceptions of his ultra-sexist views, and of the unresolved tension between Russian chauvinism and cosmopolitan internationalism in his guiding philosophy. Constructively, Tolstoy celebrates humanism; egalitarianism; mindfulness; residence; and the iconoclastic destruction of master symbols, impersonalization, and coercive institutions via homoerotic union and political struggle.

Instead of the non-consensual sadomasochism and authoritarianism encoded by labor exploitation, war, and sexual abuse, Tolstoy proposes mutual recognition, communion, reciprocal belonging, "generalized reciprocity," and "co-operative autonomy" as philosophies and life-strategies that would permit respect for the interrelated connection and independence of all humanity.[1] In mutual recognition, or humane bonding—which by definition cannot be realized through obedience, self-subordination, or repression—Eros invites interdependent participation among partners, intimacy "without demanding control," and union "without obliterating difference."[2]

Through their youthful military service in Transcaucasia, Olenin/Tolstoy discover their sympathies with the oppressed Chechens and their estrangement from the project of Tsarist expansionism, just as they find newfound loves among the Cossacks, of both same and opposite sex. In the posthumous *Hadji Murat*, the prose writer returns to the Caucasian chronotope to imagine the end of the life of the titular character, an out-of-place, courageous Avar chieftain, who launches a doomed bid to save his family and escape into the mountains. In this novella, Lev

DOI: 10.4324/9781003328964-10

Nikolaevich integrates an implicit support for self-determination of the Muslim peoples of the Caucasus region with his Christian-anarchist, anarcho-Populist, and homoerotic idealization of "natural men" as harbingers of freedom.[3]

Likewise in *War and Peace*, the author applies a dual critique of the inter-imperialist conflict between Tsarism and Bonapartism to convey a humanistic anarchist critique of bureaucratic authoritarianism and class exploitation. This anticipates the fully developed Christian-anarchist vision he will espouse in *The Kingdom of God Is Within You, Resurrection*, and other works from his later period. However, in reality, from the very start of his writing career during the Crimean War, in "The Sevastopol Sketches," the war correspondent presented the actual consequences of the bellicose decisions of States in highly realistic, tragic, and humanizing terms. *War and Peace* is but the pinnacle of Tolstoy's anti-war correspondence.

Russian Nationalism, Non-Cooperation with Evil, and Forms of Reason

In the previous chapters, we explored many of the major themes of *War and Peace* at length. These include a satire of Russia's social aristocracy; a critique of war, its parallel labor, and the authority principle; critique of the abuse of animals; examinations of the relationship between life and death; and recurrent homoeroticism and misogyny. In closing, let us take up some of the most pressing controversies and doubts we have about Tolstoy's symbol-system and thought process, as revealed in this *poema*. Our questions revolve around the author's attitudes toward Russian nationalism, non-cooperation with evil, and different forms of reason.

Firstly, while a spirit of internationalism, humanism, and anti-militarism consonant with Christian anarchism predominates in *War and Peace*, it is also true that its author promotes Slavophilism and Russian patriotism in the *poema*. In Tolstoy's defense, the novelist also celebrates Rousseauvist compassion among both Russian and French commanders toward their respective prisoners of war. Petya and the Cossacks in his detachment welcome a captive French drummer-boy, Vincent, whom they endearingly call Prince Vesenka (suggestive of весна, or spring), to eat with them as one family of "ant-brothers."[4] In like fashion, in his victory address—made shortly before dying after he was discharged and replaced, on Tolstoy's account, for having openly opposed the Tsar's drive to extend the war beyond the frontiers of the Empire—Kutuzov displays an anarcho-Populist and cosmopolitan idealization of the united sense of "majestic triumph combined with *pity for the foe* and consciousness of the justice of our cause," as felt deeply by the common soldiers and *Narod* alike.[5] Tolstoy and his spokesperson Kutuzov both recognize how the French rank-and-file troops were very often "soldiers of necessity" of peasant stock, much like the serf base of the Russian army itself, and they avoid derogating or "belittl[ing] the enemy" accordingly.[6]

Another way in which Tolstoy channels human unity is the number of allusions, implicit and explicit, he makes to Daoism and Buddhism in *War and Peace*. He does so by avowing *wu-wei*, or non-action, and integrating affirmations of compassion with depictions of *samsara, dukkha, anitya,* and *karma.* His affirmation of *wu-wei* recalls the Daoist strategy of calling on sages to sacrifice their privileges to disintegrate the artifice of imperial power, and so allow society to return to its ostensibly more cooperative and organic prior nature.[7] To be sure, such iconoclasm is consistent with the spirit of the holy fool. Indeed, one of the central conflicts of *War and Peace* revolves around the tension between the Kingdom of Caesar and the authority principle, which may be interpreted as various forms of *avidya* (ignorance), arrayed against the Kingdom of God, which is to be attained through the awakening of the mind.

Paradoxically, despite his advocacy of anti-militarist, anti-statist enlightenment, Tolstoy represses contemplation of the Russian army's deployment of over a half-million troops beyond the Empire's western borders, its vanguard role in the anti-Napoleonic campaign in 1813–1814 and the Holy Alliance in the post-war setting, and its vengeful march on and subsequent occupation of Paris. He omits how the Romanovs aimed to "establish Restoration Europe" and subsequently lord over the continent as policemen.[8] He fails to explicitly recognize, much less denounce, the Russian Empire's self-concept as a "Third Rome," following the fall of Rome and Constantinople in the fifth and fifteenth centuries, respectively.[9]

In this light, Lev Nikolaevich may have been avoiding covering events that would have required him to take up a more explicitly critical stance toward the Russian military than we find in *War and Peace.* At the least, this would have involved expanding on Andrei and Bilibin's critiques of the "direct appropriation by violence" engaged in by Russian troops. In parallel, the author evidently ignored the role played by General Barclay in both ordering the army's initial retreat into the Russian interior and spearheading the counter-attack that ultimately defeated the *Grand Armée.*[10] It is therefore apparent that Tolstoy at times uses historical sources "on his own terms," and his celebration of the *Narod*'s victory over the *Grand Armée* may point to an entrenchment of Great-Russian chauvinism that undermines his anarchist ideal.[11] While his encounter with the *Narod* informs his messianic Populism, his lack of open denunciation of the crystallization of the millenarian idea of the Imperial State in the *poema* suggests that Evelina Zaidenshnur and Alexander Gulin may have been right to interpret it as nationalistic.[12]

Secondly, we find in *War and Peace* numerous creative historical examples of individual and mass-resistance and non-cooperation with the various evils of both the story and our own world, based in authority. The emergence of resistance and disobedience speaks to the great emancipatory potential of collective action, and to Faure's point that "[p]eace will not come from on high, but from below."[13] The scenes depicting non-cooperation and the metahistorical essays proposing an anarcho-Populist interpretation of history both seek the creation of a cooperative commonwealth, based on the precept that "*Labor Omnia Vincit*" (Labor Conquers All).[14] This radical hopefulness is consistent with anti-oppression theory, which proposes that the resistance taken up by the oppressed is the harbinger of collective liberation.[15]

On Tolstoy's account, the *Grand Armée* is defeated and driven out of Russia due to four elements of mass-resistance carried out by the *Narod*—namely, the battle of Borodino, the popular abandonment of Moscow, the peasants' systematic burning of hay to starve the French military's draft animals, and the partisan and formal military struggle. At the individual, social, and political levels, Princess Marya Bolkonskaya, Natasha Rostova, and Platon Karataev proclaim and observe the Christian law of love, while Pierre commits himself first to Freemasonry. He and Prince Andrei will take advantage of Tsar Alexander's law on free agriculturalists to renegotiate the terms governing the bonded labor of the serfs "belonging" to their estates—but not seemingly go so far as to abolish their enserfment, much less endorse the abolition of classes altogether. Like the writer, at least at this time, the *poema*'s male protagonists focus more on estate management than social transformation.[16] That being said, again like the poet, they do flirt with the ideas of self-denial, and both end up engaging in revolutionary suicide: Prince Andrei, by joining the rank-and-file troops at Borodino, and Pierre, by joining the Decembrist cause.

Along these lines, Lev Nikolaevich's portrayal of the bloodthirsty peasants at the Bogucharovo manor is certainly not sympathetic or consistent with radical Populism. This lapse mirrors Tolstoy's philosophical inconsistency, his affirmation of the interests of the Russian landowning class, his distorted sense of identity, *and* his own experiences encountering resistance from the serfs of the Yasnaya Polyana manor to his paternalistic proposals to liberate them.[17] The literary critic Viktor Shklovsky is therefore right to be concerned that Tolstoy overlooks the anti-statist elements of peasant upheaval in 1812, while emphasizing its anti-French sentiments.[18] Tellingly, there is no explicit recognition in *War and Peace* of Napoleon's threat to emancipate Russia's serfs from above.[19]

In a similar vein, Pierre momentously justifies his Decembrist membership to Count Rostov by explaining that the constitutionalism sought by this rebel-society would be less destructive to their class interests than would be a repetition of the Pugachëv uprising—an outcome that could be foreseen without such political changes.[20] In this sense, we perceive the continuum linking Tolstoy's voluntarist approach to social change with Alexander I's autocratic resistance to implementing constitutional reforms and considering the abolition of serfdom; the Gandhian *Sarvodaya* ("common-welfare") movement's espousal of the redistribution of land on the terms of the landlords themselves; and confirmation of Orwin's trepidation over the limitations and even dangers of Populism as a cross-class ideology and organizing strategy.[21] Even if Pierre proclaims revolutionary suicide by joining the Decembrists, there is still considerable risk in such a top-down strategy.

Although Populism can serve the cause of unity and help promote egalitarianism, projects informed by such a spirit can simultaneously function to re-entrench boundaries between in-groups and out-groups along the lines of sex/gender, class, caste, nation, and/or race or ethnicity. Tolstoy demonstrates this in book three of *War and Peace*, when he finds nationalistic meaning in the tragic circumstances of the battle of Borodino, and Moscow's burning. In short, while many of the elements of resistance and non-cooperation depicted in the *poema* are consistent with

Tolstoy's Christian anarchism, readers must await his later works for a more consistent exposition of this prophetic philosophy.

Thirdly, Lev Nikolaevich counterposes life and death and their understandings according to different forms of reason, following Goethe's color theory, which takes after Kant's critiques. Tolstoy focuses on Eros and Thanatos, while recurrently exploring death-anxiety and grief in their existential dimensions. Ultimately, Pierre reaches a profound understanding through imagination and intuition (*Phantasie* [red] and *Verstand*/разум [blue]), whereas the Bolkonskys typify *Vernunft*/сознание (metaphysical reason, yellow), and the Rostovs *Sinnlichkeit* (sensibility, green)—this, on the individual, social, and political levels. Even so, Tolstoy appears by the *poema*'s end to endorse a harmonic (or circular) view of reason that mimics the Earth's natural cycles. The writer is evidently concerned with the "march of generations"; the circle of life; and his view of the symbiosis between war and peace, life and death, and joy and sorrow.[22]

To an extent, this dynamic uncovering of the cycles of death and resurrection over the course of the text softens the tragedies to which it gives life: the wars and invasion of Russia, the destruction of Moscow, and the deaths of Petya, Platon Karataev, Lise, Nikolai, and Andrei, standing in for those killed in the war of 1812 more broadly. Still, muses the author, if death is just another phase of existence akin to life, why must we fear it? If Petya's death is supposed to reflect some "mysterious and harmonious scheme of balance in the universe," does this not dampen its tragic nature?[23] According to the doctrine of harmonic reason, the novel's conclusion illustrating domestic equilibrium is "no more the goal of life" than the war and devastation preceding it.[24] Yes, suffering, decline, loss, and death are painful and difficult for all of us, but finitude is a fundamental element of the human condition, bounded as we are by physical and natural laws. Notably, the decomposition performed by fungi is essential for the biosphere's health.[25] As though to recognize this ecological dynamic, in Russian, the verb to die, умирать, contains the root for peace and world, мир. The truth of suffering, governing the life of all is, indeed, the first noble truth of Buddhism. Berdyaev recognizes it, as well.[26]

At the same time, in the "original" version of *War and Peace*, from 1867, neither Andrei nor Petya dies.[27] Speculatively, Lev Nikolaevich's unresolved conflicts over death-anxiety, and the demoralization he experienced after reading Schopenhauer—whose theories pose a fundamental challenge to the vital Tolstoyan ideas of "living reason" and human dignity—may well have led to his delirium in September 1869, known as the "Arzamas horror."[28] Though he spent the summer after the completion of *War and Peace* active and in good spirits, skiing, gardening, mowing, and learning ancient Greek—the last, to provide his first son Sergei with a classical education, and so that he could translate Aesop's tales for his *ABC* (Азбука)—he soon fell into a depression that could be described as having metaphorically postpartum dimensions. This was "a crisis of vocation experienced upon the completion of a major work."[29] In "Notes of a Madman" (1884), recalling this experience, the artist presents the "sense of being lost without purpose on a journey toward death in a foreign place."[30]

On the other hand, it is not necessarily true that an acknowledgment of harmonic reason betrays humanistic ethics. Though Petya, Andrei, and Platon perish, the continuation of social life afterward is no celebration of their deaths. It is just reality. Tolstoy's world in the *poema* is perpetually moving, as the stream of life is continuously flowing.[31] Even so, in *War and Peace*, similar unresolved tensions manifest in Tolstoy's thought between the artist's anarcho-Populist, Christian-anarchist, and anti-militarist normative framework, vs. his apparent belief in predestination and determinism. To an extent, this implicit endorsement of harmonic reason in *War and Peace* may speak to his affinities with the French conservative Joseph de Maistre, as with Schopenhauer, whom he discovered in 1868, in place of a strong and unambiguous commitment to Enlightenment and/or Hegelian-idealist principles of freedom, reason, and liberation. Arguably, Tolstoy's psychical masochism and impulsivity are manifesting here, undermining his self-efficacy.[32]

An uncompromising objection to harmonic reason may admittedly betray a bias in favor of linear reason, as embodied by the Bolkonskys, as well as mimic Schopenhauer, Freud, and other European theorists' own misperceptions of Buddhism as a life-negating philosophy, and Nirvana as life's renunciation. Such Orientalist, so-called Buddhologist perspectives run the considerable risk of missing the pronounced affinities that exist between Eastern Christianity and dharmic religions, including their common monastic, ascetic, and neo-Platonic features, as well as of rendering invisible the Buddhist Buryat and Kalmyk subjects of the Russian Empire.[33] Such reductiveness would furthermore overlook the affinities between Tolstoy's championing of "holy foolishness" and the philosophy of neo-Hinduist *bhakti*, a religion of loving devotion that centers the contrast between separation and unity.[34]

Though symbolized in Tolstoy's art by the image of the blowing-out of the candle that anticipates the deaths of Prince Andrei and Anna Karenina, Nirvana does not presuppose the extinction of existence, as many Western observers have claimed. Rather, it suggests life's cooling, transformation, or pacification—as experienced by Olenin in the stag's lair in *The Cossacks*. Understood as "oneness with the absolute, the bliss in experiencing one's identity with a transcendent compassion for all reality," Nirvana so closely resembles Tolstoy's desire for the Kingdom of God—the very "replacement of struggle and violence with love and accord"—that the two may by all means be considered mutual conceptual restatements of each other.[35] Siddhartha Gautama Buddha, Rousseau, Tolstoy, Ursula Le Guin, Herbert Marcuse, and the anarchistic psychoanalysts Otto Gross and Erich Fromm all concurred with the utopian proposition that collective liberation begins with inner liberation.[36]

In parallel, despite that the Daoist concept of *wu-wei* resembles masochistic non-resistance, and so threatens to "ruin the prospects which open [...] in the real world," and even to amount to suicide, the *dharma* and the *Dao* can be viewed as equally consistent with an anti-masochistic socio-political orientation. To this point, the Buddha's *dharma* teaches that "sorrow [and] evil [are] due to ignorance of the true nature of reality and a false conception of the self," while *wu-wei* suggests non-cooperation with evil. These perspectives are in turn consistent with the

Tolstoyan critique of artifice and intoxication, the classical Hindu idea of illusion (*maya*), and the Frommian concern for the various anti-social mechanisms with which one may seek to escape from freedom: namely, authoritarianism, destructiveness, and automaton conformity.[37]

This is not to overlook the gross injustices and abuses committed in the name of Buddhism, as seen especially in the 2017 genocide carried out in Myanmar/Burma by the predominantly Buddhist-run military against the Rohingya Muslim minority, much less the atrocities carried out by the army against protesters, youth, ethnic-minority communities, and workers since the February 2021 coup, including the use of scorched-earth tactics.[38] Neither is it to overlook the authoritarianism of Hindu-supremacists, as seen particularly in Occupied Kashmir and against Muslim minorities in India proper, especially since the accession of Modi's administration in 2014. We equally disavow ignoring the injustices and abuses carried out by fundamentalists in the name of Christianity or any other religion, including state and political religions.

In keeping with such a transnational, Christian-anarchist spirit, Gary Morson perceives in Tolstoy's Kutuzov a Daoist sage, and Jeff Love beholds in Platon Karataev a Master Zhuang, author of the foundational Daoist text *Zhuangzhi* (c. third century BCE). Such global associations suggest that the writer's anarcho-Populist vision, beyond its Slavophilic rootedness in the *Narod*, incorporates not only insights from the Buddhism practiced by Buryat and Kalmyk ethnic minorities within the Tsarist Empire, but also from the Daoism of China, plus Western rationalist influences, such as Kantianism and the *Vernunft*/сознание embodied by the Bolkonskys.[39]

Eros and Authority, Part III: Queer Anarchism and the Kingdom of God

Fourthly, Tolstoy includes homoerotic *and* misogynistic commentary throughout *War and Peace*, as though to convey his political-sexual preference for "free association among men."[40] Whereas expressions of homosocial or homoerotic desire by themselves cannot be compared to patriarchal domination as ethically problematic, we find that breaking the taboo on the multidimensionality of human sexuality often triggers Tolstoy into proclaiming sexism. Paradoxically, then, Lev Nikolaevich's case provides evidence for Nancy Chodorow's charge that Herbert Marcuse's vision of an Orphic Marxism, in rejecting "normal Eros," conveys an ostensible "rejection of women."[41]

This becomes clear at the beginning of *War and Peace*, when Prince Andrei expresses his preference to visit with Pierre rather than his wife late at night in the *andron* (men's quarters) after the *soirée* at Anna Pavlovna's. As if imagining himself within the homosocial and deeply homoerotic atmosphere of Plato's *Symposium*, Andrei—referring to his wife Lise—effectively repeats the physician Eryximachos' demand that the "piping-girl who has just come in may go out again, [...so] that to[night] we entertain each other with talk."[42] To accept Jeff Love's likening of Pierre to Sancho Panza, and thus of Andrei to Quixote, is edifying in this sense, considering the homophilic relationship between the two in Miguel de Cervantes' timeless novel, which affirms a "desublimated" or spiritual homosexuality.[43]

Prince Bolkonsky is perceptibly stuck in an unwanted or "official" straight marriage, and prefers to keep the company of Pierre, whom he prefers both to the artifice of high society, as to the superficiality and narcissism to which Andrei reduces the being of all women.[44] By expressing such attitudes, he conveys the sexism of his father, General Prince Nikolai Andreevich, who tries to impart upon Andrei at their separation before the War of the Third Coalition that women are a "bad business," yet "one can't unmarry."[45] Significantly, such homoerotic disregard for half of humanity echoes the extreme misogyny expressed not only by Eryximachos, Pausanias, and others from Plato's *Symposium*, but also by Schopenhauer in his 1851 essay on women. We know Tolstoy was reading this German idealist when finishing *War and Peace*.[46] Though Edward Carpenter cites the sexologist Otto de Joux's observation that gay men often serve as the "most convinced defenders" of women, this unfortunately does not apply in the case of queer Tolstoy.[47]

In parallel, the *poema* features plenty of gay and lesbian desire, as well as the creation of transient queer communes. Some instances of Tolstoy detailing humanity's polymorphously perverse sexuality within the stifling atmosphere of Tsarist Russia include the affection evinced between Captain Tushin and his "uncle," as well as Tushin and Andrei, at the battle of Schön-Grabern; between soldiers and officers for Kutuzov upon his entrance and retirement; between Tsar Alexander and the Russian army at Olmütz; between Princess Marya and Julie Karagina, and between Pierre and Andrei; by Nikolai Rostov toward Sonya, presenting in drag; by Natasha toward the skilled peasant chef Anisya Fëdorovna; by the young factory worker who approaches Pierre as they confront summary execution in occupied Moscow; by Prince Andrei's attending surgeon at Borodino, whose kiss returns Bolkonsky to life; between Bezukhov and Platon Karataev; and between Petya and the partisan Dolokhov, who intimately and courageously disguise themselves as French soldiers in the rearguard of the retreating *Grand Armée* to liberate Pierre and the other prisoners. Above all, Tolstoy's ideal gay love is conveyed in the verbal icon depicting the fleeting relationship between Petya and Dolokhov, which returns to the tantalizing bond established between Bolkonsky and Tushin at Schön-Grabern (as well as between Olenin and Lukashka in *The Cossacks*). Petya and Dolokhov collaborate in the critical task of emancipating their imprisoned compatriots and consummate their love in a kiss, but then Petya sacrifices himself leading the cavalry charge.[48] In this case, Petya exchanges a brief experience of sensual union for death, whereas Andrei held back and deferred finitude—though not for long.

Apropos, immediately upon returning to the theater of war from the abandoned Bald Hills estate, Prince Andrei watches as his men bathe collectively: "Everywhere on the bank, on the dam, and in the pond, there was healthy, white, muscular flesh." Then again, Bolkonsky is taken aback by their "dirty," or mortal, presentation. Intimating his revulsion, the prince's minions will clear the pond out of troops. Cut off from the swarm, the Stranger bathes alone. In this way, Tolstoy recurs to his sexual pleasure vs. guilt conflict, which perpetuates his erotic unhappiness.[49]

The scene, in turn, recalls the medieval Russian tradition of the *banya*, or communal bathhouse, popularly known as "the people's first doctor"—before vodka and raw garlic, that is. This ancestral homosocial space, which carried connotations of sexual union, disinhibition, pre-Oedipal relatedness with the mother, *and* the washing of corpses, was targeted for elimination by Peter I, who imported Western homonegativity to Russia.[50] Bathhouses in pre-revolutionary Russian cities were known as sites of an emerging gay subculture, where men from distinct social classes mingled for the purposes of sex work and/or erotic satisfaction.[51]

Accordingly, Tolstoy's utilization of *banya* imagery here is an unstated affirmation of Slavophilic resistance to Tsarism and an ambivalently masochistic approach to homoerotic lust. Lev Nikolaevich repeatedly portrays gay desire as animating but then subverting the desire for union and residence. More successfully than Tolstoy here, Herman Melville's novels often trace the journey of the author's ego-persona toward union with a "Dark Stranger" through rebellion against the prototypical Captain. In other words, as a gothic humanist, Melville anticipates the consummation of homoerotic desires among working men as a rejection of heteropatriarchal command structures.[52] In like manner, the observance of same-sex love was widespread among the Russian peasantry, and in his recently discovered early-nineteenth century diary, the English farmer Matthew Tomlinson normalizes same-sex attraction and behavior as natural, while denouncing its criminalization by the State.[53]

The water motif linking the pond to the *banya* imparts the political and sexual dimensions of the artist's Populist ideal. Through an anarchic sense of kenosis, Tolstoy hoped that the *Narod* would secure a bright future via an emotional and erotic approximation with ostensibly enlightened nobles, who in turn would abolish their privilege through descent.[54] An anarchist understanding of the scene can be further appreciated, if we juxtapose this and other queer chronotopes in *War and Peace* with the Athenian Pausanias's association of the repression of same-sex love, philosophy, and sports with despotism: "I suppose it is profitable to their rulers that the subjects should not be great in spirit or make strong friendships and unions, which things love [Eros] is wont to implant more than anything else."[55]

In marked contrast to the social teachings of Christian churches, which arbitrarily empower a priestly caste to regulate human sexuality, and the artificial-bourgeois utopia, which is imparted through social exclusivity, the proletarian "romantic utopia" is expressed through chance encounters and union.[56] Like Melville's sailors, who create an "erotic fraternity [...] that takes the form of a democratic union of equals," Tolstoy's bathing soldiers create a plebian "queer counterpublic" and celebrate the republican principles reportedly observed in Slavic communalism by emblematically washing away the artificiality and uselessness of Tsarism and the Orthodox Church.[57]

It is evident from such symbols, thoughts, and descriptions that the count presents conventionally attractive young Russian men as the embodiment of the "Adonis Complex" and *kalokagathia*, or the collective unification of physical and moral beauty with socio-political good.[58] Indeed, only in the wake of the overthrow of the tyrants of ancient Greece (900–500 BCE) could homoerotic and democratic cultures flourish openly. Remarkably, Tolstoy's expressions of collective queerness recall Clausewitz's "final word" on war, for in the latter's late return to the existential dimensions he had explored in youth, and his late transcendence of the strictly instrumentalist approach for which he is probably best-known, the German general proposed a trinity of *Gewalt* (violence), *Kampf* (struggle), and "the affiliation of the combatants to a cohesive community."[59] Analogously, against the Nietzschean "illusion of the superman," the critical theorist Karl Wittfogel proposed "comradeship and collective heroism as antidotes to the fetishism [of commodities]."[60]

To this very point, the gay designer C. R. Ashbee (1863–1942), who took after the utopian socialist William Morris (1834–1896), recognized how an "unconscious faith" in comrade-love, together with the "freer, more direct, and more genuine relationship between men, which is implied by it," may well have bolstered the "solidarity of labour and the modern Trade-Union movement."[61] According to the researcher Piro Subrat, intimate ties existed among the syndicalist, anti-capitalist, and LGBTQ+ movements that emerged in Spain during the transition to formal democracy, in the wake of May 1968 in Paris and the Stonewall uprising of 1969. In these terms, the interviews with queer people that were published in the left-wing magazine *Interviú* contributed to the decriminalization of same-sex relations in Spain in 1979.[62]

Intriguingly, Count Tolstoy dedicates space to considering the mutual lesbian attraction between Marya Bolkonskaya and Julie Karagina, as revealed in love letters avowedly having to do with each other's looming arranged marriages—inexorably, with men.[63] As he drew on Titov's diary as a documentary source for Pierre's gay-masonic dream diary, so Tolstoy adapted letters written between the maid of honour M. A. Volkova and her confidante V. A. Lanskaia over a six-year period beginning in 1812 as a source for this correspondence.[64] In *War and Peace*, Princess Marya blushes upon receipt of a letter from Julie, her "most intimate" childhood friend, who laments their physical separation since "last summer," and hints at their reunion and renewed partnership following a courageous mutual renunciation of conventional heterosexist marriage, otherwise known as the requisite "going behind men" (выходя/выйдя замуж). Within this context, Julie bemusedly remarks that so many ladies should approach Pierre, the new Count Bezukhov, for marriage, insinuating that he is just as queer as they (and Tolstoy).[65] In her reply, Princess Marya acknowledges her vital love for Julie, but remains distant from her suggestively bold implications, resigning herself instead to the "matrimonial plan" (план супружества) being prepared for her. Anticipating Freud's point about the link between sexual dissatisfaction and emotional unhappiness, Bolkonskaya remarks that she "look[s] on marriage [брак] as a divine institution to which we must conform."[66]

In contrast to the enlivening bonds forged among Russian soldiers, officers, and partisans, and between Julie and Marya, Napoleon makes his entrance to the *poema* discovering the fallen Prince Andrei, who is still clutching the phallic Russian standard on the Austerlitz killing fields. Bonaparte, the "absolute Stranger," has a voice the narrator likens to that of a carrion fly. Looking upon Andrei with a master's mind, he remarks, "*Voilà une belle mort!*"[67] This impulsive admission of homoerotic attraction presages Fromm's theory of necrophilia, defined as a psychopathological "passion to destroy and an attraction to everything that is dead."[68] It communicates sadism, whereby an "aggressive component of the sexual drive that has now become independent and exaggerated [...] has taken on the leading role."[69] While mistaken (considering Andrei is still alive), Napoleon's admiration for the presumed dead broadcasts Tolstoy's judgment of Bonaparte, whose demoniacal will to power demands "'passive-masochistic' surrender" from the Other.[70]

By so idealizing Bolkonsky's apparent corpse, Napoleon is shown to defy the limits of our animality, in a reflection of his mechanically narcissistic, instrumentalist attitude toward his subordinates and enemies. As Tolstoy notes in his diaries, Bonaparte "[r]ejoiced in the dead and wounded."[71] By the same token, Rodion Romanovich Raskolnikov, Dostoevsky's psychotic anti-hero in *Crime and Punishment* (1866), emulates Bonaparte's terrorism by randomly murdering the pawnbroker Alëna Ivanovna and then "strid[ing] onwards and across, without reflecting."[72] Taking into consideration Diotima's discussion with Socrates from the *Symposium*, we see that Napoleon likewise inverts the tragic bonds between classical gay couples, including Alcestis and Admestos, and Achilles and Patroclos, by lusting over a defeated enemy.[73] In his depiction of the scene, Lev Nikolaevich contrasts the unnatural, necrophilous, and cowardly Bonaparte—a slave to the world and the imperialist will—with the biophilous, heroic, and Populist prince, who, like the author, epitomizes unity and contradiction.[74]

The queer feelings expressed among the Russian officers and rank-and-file soldiers, the lesbian would-be couple Marya and Julie, and Petya and Dolokhov may well be healthy and natural, whether as an elemental part of the application of Clausewitz's trinity strategy (violence-struggle-unity) to the Russians' military campaigns, as natural expressions of polymorphously perverse sexuality, or a bit of both. However, when same-sex lust is experienced and expressed by Bonaparte, it reveals his affinities with death, bureaucracy, and militarism. Since Napoleon lacks Andrei's power of love, creativity, and humanist affirmation of life, he perversely seeks out meaning through the "negative transcendence" of militarist destruction, bureaucratic despotism, and the overall objectification of human life.[75] In the links here implicitly drawn by the writer between necrophilia and authoritarianism, considering the ubiquity of masses of slaughtered and maimed soldiers in the chronotope, we can apprehend the historical continuities between the malignant aggression mandated by Bonaparte and Hitler, as commonly autocratic, imperialist invaders of Russia and the Soviet Union who were "below awareness" of the sins they committed.[76]

In psychodynamic terms, the sadistic oppressor is symbiotically dependent upon the willing masochist, who "kneels down like the camel and wishes to be well laden," in the words of Nietzsche.[77] Both sadist and masochist are paradoxically enlivened by the latter's erotic and political self-subordination, while one's destructiveness externalized toward an Other is indissolubly tied to self-destructive impulses.[78] As detailed in *War and Peace*, the political and erotic energies of such "bad gays" as Napoleon and Alexander support this hypothesized psychodynamic.[79]

Andrei Nikolaevich's remaining time, between surviving Austerlitz and succumbing after Borodino, serves as a psychosexual journey of self-discovery, through which Bolkonsky awakens from enthrallment to the "Napoleon myth," otherwise known as "great man" theory; disavows the "mind of the master," which enslaves self and Other; and embraces "new fundamental fantas[ies]" of "repair[ing] the universe" and spiritually uniting with his fellow men.[80] His fateful request to transfer from the high command to fight alongside rank-and-file soldiers before the battle of Borodino crystallizes his newfound queer-anarchist understanding. Like Buddha, Prince Andrei seeks to overcome his estrangement from existence through connecting with others, and seeking both residence and a freedom that would overcome the will to power *and* the imperialistic will through the self-managed development of personality. Indeed, the plot of *War and Peace* attests to the ideas of mutual love and non-cooperation with evil being destituent strategies that prefigure collective emancipation.[81] Against despotic authority, the spiritual aristocrats Andrei, Pierre, Marya, Natasha, Petya, and Platon are beautiful people who stand for the egalitarian legacy of a non-repressive civilization and the Kingdom of God (see Figure 10.1).

Closing Thoughts on Tolstoy's Blatant Sexism and Unconscious Feminism

In closing, we must say that, in light of the otherwise progressive and humanistic vision which Lev Nikolaevich advances in *War and Peace*, it is disgraceful for him to propagate misogyny in the *poema* as he does. His backwardness on the woman question is in keeping with his philosophical mentors, considering the extreme sexism of Rousseau's *Emile, or on Education* (1762) and Proudhon's *Pornocracy, or Women in Modern Times* (1875). Disconcertingly, the Russian prose poet's sexism transmits his identification with Russia's status as "a male chauvinist nation in the extreme," whose *muzhiki* had traditionally revered the Tsar precisely for his toxic masculinity.[82] Tolstoy often describes female characters in *War and Peace* as silly and child-like—namely, Princess

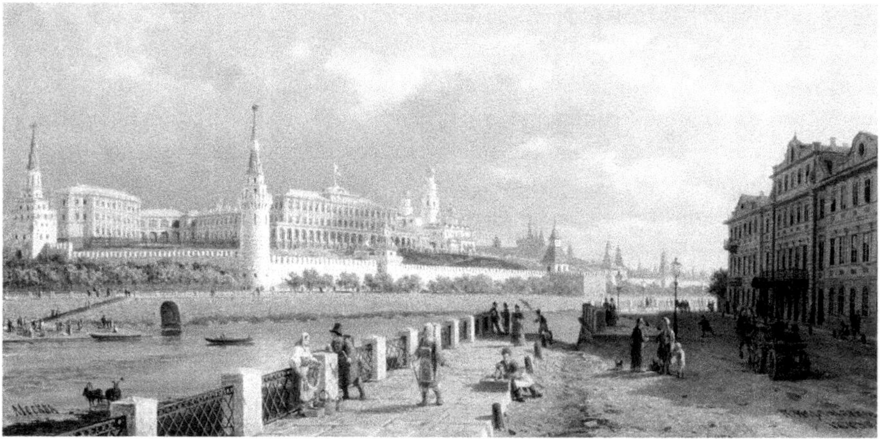

FIGURE 10.1 Peter Vereshchagin, *View of the Moscow Kremlin* (1879)

Katerina Semëvna, Lise, and Hélène Kuragina—and literally compares Sonya to a "pretty, half-grown kitten."[83]

However, mirroring her origin in the poet's emotional memory of his mother, Princess Marya Bolkonskaya is one of the few exceptions to such gross sexism. Lev Nikolaevich portrays her as intelligent and heartfelt, a champion of loving one's neighbor, an advocate of non-resistance and forgiveness, and an aristocrat with compassion for the serfs. As the Slavist Edwina Cruise rightly observes, "her spiritual aspirations propel her into a realm of cerebration otherwise reserved [by Tolstoy] for male characters," in a reflection of the poet's greater interest in men.[84] Whereas Natasha will serve as Andrei's nurse, in an intertextual foreshadowing of Kitty's serving the same role for the dying Nikolai Levin in *Anna Karenina*, Marya's intellectual acumen and contemplativeness allow her to reflect on questions of life and death, for which Tolstoy's other female characters typically show little interest.

To be sure, Lev Nikolaevich associates Natasha's approximation to Anatole in the dim opera house in book two with narcissism, artifice, and a lack of insight. Even worse, the author appears to blame the inexperienced Natasha herself for this near-miss, rather than hold Kuragin to account. Does he not see that the overwhelmingly artificial world in which Rostova is enmeshed blunts her "living reason"?[85] At times, Tolstoy comes close to parroting the sexists of today who resist the #MeToo movement by casting aspersion on victims of abuse, in place of calling for the investigation of sexual assault and intimate partner violence, much less challenging toxic masculinity.

The artist's lapses in this sense are all the more disturbing, when we consider two specific expressions of intent to harm women made in *War and Peace*: namely, the threat Prince Nesvitsky makes, in the presence of his comrades, to violate nuns in a hillside convent as the Russian military crosses the Enns River—evincing a sublimated homoeroticism, plus an Oedipal repudiation of femininity—as well as Pierre's threat to murder Hélène for defying him over his duel with Dolokhov.[86] Such death threats are all the more worrisome in light of the femicidal protagonist Pozdnyshev from Count Tolstoy's later work, "The Kreutzer Sonata" (1889), who will harass and kill his wife out of jealousy and paranoia.[87] Hélène herself dies in mysterious circumstances suggestive of either a fatal attempt at abortion, or complications from a sexually transmitted infection. To consider that Lev Nikolaevich removed Pierre and Andrei's mothers from the final draft of *War and Peace*, and that he exhibits Lise's maternal mortality and Hélène's death through sex, transmits the count's misogynistic hatred of mothers.[88]

Deplorably, this contemptible attitude toward women is not dynamic over the course of *War and Peace*. This is not to claim that Tolstoy ignores violence against women in the War of 1812: he does not, entirely, and he portrays it as being perpetrated by the occupying French and allied military, as well as by Russian men.[89] Pierre is imprisoned for trying to rescue a Caucasian woman and her family from the French. Then again, the novel's finale illustrates family "happiness" through Natasha's traditionalist internalization of her supposed duties as obedient wife, committed mother, and domestic slave. Sadly, the young woman appears "oblivious" to the similarities between the marital bond and "a straitjacket."[90] Henceforth, her husband Pierre will reap the benefits from this domestic despotism that bases itself on the "taming" of Natasha's sensuality and curiosity.[91] In like manner, even his imagined participation in the homosocial Decembrist movement may be taken to further signal his misogyny, considering that, "from beginning to end, [the conspiracy] had been a man's affair." Its societies envisioned life in the future as inexorably traditional, and sought a constitutionalism that would have disenfranchised women.[92]

No surprise, then, that Inessa Armand (1874–1920), the first director of the Zhenotdel, or Women's Department within the Soviet Central Committee (founded in 1919), was appalled when reading in *War and Peace* at the age of 15 that Natasha had only become human upon her marriage to Pierre. Likewise, Tolstoy's younger contemporary critics had decried the *poema*'s affirmation of traditional family values.[93] This problem returns blatantly in *Anna Karenina* and "The Kreutzer Sonata," to such an extent that it can be concluded that—their vast differences on war, religion, labor, and the State to the side—Tolstoy and Stalin actually approached the Tsars and the Orthodox Church in their rank misogyny.[94] Such sexist affinities are not unrelated to the continuities Evelina Zaidenshnur perceives between the "patriotic spirit" of *War and Peace* and Stalin's effective appeal to Tsarist principles of Orthodoxy, autocracy, and nationality during the "Great Patriotic War" against the Nazi invaders.[95]

Whereas David Holbrook reads in the *poema*'s finale the essence of sexist propaganda that would confine "women to the nursery and deprive them of any cultural or intellectual life," in it we can also discern further affirmation of harmonic reason and the passing of time and of the generations.[96] In *War and Peace*, Count Tolstoy contrives an opposition between "clever women" and "real women," forgetting how General Prince Nikolai Bolkonsky had encouraged his daughter Marya to study mathematics in his library. As such, the literary character converges with Mikhail Bakunin's father, Alexander Mikhailovich (1768–1854), and the noted proto-feminist surgeon Nikolai Pirogov (1810–1881), in emphasizing the importance of women's education. The real-life Nikolai Sergeivich Volkonsky oversaw his daughter Marya's study of mathematics, astronomy, government, classics, and agriculture at Yasnaya Polyana, precisely to avoid her falling into the trap of the dehumanizing ideals of "silly ladies" or "dolls," to which the Russian landowning classes demanded that upper-class women conform.[97]

As a consequence, Tolstoy/Bolkonsky implicitly second Mary Wollstonecraft's (1759–1797) argument that women must "be allowed to found their virtue on knowledge." In effect, this completes the circle linking women's self-help, philanthropy, and education with Tolstoy's queer critique of hyper-masculinity. Still, while Tolstoy's "double attitude" to Freud's hypothesized Oedipus complex encodes respect for polymorphously perverse sexuality, care ethics, and an implicit feminism, it paradoxically also manifests as rank misogyny, especially of the homoerotic variety.[98] Biographically speaking, despite the sexism he imparts in many of his volumes, women's education would nevertheless prove highly beneficial for Lev Nikolaevich's own artistic creativity, and continuous engagement with the memory of his mother proved critical to the espousal of his queer, Christian-anarchist vision.[99]

Notes

1 Chancer 1992: 74–8; 2020; Gustafson 1986: 8; Benjamin 192; Colling 41; Carter 273n20.
2 Benjamin 40–8, 220; Ginzberg 86.
3 Evtuhov et al. 403–4. In this sense, consider the Russian officer Vladimir Alexeevich Poltoratsky's reaction to meeting Hadji Murat: he "had never expected this fearsome mountaineer to be like that. He had expected to see a gloomy, dry, alien man, and before him was a most simple man, who smiled such a kindly smile that he seemed not alien, but a long-familiar friend" (Tolstoy 2009b: 27).
4 Tolstoy 2010: 1126–7, 1144–5, 1181–2.
5 *Ibid* 1172 (emphasis added), 1186.
6 Forrest 60–4.
7 Rapp; Green.
8 Foster J 29, 113.
9 Proposed by the monk Filofei to Grand Prince Ivan III (r. 1462–1505), this messianic idea of Moscow as the Third Rome took off with Ivan IV's vanquishing of the Kazan khanate in 1552 (Berdyaev 1966: 10; Evtuhov et al. 126–8).
10 Gerth and Mills 217; Lieven 2012: 16–17.
11 Ungurianu 36; Love 2007; Rancour-Laferriere 1995.
12 Berdyaev 1966.
13 Faure 259.
14 Gindin 230.
15 Dong and Temple.
16 Zorin 112.
17 Evtuhov et al. 373.
18 Ungurianu 38.
19 McConnell 75.
20 The *Pugachëvshchina*, named for its leader, Yemelyan Pugachëv, was a vast peasant revolt which raged from 1773–1774, proclaiming the abolition of serfdom and the expropriation of land (Evtuhov et al. 286–8). Bezukhov's comments appear to mimic a speech given by Tsar Alexander II in Moscow in March 1856, which itself echoed the *philosophe* Alexander Radishchev's conclusion in *Journey from St. Petersburg to Moscow* (Bartlett 2011: 127; Yarmolinsky).
21 Tarasulo; Tolstoy 2010: 1259; Clark 2013; Orwin 2002a: 52.
22 Clay 211–12.
23 Orwin 1993: 146.
24 *Ibid* 107.
25 Furci.
26 Gustafson 1986: 391; Milivojevic 1993: 64; Clay 212; Rancour-Laferriere 1995: 55.
27 McLean 2008: 84–5.
28 Orwin 1993: 155–6.
29 Bartlett 2011: 180–90; Gustafson 1986: 193.
30 Gustafson 1986: 194.
31 Samet 164; Maude 1987a: 418.
32 Rancour-Laferriere 1998: 156; Békés et al.; Kaufman and Paul.
33 Gustafson 1988: 25; Gustafson 1999: 125; Morgachëv 171.
34 Milivojevic 1991: 99–100.
35 Gustafson 1986: 444; 1999: 124. Supporting evidence for this view includes the fact that the Sermon on the Mount, which serves as the basis of Tolstoy's Christian anarchism, largely reinforces prior lessons preached by Laozi, Buddha, and Socrates (Reitz 104).
36 Pietikainen 14–20, 29, 194; Heuer; Le Guin; Marcuse 1980.
37 Freud 1995: 283; Denner 2001: 15; Milivojevic 1991: 103; 1993: 69–72; Fromm 1969.
38 Tatum; Lin; Kyaw and Ratcliffe.
39 Morson 2012: 82; Love 2012: 93; Gustafson 1999: 125.
40 Chitty 87.

41 Chitty 87; Chodorow 1991: 140. There appears to be some evidence for this dynamic from contemplation of gender relations in classical Greece, especially among the Dorians, who imposed women's seclusion, just as they institutionalized pederasty (Carpenter 1919; Chitty 58).
42 Plato 2015: 77. In his diaries, Tolstoy similarly expresses the view that "the society of women [is] an inevitable evil of social life" that he must avoid as much as possible (Maude 1987a: 43).
43 Love 2012: 85; Smith P 227; Bullock.
44 Samet 166–7; Tolstoy 2010: 30–1.
45 Tolstoy 2010: 117.
46 Plato 2015; Schopenhauer; Orwin 1993: 156.
47 Carpenter 1912: 33–4.
48 Tolstoy 2010: 1127–38.
49 *Ibid* 755–6; Newlin 372; Békés et al; Freud 1995.
50 Karlinsky; Figes 2002: 46–7; Rancour-Laferriere 1995: 189–200.
51 Healey 26–35.
52 Johansson 1990h; Johnson.
53 Karlinsky; Coughlan.
54 Zorin 39–40. Of course, to reiterate, that Prince Andrei fails to connect erotically with his fellow men in both cases underlines Tolstoy's masochism. A similar analysis could be made of Olenin's sexual alienation in *The Cossacks*.
55 Plato 2015: 83.
56 Fone 12; Gilman-Opalsky 225.
57 Johansson 1990h: 799; Chitty 180–7; Walicki 1991.
58 Lanzieri and Hildebrant 282.
59 Herberg-Rothe 159.
60 Smith D 142.
61 Ashbee 160–1.
62 Moreira; Subrat.
63 In Russian, the verb "marry" for a woman marrying a male partner, выходить/выйти замуж, literally means, "to go behind the man." For a man marrying a female partner, the verb is жениться, which translates roughly as, "to take a woman."
64 Shcherbakov 81.
65 The adjective in the original Russian is ничтожный, which can be translated as "unworthy of attention" (Толстой 2012a: 83).
66 Tolstoy 2010: 95–99, 101; Толстой 2012a: 86; Freud 1995.
67 Tolstoy 2010: 310–12; Gustafson 1986: 228–9. "What a beautiful death!"
68 Cortina 395.
69 Freud 2016: 71–2.
70 Benjamin 144; Berdyaev 2009.
71 Becker 85; Tolstoy 1985: 165.
72 McCall; Dostoevsky 2003: 495, 586.
73 Plato 2015: 112.
74 Fuchs; Berdyaev 2009.
75 Cortina 396; Fuchs 6–11.
76 Friedman 311–14; Bulgakov 36.
77 Shestov.
78 Chancer 1992: 48; Benjamin 60–2; Fromm 1947: 225; Fromm 1969.
79 Staples.
80 Love 2012: 86; Gustafson 1986: 43–62; Berdyaev 2009; Clark 2019: 249; Hall 202.
81 Атабекян 153.
82 Rancour-Laferriere 1995: 130; Figes and Kolonitskii 14–17.
83 Tolstoy 2010: 43, 71–8, 112, 470.
84 Cruise 199.
85 Orwin 1993: 158.

86 Tolstoy 2012: 147, 210, 220; Rancour-Laferriere 1985: 350.
87 Zorin 132.
88 Rancour-Laferriere 1998: 3, 101.
89 By the French, explicitly in the public abuse of a "Georgian or Armenian" woman by a French occupier in Moscow, resulting in Pierre's heroic response, drawing on his experience as a brawler, which leads to his captivity; by the Russians, in the femicide committed by a Smolensk innkeeper against his mistress after she urges him to help evacuate with her children (Tolstoy 2010: 746, 997–9).
90 Cruise 200.
91 LeBlanc 1993: 8.
92 Stites 1990: 115–16.
93 *Ibid* 255; Bartlett 2011: 178.
94 Healey.
95 McLean 2008: 83; Evtuhov et al. 712–13.
96 Holbrook 145.
97 Tolstoy 2010: 95–6, 1203; Bartlett 2011: 27–8, 151.
98 Freud 1961a.
99 Stites 1990: 32–3, 64–8; Bartlett 2011: 24.

BIBLIOGRAPHY

Атабекян, Александр Моисеевич 2015. *Против власти*. Moscow: Editorial URSS.

Громова-Опульская, Л. Д. 2000. *Комментарии: Толстой, Л. Н. Полное собрание сочинений: В 100 т.* Moscow: Наука.

КВПУ (Конфедерація вільних профспілок України) 2020. "Employer Filed a Lawsuit against Miners Protesting Underground for 37 days." *КВПУ*, 9 October. Available online: https://kvpu.org.ua/en/news/4319-employer-filled-a-lawsuit-against-miners-protesting-underground-for-37-days. Accessed 31 October 2020.

Книжный чел 2020. "Николай Усков: книги по истории России и мира, писатели и цари." Available online: https://youtu.be/xgG48PCw1hs. Accessed 14 May 2021.

Кон, Игорь С. 2003. *Лунный свет на заре: Лики и маски однополой любви*. Moscow: Olimp.

Леонтьев, Ярослав 2021. "Последние из могикан—анархистка Татьяна Гарасева и кронштадтский матрос Иван Ермолаев." Available online: www.youtube.com/watch?v=EYkHQwSR288. Accessed 24 March 2021.

Матонин, Евгений 2016. *Яков Блюмкин. Ошибка резидента*. Moscow: Youth Guard.

Никитина, Нина 2007. *Повседневная жизнь Льва Толстого Ясной Поляне*. Moscow: Youth Guard.

Первый канал 2001. "В Шелковском районе Чечни в станице Старогладовской каким-то чудом уцелел музей Льва Толстого." *Первый канал*, 30 April. Available online: www.1tv.ru/news/2001-04-30/281290-v_shelkovskom_rayone_chechni_v_stanitse_starogladovskoy_kakim_to_chudom_utselel_muzey_lva_tolstogo. Accessed 24 December 2019.

Петлянова, Нина 2022. "Президент, меняйте курс!" *Novaya Gazeta*, 28 March. Available online: https://novayagazeta.ru/articles/2022/03/28/prezident-meniaite-kurs. Accessed 14 May 2022.

Шевелев, Алексей 2019. "'У ней одна цель': почему Лев Толстой ненавидел женщин." *Газета.Ru*, 9 September. Available online: www.gazeta.ru/culture/2019/09/09/a_12638479.shtml. Accessed 26 September 2021.

Толстой, Лев Николаевич 1928–1964. *Полное собрание сочинений*, 90 vols. Moscow: Издательство «Художественная литература».

Толстой, Лев Николаевич 2012a. *Война и Мир. Тома* 1 и 2. London: The Planet.

Толстой, Лев Николаевич 2012b. *Война и Мир. Тома* 3 и 4. London: The Planet.

Толстой, Лев Николаевич 2021. *Дневники*. Available online: http://tolstoy-lit.ru/tolstoy/dnevniki/index.htm. Accessed 17 October 2021.

Зверев, Алексей и Владимир Туниманов 2006. *Лев Толстой*. Moscow: Молодая гвардия.

Abellán, Liam Jackson 2020. "At the Open Grave: Dealing with the Legacy of Franco's Terror in Today's Spain." *Open Democracy*, 8 December. Available online: www.opendemocracy.net/en/can-europe-make-it/at-the-open-grave-dealing-with-the-legacy-of-francos-terror-in-todays-spain/. Accessed 11 December 2020.

Abromeit, John 2017. "Transformations of Producerist Populism in Western Europe." *Transformations of Populism in Europe and the Americas: History and Recent Tendencies*. Ed. John Abromeit, York Norman, Gary Marotta, Bridget María Chesterton. London: Bloomsbury. 367–413.

Adib-Moghaddam, Arshin 2020. "Bani Adam: The 13th-Century Persian Poem that Shows Why Humanity Needs a Global Response to Coronavirus." *The Conversation*, 27 March. Available online: https://theconversation.com/bani-adam-the-13th-century-persian-poem-that-shows-why-humanity-needs-a-global-response-to-coronavirus-134836. Accessed 19 November 2020.

Adorno, Theodor W. 2005. *Minima Moralia: Reflections on a Damaged Life*. Trans. E. F. N. Jephcott. London: Verso.

Adorno, Theodor W. and Max Horkheimer 2002. *Dialectic of Enlightenment*. Trans. Edmund Jephcott. Redwood City, CA: Stanford University Press.

Adorno, Theodor W. *et al.* 1950. *The Authoritarian Personality*, vol. 1. New York: Harper & Row.

Ahmed, Asiya 2022. "How Ukraine's LGBTIQ Community Is Rallying to Resist Russian Invasion." *Open Democracy*, 2 March. Available online: www.opendemocracy.net/en/5050/ukraine-lgbtiq-community-rallying-resist-russia-invasion/. Accessed 21 May 2022.

Aldris, Aisha 2021. "In Exile, in Danger and in Music: How Amir Al-Muarri Is Using Rap as a Form of Political Resistance against the Syrian Regime." *The New Arab*, 15 October. Available online: https://english.alaraby.co.uk/features/amir-al-muarri-translating-syrian-trauma-rap-music. Accessed 19 October 2021.

Al-Kateab, Waad and Edward Watts 2019. *For Sama*. Channel 4/ITN Productions. Available online: www.pbs.org/wgbh/frontline/film/for-sama/. Accessed 23 November 2019.

Alliez, Éric and Maurizio Lazzarato 2018. *Wars and Capital*. South Pasadena, CA: Semiotext(e).

Al Yafai, Faisal 2021. "The Hidden Face of Nawal El Saadawi." *Frontlines*, 23 March. Available online: https://newlinesmag.com/review/the-hidden-face-of-nawal-el-saadawi. Accessed 26 March 2021.

Anderson, Elizabeth 2017. *Private Government: How Employers Rule Our Lives (and Why We Don't Talk about It)*. Princeton, NJ: Princeton University Press.

Anemone, Anthony 1993. "Gender, Genre, and the Discourse of Imperialism in Tolstoy's *The Cossacks*." *Tolstoy Studies Journal*, vol. 6. 47–63.

Artukoglu, Bekir B. and Natalia Szejko 2019. "Tarkovsky's *Stalker*: Existentialism and Mental Health." *The Lancet Psychiatry*, vol. 7, issue 1. 24–26.

Ashbee, C. R. 1894. *A Few Chapters in Workshop Re-Construction and Citizenship*. London: Guild and School of Handicraft.

Aslan, Reza 2013. *Zealot: The Life and Times of Jesus of Nazareth*. New York: Random House.

Atterbury, Lyn 1984. "Nicholas Berdyaev, Orthodox Nonconformist." *Third Way*. Available online: www.chebucto.ns.ca/Philosophy/Sui-Generis/Berdyaev/essays/thirdway.htm. Accessed 28 October 2020.

Aubin, Sophian 2021. "Syria War: Ten Years On, Syrian Christians Say Assad 'Has Taken Us Hostage.'" *Middle East Eye*, 14 March. Available online: www.middleeasteye.net/news/syria-war-anniversary-christians-assad-manipulation. Accessed 26 May 2021.

Babel, Isaac 2014. *Red Cavalry*. Trans. Boris Dralyuk. London: Pushkin Press.

Bakunin, Mikhail 1867. "Federalism, Socialism, Anti-Theologism." Available online: www.marxists.org/reference/archive/bakunin/works/various/reasons-of-state.htm. Accessed 26 May 2021.

Bakunin, Mikhail 1973. *Selected Writings*. London: Jonathan Cape Ltd.

Bakunin, Mikhail 2005. *Statism and Anarchy*. Trans. and ed. Marshall Shatz. Cambridge: Cambridge University Press.

Balan, Neil 2016. "War." *Keywords for Radicals*. Ed. Kelly Fritsch *et al.* Chico, CA: AK Press. 463–468.

Balasubramanian, Radha 2011. "Research Notes: Leo Tolstoy from 1901–2010 in Two Leading English-Language Newspapers in India." *Tolstoy Studies Journal*, vol. 23. 61–69.

Baldwin, James 1985. *The Price of the Ticket: Collected Nonfiction, 1948–1985*. New York: St. Martin's Press.

Ballou, Kathryn A. and Kandace J. Landreneau 2010. "The Authoritarian Reign in American Health Care." *Policy, Politics, & Nursing Practice*, vol. 11, issue 1. 71–79.

Banister, Jeffrey M. 2014. "Are you Wittfogel or against Him? Geophilosophy, Hydro-Sociality, and the State." *Geoforum*, vol. 57. 205–214.

Barnes *et al.* 2022. "US Intelligence Is Helping Ukraine Kill Russian Generals, Officials Say." *New York Times*, 4 May. Available online: www.nytimes.com/2022/05/04/us/politics/russia-generals-killed-ukraine.html. Accessed 4 May 2022.

Bartlett, Rosamund 2011. *Tolstoy: A Russian Life*. New York: Houghton Mifflin.

Bartlett, Rosamund 2014. "What the Bees do in Anna Karenina and Other Works by Tolstoy: A Study in Three Parts." *Tolstoy Studies Journal*, vol. 26. 1–18.

Batty, David 2020a. "Holocaust Survivor's Daughter Takes Historian to Court over Claim of Lesbian Liaison with Nazi Guard." *Guardian*, 8 October. Available online: www.theguardian.com/education/2020/oct/08/survivors-daughter-sues-historian-claim-lesbian-liaison-nazi-guard. Accessed 9 October 2020.

Batty, David 2020b. "Court Fines Historian over Claims of Holocaust Survivor's Lesbian Affair." *Guardian*, 21 December. Available online: www.theguardian.com/education/2020/dec/21/court-fines-historian-over-claims-holocaust-survivor-lesbian-affair. Accessed 21 December 2020.

Becker, Ernest 1973. *The Denial of Death*. Free Press: New York.

Beiner, Robert 2018. *Dangerous Minds: Nietzsche, Heidegger, and the Return of the Far Right*. Philadelphia, PA: University of Pennsylvania Press.

Békés, Vera *et al.* 2016. "Psychological Masochism: A Systematic Review of the Literature on Conflicts, Defenses, and Motives." *Psychotherapy Research*. doi:10.1080/10503307.2016.1189618.

Bekiempis, Victoria 2020. "Ghislaine Maxwell Requests Bail Release Due to 'Unprecedented' Covid-19 Risks." *Guardian*, 10 July. Available online: www.theguardian.com/us-news/2020/jul/10/ghislaine-maxwell-bail-release-covid-19-jeffrey-epstein. Accessed 10 July 2020.

Bell, David A. 2020. "Fascism or Caesarism? How Napoleon, not Hitler, Exemplifies an Enduring Threat to Modern Democracies." *Public Seminar*. Available online: https://publicseminar.org/2020/08/fascism-or-caesarism/. Accessed 27 August 2020.

Bellamy, Christopher 2001a. "Borodino, Battle of." *The Oxford Companion to Military History*. Ed. Richard Holmes. Oxford: Oxford University Press. 142.

Bellamy, Christopher 2001b. "Cossacks." *The Oxford Companion to Military History*. Ed. Richard Holmes. Oxford: Oxford University Press. 229–230.

Bellamy, Christopher 2001c. "Moscow, Battle of." *The Oxford Companion to Military History*. Ed. Richard Holmes. Oxford: Oxford University Press. 602.

Benjamin, Jessica 1988. *The Bonds of Love: Psychoanalysis, Feminism, and the Problem of Domination*. New York: Pantheon.

Berdyaev, Nicolas 1966. *The Origin of Russian Communism*. Ann Arbor, MI: University of Michigan Press.

Berdyaev, Nicolas 2009. *Slavery and Freedom*. San Rafael, CA: Semantron Press.

Bergamini, John D. 1974. *The Spanish Bourbons: The History of a Tenacious Dynasty*. New York: Putnam.

Berger, Eric 2022. "'It's a War Zone': Healthcare Workers Show Signs of Stress Similar to Combat Veterans." *Guardian*, 19 January. Available online: www.theguardian.com/world/2022/jan/19/healthcare-workers-post-traumatic-stress-disorder-pandemic-covid. Accessed 19 January 2022.

Berlin, Isaiah 1978. *Russian Thinkers*. London: Penguin.

Berlin, Isaiah 1999. *The Roots of Romanticism*. 2nd ed. Ed. Henry Hardy. Princeton, NJ: Princeton University Press.

Bernardini, David 2021. "A Different Antifascism: An Analysis of the Rise of Nazism as Seen by Anarchists during the Weimar Period." *History of European Ideas*. doi:10.1080/01916599.2021.1963629.

Blais, Donald 1997. *Passion and Pathology in Teresa of Avila's Mystical Transformation*. Ottawa: National Library of Canada.

Bloom, Harold 2009. *Leo Tolstoy*. New York: Infobase Publishing.

Bondarchuk, Sergei 1966–1967. *War and Peace*. Moscow: Mosfilm.

Bookchin, Murray 2018. "The Kronstadt Uprising: Introduction by Murray Bookchin." *1917: Revolution in Russia and Its Aftermath*. Eds. Dan Georgakas *et al.* Montréal: Black Rose Books. 317–326.

Borshchevskaya, Anna 2022. *Putin's War in Syria: Russian Foreign Policy and the Price of America's Absence*. London: I. B. Tauris.

Bosworth, C. E. 2001. "Shamyl." *The Oxford Companion to Military History*. Ed. Richard Holmes. Oxford: Oxford University Press. 827.

Bounds, Philip 2019. "Review of *Radical Utopianism and Cultural Studies: On Refusing to be Realistic* by John Storey." *Marx and Philosophy*, 4 December. Available online: https://marxandphilosophy.org.uk/reviews/17533_radical-utopianism-and-cultural-studies-on-refusing-to-be-realistic-by-john-storey-reviewed-by-philip-bounds. Accessed 1 March 2020.

Bronowski, Yoram 2001. "Yes, He Was a Male, This Chauvin." *Ha'aretz*, 21 September. Available online: www.haaretz.com/1.5403757. Accessed 23 July 2021.

Browne, Paul Leduc 2020. "'Symbolic Violence: Conversations with Bourdieu' by Michael Burawoy Reviewed by Paul Leduc Browne." *Marx and Philosophy*, 30 October. Available online: https://marxandphilosophy.org.uk/reviews/18425_symbolic-violence-conversations-with-bourdieu-by-michael-burawoy-reviewed-by-paul-leduc-browne/. Accessed 7 November 2020.

Buck-Morss, Susan 2005. *Hegel, Haiti, and Universal History*. Pittsburgh, PA: University of Pittsburgh.

Bulgakov, Sergei 1994. "Heroism and Asceticism: Reflections on the Religious Nature of the Russian Intelligentsia." *Vekhi: Landmarks*. Trans. Marshall E. Shatz and Judith E. Zimmerman. New York: Routledge. 17–49.

Bullock, Philip Ross. "'That's Not the Only Reason We Love Him': Chaikovsky Reception in Post-Soviet Russia." *Soviet and Post-Soviet Sexualities*. Ed. Richard C. M. Mole. London: Routledge. 103–128.

Burdyga, Igor 2020. "These Miners Protested for 43 Days Underground: Then They Were Betrayed." *Open Democracy*, 3 December. Available online: www.opendemocracy.net/en/odr/kryvyi-rih-miners-protest-2020/. Accessed 5 December 2020.

Burgen, Stephen 2021. "'Iconic Gay Image': History of Sailors and Sex Explored in Barcelona Exhibition." *Guardian*, 29 June. Available online: www.theguardian.com/artanddesign/2021/jun/29/fluid-desires-sailors-sexual-chemistry-depicted-in-barcelona. Accessed 13 July 2021.

Buruma, Ian and Avishai Margalit 2004. *Occidentalism: The West in the Eyes of its Enemies*. New York: Penguin.

Byrd, Dustin J. 2017. "Ali Shariati and Critical Theory: From Black Affirmation to Red Negation." *Ali Shariati and the Future of Social Theory*. Eds. Dustin J. Byrd and Seyed Javad Miri. Chicago, IL: Haymarket Books. 98–127.

Byrd, Dustin J. and Seyed Javad Miri 2017. "Introduction." *Ali Shariati and the Future of Social Theory*. Eds. Dustin J. Byrd and Seyed Javad Miri. Chicago, IL: Haymarket Books. 1–8.

Campbell, Mel. "We Spend So Much Time Staring at Our Phones: What Do We Miss When We Don't Look Up?" *Guardian*, 19 November. Available online: www.theguardian.com/film/2019/nov/20/we-spend-so-much-time-staring-at-our-phones-what-do-we-miss-when-we-dont-look-up. Accessed 23 November 2019.

Capra, Fritjof 2010. *The Tao of Physics: An Exploration of the Parallels between Modern Physics and Eastern Mysticism*. Boston, MA: Shambhala.

Carlo, Andrea 2021. "Why It Took Decades for LGBTQ Stories to Be Included in Holocaust History." *Time*, 7 April. Available online: https://time.com/5953047/lgbtq-holocaust-stories. Accessed 22 August 2021.

Carpenter, Edward 1912. *The Intermediate Sex: A Study of Some Transitional Types of Men and Women*. New York: Mitchell Kennerley.

Carpenter, Edward 1919. *Intermediate Types Among Primitive Folk: A Study in Social Evolution*. 2nd ed. London: George Allen and Unwin.

Carter, Alan 1988. *Marx: A Radical Critique*. Boulder, CO: Westview Press.

Cera, Agostino 2019. "*The Performance Paradigm: A Marcusean Hermeneutics of the Present Dark Times*." Presentation given at the International Herbert Marcuse Society conference, University of California Santa Barbara, 11 October.

Cervantes, Miguel de 2000. *The Ingenious Don Quixote de la Mancha*. Trans. John Rutherford. New York: Penguin.

Chancer, Lynn S. 1992. *Sadomasochism in Everyday Life: The Dynamics of Power and Powerlessness*. New Brunswick, NJ: Rutgers University Press.

Chancer, Lynn S. 2020. "Feminism, Humanism, and Erich Fromm." *Erich Fromm's Critical Theory: Hope, Humanism, and the Future*. Eds. Kieran Durkin and Joan Braune. London: Bloomsbury Academic. 96–107.

Chausovsky, Eugene 2021. "The City of Kazan and Russia's Non-Slavic Future." *Newlines Magazine*, 9 February. Available online: https://newlinesmag.com/reportage/the-city-of-kazan-and-russias-non-slavic-future/. Accessed 11 February 2021.

Chekhov, Anton 1999. *Peasants and Other Stories*. Trans. Constance Garnett. New York: New York Review of Books.

Chekhov, Anton 2004. *Letters of Anton Chekhov*. Trans. Constance Garnett. Chapel Hill, NC: Project Gutenberg.

Chernyshevsky, Nikolai 1989. *What Is to Be Done?* Trans. Michael R. Katz. Ithaca, NY: Cornell University Press.

Child, Ben 2021. "Future Lord of the Rings Films Should Acknowledge the Book's Queer Leanings." *Guardian*, 2 July. Available online: www.theguardian.com/film/2021/jul/02/

future-lord-of-the-rings-films-should-acknowledge-the-books-queer-leanings. Accessed 26 July 2021.
Child, John 2009. "Challenging Hierarchy." *The Oxford Handbook of Critical Management Studies*. Eds. Mats Alvesson *et al.* Oxford: Oxford University Press. 501–514.
Chitty, Christopher 2020. *Sexual Hegemony: Statecraft, Sodomy, and Capital in the Rise of the World System*. Durham, NC: Duke University Press.
Chodorow, Nancy 1991. *Feminism and Psychoanalytic Theory*. New Haven, CT: Yale University Press.
Chodorow, Nancy 1999. *The Power of Feelings*. New Haven, CT: Yale University Press.
Chouliaraki, Lilie 2006. *The Spectatorship of Suffering*. London: Sage.
Christoyannopoulos, Alexandre 2006. "Tolstoy the Peculiar Christian Anarchist." Available online: https://archive.org/details/TolstoyThePeculiarChristianAnarchist/page/n1/mode/2up. Accessed 28 September 2022.
Christoyannopoulos, Alexandre 2010. "'Bethink Yourselves or You Will Perish': Leo Tolstoy's Voice a Centenary after His Death." *Anarchist Studies*, vol. 18, issue 2. 11–18.
Christoyannopoulos, Alexandre 2011. *Christian Anarchism: A Political Commentary on the Gospel*. Exeter: Imprint Academic.
Chulov, Martin 2022. "Syria's Barrel Bomb Experts in Russia to Help with Potential Ukraine Campaign." *Guardian*, 22 May. Available online: www.theguardian.com/world/2022/may/22/syrias-barrel-bomb-experts-in-russia-to-help-with-potential-ukraine-campaign. Accessed 23 May 2022.
Clark, John P. 2013. *The Impossible Community: Realizing Communitarian Anarchism*. New York: Bloomsbury.
Clark, John P. 2019. *Between Earth and Empire: From the Necrocene to the Beloved Community*. Oakland, CA: PM Press.
Clark, John P. 2021. "Élisée Reclus: The Making of a Communard." *ROAR Magazine*, 18 March. Available online: https://roarmag.org/essays/elisee-reclus-paris-commune. Accessed 25 March 2021.
Clarke, Samuel 2020. "無爲: 'Wu Wei' and Anarchy as Order." *The Commoner*, 18 April. Available online: www.thecommoner.org.uk/wu-wei-and-anarchy-as-order/. Accessed 27 October 2020.
Clay, George R. 2002. "Tolstoy in the Twentieth Century." *The Cambridge Companion to Tolstoy*. Ed. Donna Tussing Orwin. Cambridge: Cambridge University Press. 206–221.
CNT 2021. "The Kurdish Myth—Critique of Abdullah Ocalan's Political Project." Trans. Monica Jornet. *Anarchist Communist Group*. Available online: www.anarchistcommunism.org/2021/03/01/discussion-abdullah-ocalan-and-the-kurdish-myth/. Accessed 2 March 2021.
Cocker, Mark 2020. "Laurence C Smith's *Rivers of Power:* How Water Shapes Our World." *New Statesman*, 10 July. Available online: www.newstatesman.com/culture/books/2020/07/laurence-c-smith-s-rivers-power-how-water-shapes-our-world. Accessed 1 November 2020.
Cohn, Jesse 2014. *Underground Passages: Anarchist Resistance Culture, 1848–2011*. Oakland, CA: AK Press.
Colling, Sarat 2021. *Animal Resistance in the Global Capitalist Era*. East Lansing, MI: Michigan State University Press.
Cookson, Richard *et al.* 2021. "The Inverse Care Law Re-Examined: A Global Perspective." *The Lancet*. doi:10.1016/S0140-6736(21)00243-9.
Cornett, Carlton W. and Ross A. Hudson 1986. "Psychoanalytic Theory and Affirmation of the Gay Lifestyle: Are They Necessarily Antithetical?" *Journal of Homosexuality*, vol. 12, issue 1. 97–108.
Cortina, Mauricio 2015. "The Greatness and Limitations of Erich Fromm's Humanism." *Contemporary Psychoanalysis*, vol. 51, issue 3. 388–422.

Coughlan, Sean 2021. "The 200-Year-Old Diary that's Rewriting Gay History." *BBC News*, 10 February. Available online: www.bbc.com/news/education-51385884. Accessed 15 February 2021.

Croll, Neil 2004. "The Role of M. N. Tukhachevskii in the Suppression of the Kronstadt Rebellion." *Revolutionary Russia*, vol. 17, issue 2. 1–48.

Cruise, Edwina 2002. "Women, Sexuality, and the Family in Tolstoy." *The Cambridge Companion to Tolstoy*. Ed. Donna Tussing Orwin. Cambridge: Cambridge University Press. 191–205.

Cunliffe, Barry 2017. "*Against the Grain* by James C Scott Review—The Beginning of Elites, Tax, Slavery." *Guardian*, 25 November. Available online: www.theguardian.com/books/2017/nov/25/against-the-grain-by-james-c-scott-review. Accessed 14 November 2021.

Currie, Kate 1984. "The Asiatic Mode of Production: Problems of Conceptualising State and Economy." *Dialectical Anthropology*, vol. 8. 251–268.

Danaher, David 1998. "The Function of Pain in Tolstoy's The Death of Ivan Il'ich." *Tolstoy Studies Journal*, vol. 10. 20–28.

Dare, Natali 2021. "Taking a Pen as her Sword and Challenging the Patriarchy: Nawal El Saadawi's Phenomenal Legacy." *The New Arab*, 6 April. Available online: https://english.alaraby.co.uk/english/society/2021/4/6/the-phenomenal-legacy-of-nawal-el-saadawi. Accessed 6 April 2021.

Darrow, Clarence S. and Arthur M. Lewis 2003. *Marx versus Tolstoy: A Debate*. Honolulu, HI: University Press of the Pacific.

Darwin, Charles 1981. *The Descent of Man, and Selection in Relation to Sex*. Princeton, NJ: Princeton University Press.

Darwin, Charles 1987. *Charles Darwin's Notebooks, 1836–1844. Geology, Transmutation of Species, Metaphysical Enquiries*. Transcribed and ed. P. H. Barrett *et al.* London: British Museum.

de Kuyper, Eric 1993. "The Freudian Construction of Sexuality: The Gay Foundations of Heterosexuality and Straight Homophobia." *Journal of Homosexuality*, vol. 24, issues 3–4. 137–144.

de Lauretis, Teresa 2017. "The Queerness of the Drive." *Journal of Homosexuality*, vol. 64, issue 14. 1913–1929.

Denner, Michael 2001. "Tolstoyan Nonaction: The Advantage of Doing Nothing." *Tolstoy Studies Journal*, vol. 13. 8–22.

Denner, Michael 2011. "Use Tolstoy to Find Your Way…" *Tolstoy Studies Journal*, vol. 23. 93–99.

Desai, Ashwin and Goolam H. Vahed 2015. *The South African Gandhi: Stretcher-Bearer of Empire*. Stanford, CA: Stanford University Press.

DeYoung, Colin G. 2012. "From Madness to Genius: The Openness/Intellect Trait Domain as a Paradoxical Simplex." *Journal of Research in Personality*, vol. 46. 63–78.

Dinerstein, Ana Cecilia 2019. "Basic Income Bows to the Master." *Open Democracy*, 18 September. Available online: www.opendemocracy.net/en/beyond-trafficking-and-slavery/basic-income-bows-master/. Accessed 15 December 2019.

Dodds, Rosie 2021. "Borderline Personality Disorder: My Greatest Asset." *The Lancet Psychiatry*, vol. 8, issue 3. 188–190.

Dodson, Kevin E. 2019. "Review of *The New Faces of Fascism: Populism and the Far Right* by Enzo Traverso." *Marx and Philosophy*, 18 December. Available online: https://marxandphilosophy.org.uk/reviews/17571_the-new-faces-of-fascism-populism-and-the-far-right-by-enzo-traverso-reviewed-by-kevin-e-dodson/. Accessed 18 December 2019.

Donaldson, Stephen 1990a. "Rape of Males." *The Encyclopedia of Homosexuality*. Ed. Wayne R. Dynes. New York: Garland Press. 1094–1098.

Donaldson, Stephen 1990b. "Working Class, Eroticization of." *The Encyclopedia of Homosexuality*. Ed. Wayne R. Dynes. New York: Garland Press. 1405–1406.

Dong, Doris and Beverley Temple 2011. "Oppression: A Concept Analysis and Implications for Nurses and Nursing." *Nursing Forum*, vol. 24, issue 3. 169–176.

Donskov, A. A. 2001. "Review of Peter Brock and John L. Keep, eds. *Life in a Penal Battalion of the Imperial Russian Army: The Tolstoyan N. T. Iziumcheko's Story*." *Tolstoy Studies Journal*, vol. 6. 136–137.

Dostoevsky, Fyodor 1990. *The Brothers Karamazov*. Trans. Richard Pevear and Larissa Volokhonsky. New York: Farrar, Straus, and Giroux.

Dostoevsky, Fyodor 2003. *Crime and Punishment*. Trans. David McDuff. London: Penguin.

Dragunovsky, Yakov 1993. *From the Papers of Yakov Dragunovsky*. Trans. William Edgerton. Bloomington, IN: Indiana University Press. 181–246.

Du Bois, W. E. B. 1987. *W. E. B. Du Bois: Writings*. Ed. Nathan Huggins. New York: Library of America.

Dunne, Tim and Brian C. Schmidt 2005. "Realism." *The Globalization of World Politics*, 3rd ed. Eds. John Baylis, Steve Smith, and Patricia Owens. Oxford: Oxford University Press. 161–183.

Durkin, Kieran 2020. "Introduction." *Erich Fromm's Critical Theory: Hope, Humanism, and the Future*. Eds. Kieran Durkin and Joan Braune. London: Bloomsbury Academic. 1–19.

Dynes, Wayne R. 1990a. "Androphilia." *The Encyclopedia of Homosexuality*. Ed. Wayne R. Dynes. New York: Garland Press. 58.

Dynes, Wayne R. 1990b. "Asceticism." *The Encyclopedia of Homosexuality*. Ed. Wayne R. Dynes. New York: Garland Press. 82–84.

Dynes, Wayne R. 1990c. "Beauty Competitions." *The Encyclopedia of Homosexuality*. Ed. Wayne R. Dynes. New York: Garland Press. 121–122.

Dynes, Wayne R. 1990d. "Birds and Avian Symbolism." *The Encyclopedia of Homosexuality*. Ed. Wayne R. Dynes. New York: Garland Press. 142–143.

Dynes, Wayne R. 1990e. "Blüher, Hans." *The Encyclopedia of Homosexuality*. Ed. Wayne R. Dynes. New York: Garland Press. 154–155.

Dynes, Wayne R. 1990f. "Camp." *The Encyclopedia of Homosexuality*. Ed. Wayne R. Dynes. New York: Garland Press. 189–190.

Dynes, Wayne R. 1990g. "Color Symbolism." *The Encyclopedia of Homosexuality*. Ed. Wayne R. Dynes. New York: Garland Press. 249–250.

Dynes, Wayne R. 1990h. "Dionysus." *The Encyclopedia of Homosexuality*. Ed. Wayne R. Dynes. New York: Garland Press. 318–320.

Dynes, Wayne R. 1990i. "Fiedler Thesis." *The Encyclopedia of Homosexuality*. Ed. Wayne R. Dynes. New York: Garland Press. 398–399.

Dynes, Wayne R. 1990j. "Ganymede." *The Encyclopedia of Homosexuality*. Ed. Wayne R. Dynes. New York: Garland Press. 454–455.

Dynes, Wayne R. 1990k. "Homophile." *The Encyclopedia of Homosexuality*. Ed. Wayne R. Dynes. New York: Garland Press. 552.

Dynes, Wayne R. 1990l. "Hemingway." *The Encyclopedia of Homosexuality*. Ed. Wayne R. Dynes. New York: Garland Press. 524.

Dynes, Wayne R. 1990m. "Latent Homosexuality." *The Encyclopedia of Homosexuality*. Ed. Wayne R. Dynes. New York: Garland Press. 677–678.

Dynes, Wayne R. 1990n. "Polymorphous Perverse." *The Encyclopedia of Homosexuality*. Ed. Wayne R. Dynes. New York: Garland Press. 1022–1023.

Dynes, Wayne R. 1990o. "Utopianism." *The Encyclopedia of Homosexuality*. Ed. Wayne R. Dynes. New York: Garland Press. 1356–1357.

Eagleton, Terry 2009. *Reason, Faith, and Revolution: Reflections on the God Debate*. New Haven, CT: Yale University Press.

Edwards, Robert 1993. "Tolstoy and Alice B. Stockham: The Influence of 'Tokology' on *The Kreutzer Sonata*." *Tolstoy Studies Journal*, vol. 6. 87–102.

Efird, Robert O. 2014. "The Holy Fool in Late Tarkovsky." *Journal of Religion and Film*, vol. 18, issue 1. 1–25.

Eisenberg, Daniel 1990. "Fantasies." *The Encyclopedia of Homosexuality*. Ed. Wayne R. Dynes. New York: Garland Press. 386–387.

Eisler, Riane 1987. *The Chalice and the Blade: Our History, Our Future*. New York: HarperCollins.

Emerson, Caryl 2002. "Leo Tolstoy and the Rights of Music under Stalin (Another Look at Prokofiev's Party-Minded Masterpiece, *War and Peace*)." *Tolstoy Studies Journal*, vol. 14. 1–14.

Engel, Stephanie 1980. "Femininity as Tragedy, Re-Examining the New Narcissism." *Socialist Review*, vol. 53. 77–104.

Erwin-Jansen, Peter 2017. "The Desire for Community." *Transvaluation of Values and Radical Social Change: Five New Lectures, 1966–1976*. Eds. Peter-Erwin Jansen, Sarah Surak, and Charles Reitz. Toronto: International Herbert Marcuse Society. 101–116.

Essig, Laurie and Alexander Kondakov 2019. "A Cold War for the Twenty-First Century: Homosexualism vs. Heterosexualism." *Soviet and Post-Soviet Sexualities*. Ed. Richard C. M. Mole. London: Routledge. 79–102.

Evtuhov, Catherine *et al.* 2004. *A History of Russia: Peoples, Legends, Events, Forces*. Boston, MA: Houghton Mifflin.

Falk, Candace 1984. *Love, Anarchy and Emma Goldman: A Biography*. New York: Holt, Rinehart and Winston.

Faure, Sébastien 2019. *The Anarchist Encyclopedia (Abridged)*. Trans. Mitchell Abidor. Chico, CA: AK Press.

Feldman, Abraham Bronson 1962. *Stalin: Red Lord of Russia, 1879–1953*. Philadelphia, PA: Mercury Books.

Ferguson, Ann 2018. "Socialist-Feminist Transitions and Visions." *Radical Philosophy Review*, vol. 21, issue 1. 177–200.

Feuer, Kathryn B. 1996. *Tolstoy and the Genesis of War and Peace*. Eds. Robin Feuer Miller and Donna Tussing Orwin. Ithaca, NY: Cornell University Press.

Fiedler, Leslie 1999. *A New Fiedler Reader*. Amherst, NY: Prometheus Books.

Figes, Orlando 1996. *A People's Tragedy: The Russian Revolution, 1891–1924*. New York: Penguin.

Figes, Orlando 2002. *Natasha's Dance: A Cultural History of Russia*. New York: Metropolitan Books.

Figes, Orlando and Boris Kolonitskii 1999. *Interpreting the Russian Revolution: The Language and Symbols of 1917*. New Haven, CT: Yale University Press.

Fink, Andreas *et al.* 2014. "Creativity and Psychopathology: Are There Similar Mental Processes Involved in Creativity and in Psychosis-Proneness?" *Frontiers in Psychology*. https://doi.org/10.3389/fpsyg.2014.01211.

Fischer, Thomas *et al.* 2021. "Abusive Supervision: A Systematic Review and Fundamental Rethink." *The Leadership Quarterly*, vol. 32, issue 6. https://doi.org/10.1016/j.leaqua.2021.101540.

Fisher, Richard 2020. "Humanity Is Stuck in Short-Term Thinking: Here's How We Escape." *MIT Technology Review*, 21 October. Available online: www.technologyreview.com/2020/10/21/1009443/short-term-vs-long-term-thinking/. Accessed 26 October 2020.

Fone, Byrne R. S. 1998. "Eros in Arcadia: Greek Literature." *The Columbia Anthology of Gay Literature*. Ed. Byrne R. S. Fone. New York: Columbia University Press. 11–15.

Fontesse, Sullivan *et al.* 2019. "Dehumanization of Psychiatric Patients: Experimental and Clinical Implications in Severe Alcohol-Use Disorders." *Addictive Behaviors*, vol. 89. 216–223.

Forrest, Alan 2012. "The French at War: Representations of the Enemy." *Tolstoy on War*. Eds. Rick McPeak and Donna Tussing Orwin. Ithaca, NY: Cornell University Press. 59–73.

Foster, John Burt, Jr. 2013. *Transnational Tolstoy: Between the West and the World*. New York: Bloomsbury.

Foster, Roger 2020. "Erich Fromm and the Prospects for Renewing Critical Theory in the Neoliberal Era." *Erich Fromm's Critical Theory: Hope, Humanism, and the Future*. Eds. Kieran Durkin and Joan Braune. London: Bloomsbury Academic. 75–95.

Fournier, August 1904. *Napoleon the First*. New York: H. Holt and Company.

Frank, Simon 1994. "The Ethic of Nihilism: A Characterization of the Russian Intelligentsia's Moral Outlook." *Vekhi: Landmarks*. Trans. Marshall E. Shatz and Judith E. Zimmerman. New York: Routledge. 131–155.

Freire, Paulo 2000. *Pedagogy of the Oppressed*. Trans. Myra Bergman Ramos. New York: Continuum.

French, Howard W. 2021. "Built on the Bodies of Slaves: How Africa Was Erased from the History of the Modern World." *Guardian*, 12 October. Available online: www.theguardian.com/news/2021/oct/12/africa-slaves-erased-from-history-modern-world. Accessed 13 October 2021.

Freud, Sigmund 1953. "Creative Writers and Daydreaming." *Collected Papers*, vol. 4. Trans. Joan Riviere *et al.* Ed. Ernest Jones. New York: Basic Books. 419–428.

Freud, Sigmund 1961a. "Dostoevsky and Parricide." *The Standard Edition of the Complete Psychological Works of Sigmund Freud*, vol. XXI. Trans. James Strachey and Anna Freud. London: Hogarth. 175–196.

Freud, Sigmund 1961b. *Leonardo da Vinci and a Memory of His Childhood*. Trans. Alan Tyson. Ed. James Strachey. New York: W. W. Norton & Co.

Freud, Sigmund 1964. "New Introductory Lectures." *The Standard Edition of the Complete Psychological Works of Sigmund Freud*, vol. XXII. Trans. James Strachey and Anna Freud. London: Hogarth.

Freud, Sigmund 1995. "The Economic Problem of Masochism." *Essential Papers on Masochism*. Ed. Margaret Ann Fitzpatrick Hanly. New York: New York University Press. 274–283.

Freud, Sigmund 2013. *Psycho-Analytic Notes on an Autobiographical Account of a Case of Paranoia (Dementia Paranoides)*. Redditch: Read Books Ltd.

Freud, Sigmund 2016. *Three Essays on the Theory of Sexuality*. Trans. Ulrike Kistner. London: Verso.

Friedman, Lawrence 2013. *The Lives of Erich Fromm: Love's Prophet*. With assistance from Anke M. Schreiber. New York: Columbia University Press.

Fromm, Erich 1947. *Man for Himself: An Inquiry into the Psychology of Ethics*. New York: Henry Holt.

Fromm, Erich 1968. *The Revolution of Hope*. New York: Harper and Row.

Fromm, Erich 1969. *Escape from Freedom*. New York: Avon Books.

Fromm, Erich 1973. *The Anatomy of Human Destructiveness*. New York: Henry Holt.

Fromm, Erich 1994. *Escape from Freedom*. New York: Henry Holt.

Fromm, Erich 2006. *The Art of Loving*. New York: Harper Collins.

Fuchs, Christian 2020. "Erich Fromm and the Critical Theory of Communication." *Humanity and Society*, vol. 44, issue 3. 298–325.

Fudge, Judy 2020. "Twenty Years after Palermo, Can We Stop Discussing Labour Exploitation and Start Fixing It?" *Open Democracy*, 19 November. Available online: www.opendemocracy.net/en/beyond-trafficking-and-slavery/twenty-years-after-palermo-can-we-stop-discussing-labour-exploitation-and-start-fixing-it/. Accessed 19 November 2020.

Furci, Giuliana 2021. "The Earth's Secret Miracle Worker Is Not a Plant or an Animal: It's Fungi." *Guardian*, 11 November. Available online: www.theguardian.com/commentisfree/2021/nov/11/fungi-earth-secret-miracle-weapon. Accessed 12 November 2021.

Furner, James 2019. *Marx on Capitalism: The Interaction-Recognition-Antinomy Thesis*. Chicago, IL: Haymarket Books.

Gandesha, Samir 2020. "The Left Contra Critique?" *Open Democracy*, 13 March. Available online: www.opendemocracy.net/en/left-contra-critique/. Accessed 12 April 2020.

Garner, Ian 2022. "'We've Got to Kill Them': Responses to Bucha on Russian Social Media Groups." *Journal of Genocide Research*. doi:10.1080/14623528.2022.2074020.

Gates, David 2001. "Napoleonic Wars." *The Oxford Companion to Military History*. Ed. Richard Holmes. Oxford: Oxford University Press. 623–627.

Gerth, Hans and C. Wright Mills 1954. *Character and Social Structure: The Psychology of Social Institutions*. Routledge: London.

Gettone, Evelyn 1990. "Woolf, Virginia." *The Encyclopedia of Homosexuality*. Ed. Wayne R. Dynes. New York: Garland Press. 1404–1405.

Giammarinaro, Maria Grazia 2020. "Are Our Laws Cut Out for Addressing Systemic Exploitation?" *Open Democracy*, 18 November. Available online: www.opendemocracy.net/en/beyond-trafficking-and-slavery/are-our-laws-cut-out-addressing-systemic-exploitation/. Accessed 19 November 2020.

Giddens, Anthony 1971. *Capitalism and Modern Social Theory: An Analysis of the Writings of Marx, Durkheim and Max Weber*. Cambridge: Cambridge University Press.

Gilman-Opalsky, Richard 2020. *The Communism of Love*. Chico, CA: AK Press.

Gindin, Sam 2016. "Labor." *Keywords for Radicals*. Ed. Kelly Fritsch *et al.* Chico, CA: AK Press. 223–230.

Ginzberg, Ruth 1992. "Audre Lorde's (Nonessentialist) Lesbian Eros." *Hypatia*, vol. 7, issue 4. 73–90.

Goodwin, James 2010. *Confronting Dostoevsky's Demons: Anarchism and the Specter of Bakunin in Twentieth-Century Russia*. New York: Peter Lang.

Graeber, David 2018. *Bullshit Jobs*. New York: Simon and Schuster.

Graeber, David and David Wengrow 2021. "Unfreezing the Ice Age: The Truth about Humanity's Deep Past." *Guardian*, 19 October. Available online: www.theguardian.com/news/2021/oct/19/unfreezing-the-ice-age-the-truth-about-humanitys-deep-past. Accessed 22 October 2021.

Graham, Robert 2015. *We Do Not Fear Anarchy; We Invoke It*. Oakland, CA: AK Press.

Grand Lodge of British Columbia and Yukon 2007. "Freemasonry and Nineteenth-Century Revolution." Available online: http://freemasonry.bcy.ca/history/revolution/. Accessed 18 October 2019.

Grant, Adam M. and Wade-Benzoni, Kimberly A. 2009. "The Hot and Cool of Death Awareness at Work: Mortality Cues, Aging, and Self-Protective and Prosocial Motivations." *The Academy of Management Review*, vol. 34, issue 4. 600–622. https://doi.org/10.5465/AMR.2009.44882929.

Gregg, Richard 1988. "Roundtable: Richard F. Gustafson, *Leo Tolstoy. Resident and Stranger*." *Tolstoy Studies Journal*, vol. 1. 16–18.

Griffin, Horace 2000. "Their Own Received Them Not: African American Lesbians and Gays in Black Churches." *Theology & Sexuality*, vol. 2000, issue 12. 88–100.

Griffith, Erin 2019. "Why Are Young People Pretending to Love Work?" *New York Times*, 26 January. Available online: www.nytimes.com/2019/01/26/business/against-hustle-culture-rise-and-grind-tgim.html. Accessed 30 August 2021.

Grodetskaya, A. G. 2008. “Review Article: The Living Life in Eternity: The New Tolstoy Biography from *Lives of Extraordinary People*.” Trans. David Houston. *Tolstoy Studies Journal*, vol. 20. 97–101.

Gromova-Opul’skaia, L. D. 2000. “The Departure and Death of Lev Tolstoy.” *Tolstoy Studies Journal*, vol. 12. 79–83.

Grubačić, Andrej and Denis O’Hearn 2016. *Living at the Edges of Capitalism: Adventures in Exile and Mutual Aid*. Oakland, CA: University of California Press.

Guardian 2022. “The *Guardian* View on the Russian Orthodox Church: Betrayed by Putin’s Patriarch.” *Guardian*, 3 April. Available online: www.theguardian.com/commentisfree/2022/apr/03/the-guardian-view-on-the-russian-orthodox-church-betrayed-by-putins-patriarch. Accessed 3 April 2022.

Guevara, Ernesto “Che” 1996. *The Motorcycle Diaries: A Journey around South America*. Trans. Ann Wright. New York: Verso.

Gustafson, Richard F. 1986. *Leo Tolstoy: Resident and Stranger*. Princeton, NJ: Princeton University Press.

Gustafson, Richard F. 1988. “Roundtable: Richard F. Gustafson, *Leo Tolstoy. Resident and Stranger*.” *Tolstoy Studies Journal*, vol. 1. 23–26.

Gustafson, Richard F. 1999. “Review: Dragan Milivojevic, *Leo Tolstoy and the Oriental Religious Heritage*.” *Tolstoy Studies Journal*, vol. 11. 123–125.

Habermas, Jürgen 1981. *The Theory of Communicative Action*, vol. 1: *Reason and the Rationalization of Society*. Trans. Thomas McCarthy. Boston, MA: Beacon.

Habermas, Jürgen 2014. *The Structural Transformation of the Public Sphere*. Cambridge: Cambridge University Press.

Hájková, Anna 2021. “Between Love and Coercion: Queer Desire, Sexual Barter and the Holocaust.” *German History*, vol. 39, issue 1. 112–133.

Hall, Jonathan 2020. *Reaction Formations: Dialogism, Ideology, and Capitalism Culture*. Chicago, IL: Haymarket Books.

Hamburg, G. M. 2010. “Marriage, Estate Culture and Public Life in Sofia Andreyevna Tolstaya’s My Life.” *Tolstoy Studies Journal*, vol. 22. 122–135.

Harding, Luke 2022. “‘We Are a Huge Amount of Ants’: The United Front of Ukrainian Volunteers.” *Guardian*, 2 March. Available online: www.theguardian.com/world/2022/mar/02/ukrainian-volunteers-united-front-against-russia-invasion. Accessed 10 April 2022.

Hardt, Michael and Kathi Weeks 2020. “Exploitation Is the Rule, Not the Exception.” *Open Democracy*, 17 November. Available online: www.opendemocracy.net/en/beyond-trafficking-and-slavery/exploitation-rule-not-exception/. Accessed 18 November 2020.

Harris, Jane Gary 1991. “A Humanist Reading of Tolstoy: The Writings of Petr M. Bitsilli.” *Tolstoy Studies Journal*, vol. 4. 73–95.

Healey, Daniel 2001. *Homosexual Desire in Revolutionary Russia: The Regulation of Sexual and Gender Dissent*. Chicago, IL: University of Chicago Press.

Hegel, George WilhelmFriedrich 1806. “Hegel to Niethammer: October 13, 1806.” Available online: www.marxists.org/reference/archive/hegel/works/letters/1806-10-13.htm. Accessed 2 March 2020.

Hekma, Gert 1990. “Homosociality.” *The Encyclopedia of Homosexuality*. Ed. Wayne R. Dynes. New York: Garland Press. 560–561.

Heller, Agnes 1990. “Freedom and Happiness in Kant’s Political Philosophy.” *Graduate Faculty Philosophy Journal*, vol. 13, issue 2. 115–131.

Herzen, Alexander 1973. *My Past and Thoughts*. Trans. Constance Garnett. Berkeley, CA: University of California Press.

Heuer, Gottfried 2017. *Freud’s “Outstanding” Colleague/Jung’s “Twin Brother*.”London: Routledge.

Hillman, James 2004. *A Terrible Love of War*. New York: Penguin.

Ho, Vivian 2020. "'Everyone Tested Positive': Covid Devastates Agriculture Workers in California's Heartland." *Guardian*, 8 August. Available online: www.theguardian.com/us-news/2020/aug/08/california-covid-19-central-valley-essential-workers. Accessed 8 August 2020.

Hoare, Philip 2021. "Sperm Whales in 19th Century Shared Ship Attack Information." *Guardian*, 17 March. Available online: www.theguardian.com/environment/2021/mar/17/sperm-whales-in-19th-century-shared-ship-attack-information. Accessed 26 March 2021.

Holbrook, David 1997. *Tolstoy, Woman, and Death: A Study of War and Peace and Anna Karenina*. Madison, NJ: Fairleigh Dickinson University Press.

Holmes, Richard 2001. "Salamanca, Battle of." *The Oxford Companion to Military History*. Ed. Richard Holmes. Oxford: Oxford University Press. 802.

Homer 1998. "Zeus and Ganymede." Trans. E. V. Rieu. *The Columbia Anthology of Gay Literature*. Ed. Byrne R. S. Fone. New York: Columbia University Press. 16.

Honneth, Axel 2017. *The Idea of Socialism*. Trans. Joseph Ganahl. Cambridge: Polity.

Horner, Tom 1990. "Jesus." *The Encyclopedia of Homosexuality*. Ed. Wayne R. Dynes. New York: Garland Press. 637–639.

Houser, Ward 1990. "Dance." *The Encyclopedia of Homosexuality*. Ed. Wayne R. Dynes. New York: Garland Press. 291–292.

Hrdy, Sarah Blaffer 2009. *Mothers and Others: The Evolutionary Origins of Mutual Understanding*. Cambridge, MA: Harvard University Press.

Hudis, Peter 2013. *Marx's Concept of the Alternative to Capitalism*. Chicago, IL: Haymarket Books.

Huetteman, Emmarie 2020. "US Hospitals Pressure Healthcare Staff to Work Even If They Have Covid Symptoms." *Guardian*, 13 August. Available online: www.theguardian.com/us-news/2020/aug/13/us-nurses-doctors-covid-19-symptoms-working. Accessed 13 August 2020.

Hyde, Rob 2021. "The Slow Road to Atonement." *The Lancet*, vol. 398, issue 10295. 105–108.

Irwin, William 2013. "Death by Inauthenticity: Heidegger's Debt to Ivan Il'ich's Fall." *Tolstoy Studies Journal*, vol. 25. 15–21.

Jackson, Robert Louis 2003. "Scenes from the Apocalypse in Tolstoy's *War and Peace*: The Lion of Judah." *Tolstoy Studies Journal*, vol. 15. 25–33.

Jahn, Gary R. 2002. "Tolstoy as a Writer of Popular Literature." *The Cambridge Companion to Tolstoy*. Ed. Donna Tussing Orwin. Cambridge: Cambridge University Press. 113–126.

Jakim, Boris 2009. "A Brief Overview of Nikolai Berdyaev's Life and Works." *Slavery and Freedom*. San Rafael: Semantron Press. 269–275.

James, C. L. R. 1989. *The Black Jacobins*. New York: Vintage.

Jameson, Fredric 2005. *Archaeologies of the Future: The Desire Called Utopia and Other Science Fictions*. New York: Verso.

Jansen, Robert S. 2011. "Populist Mobilizations: A New Theoretical Approach to Populism." *Sociological Theory*, vol. 29, issue 2. 75–96.

Jay, Martin 2021. "Marcuse and the Weaponization of 'Free Speech.'" Keynote address at the International Herbert Marcuse Society conference, University of Arizona, 9 October.

Johansson, Warren 1990a. "Authoritarian Personality." *The Encyclopedia of Homosexuality*. Ed. Wayne R. Dynes. New York: Garland Press. 99–100.

Johansson, Warren 1990b. "Fascist Perversion, Belief in." *The Encyclopedia of Homosexuality*. Ed. Wayne R. Dynes. New York: Garland Press. 390–391.

Johansson, Warren 1990c. "Freemasonry." *The Encyclopedia of Homosexuality*. Ed. Wayne R. Dynes. New York: Garland Press. 429–430.

Johansson, Warren 1990d. "Freudian Concepts." *The Encyclopedia of Homosexuality*. Ed. Wayne R. Dynes. New York: Garland Press. 432–437.

Johansson, Warren 1990e. "Injustice Collecting." *The Encyclopedia of Homosexuality*. Ed. Wayne R. Dynes. New York: Garland Press. 601.

Johansson, Warren 1990f. "Intermediate Stages, Sexual." *The Encyclopedia of Homosexuality*. Ed. Wayne R. Dynes. New York: Garland Press. 608–609.

Johansson, Warren 1990g. "Kuzmin, Mikhail Alekseevich." *The Encyclopedia of Homosexuality*. Ed. Wayne R. Dynes. New York: Garland Press. 670–671.

Johansson, Warren 1990h. "Melville." *The Encyclopedia of Homosexuality*. Ed. Wayne R. Dynes. New York: Garland Press. 798–799.

Johansson, Warren 1990i. "Military." *The Encyclopedia of Homosexuality*. Ed. Wayne R. Dynes. New York: Garland Press. 814–817.

Johansson, Warren 1990j. "Monasticism." *The Encyclopedia of Homosexuality*. Ed. Wayne R. Dynes. New York: Garland Press. 828–831.

Johansson, Warren 1990k. "Napoleon Bonaparte." *The Encyclopedia of Homosexuality*. Ed. Wayne R. Dynes. New York: Garland Press. 874–875.

Johansson, Warren 1990l. "Particular Friendships." *The Encyclopedia of Homosexuality*. Ed. Wayne R. Dynes. New York: Garland Press. 950–951.

Johansson, Warren 1990m. "Pederasty." *The Encyclopedia of Homosexuality*. Ed. Wayne R. Dynes. New York: Garland Press. 959–964.

Johansson, Warren 1990n. "Plato." *The Encyclopedia of Homosexuality*. Ed. Wayne R. Dynes. New York: Garland Press. 1000–1002.

Johansson, Warren 1990o. "Röhm, Ernst." *The Encyclopedia of Homosexuality*. Ed. Wayne R. Dynes. New York: Garland Press. 1111–1112.

Johansson, Warren 1990p. "Rozanov, Vasilii Vasil'evich." *The Encyclopedia of Homosexuality*. Ed. Wayne R. Dynes. New York: Garland Press. 1130–1132.

Johansson, Warren 1990q. "Tchaikovsky, Peter Il'yich." *The Encyclopedia of Homosexuality*. Ed. Wayne R. Dynes. New York: Garland Press. 1279–1280.

Johansson, Warren 1990r. "Uranianism." *The Encyclopedia of Homosexuality*. Ed. Wayne R. Dynes. New York: Garland Press. 1352–1353.

Johansson, Warren 1990s. "Voltaire." *The Encyclopedia of Homosexuality*. Ed. Wayne R. Dynes. New York: Garland Press. 1378–1380.

Johns, Steven 2014. "The Christmas Truce, 1914." *Libcom*, 22 December. Available online: https://libcom.org/history/christmas-truce-1914-steven-johns. Accessed 15 December 2019.

Johnson, Daniel 2021. "American Gothic; or, What Melville Can Teach Us." *New Politics*, Summer. Available online: https://newpol.org/issue_post/american-gothic-or-what-melville-can-teach-us. Accessed 13 October 2021.

Jones, Garrett 2001. *Alfred and Arthur: An Historic Friendship*. Hertford: Authors OnLine.

Jones, Owen 2022. "Why Homophobia against Straight Men Matters." *Guardian*, 17 May. Available online: www.theguardian.com/commentisfree/2022/may/17/homophobia-against-straight-men-lgbtq. Accessed 18 May 2022.

Kant, Immanuel 1784. "Idea for a Universal History from a Cosmopolitan Point of View." Available online: www.marxists.org/reference/subject/ethics/kant/universal-history.htm. Accessed 30 November 2020.

Kant, Immanuel 1991. *Political Writings*. Ed. Hans Reiss. Cambridge: Cambridge University Press.

Kant, Immanuel 2004. *Critique of Practical Reason*. Trans. Thomas Kingsmill Abbott. Mineola, NY: Dover.

Kant, Immanuel 2007. *Critique of Pure Reason*. Trans. and ed. Marcus Weiglet. London: Penguin.

Kaplan, Mark S. *et al.* 2012. "Estimating the Risk of Suicide Among US Veterans: How Should We Proceed From Here?" *American Journal of Public Health*, vol. 102, issue S1. S21–S23. Available online: www.ncbi.nlm.nih.gov/pmc/articles/PMC3496465/. Accessed 31 October 2020.

Karlinsky, Simon 1990. "Russia and USSR." *The Encyclopedia of Homosexuality*. Ed. Wayne R. Dynes. New York: Garland Press. 1133–1138.

Katz, Michael R. and William G. Wagner 1989. "Chernyshevsky, *What Is To Be Done?* and the Russian Intelligentsia." *What Is To Be Done?* Trans. Michael R. Katz. Ithaca, NY: Cornell University Press.

Kaufman, Scott Barry and Elliot S. Paul 2014. "Creativity and Schizophrenia Spectrum Disorders across the Arts and Sciences." *Frontiers in Psychology*, 3 November.https://doi.org/10.3389/fpsyg.2014.01145.

Kaur, Gunisha 2021. "From Torture to Ultraviolence: Medical and Legal Implications." *The Lancet*, 6 April. https://doi.org/10.1016/S0140-6736(21)00222-1.

Kautsky, Karl 1953. *The Foundations of Christianity*. Trans. Henry F. Mins. New York: Russell and Russell. Available online: www.marxists.org/archive/kautsky/1908/christ/index.htm. Accessed 5 May 2021.

Keeney, Charles B. 2021. "A Century Ago, West Virginia Miners Took Up Arms against King Coal." *Jacobin*, 23 June. Available online: https://jacobinmag.com/2021/06/battle-of-blair-mountain-red-necks-labor-uprising-west-virginia-charles-b-keeney-interview. Accessed 24 August 2021.

Ken, Teo Lee 2017. "Ali Shariati and Ethical Humanism: Conceiving a Perspective of Liberative Social Ethics." *Ali Shariati and the Future of Social Theory*. Eds. Dustin J. Byrd and Seyed Javad Miri. Chicago, IL: Haymarket Books. 128–156.

Kennedy, Hubert 1995. "Johann Baptist von Schweitzer: The Queer Marx Loved to Hate." *Journal of Homosexuality*, vol. 29, issue 2–3. 69–96.

Kentish, Jane 1987. "Introduction." *A Confession and Other Religious Writings*. Trans. Jane Kentish. London: Penguin Books. 7–15.

Khayar, Ibrahim 2020. "Tools for a Political Psychiatry." *Radical Philosophy Review*, vol. 2, issue 8. Available online: www.radicalphilosophy.com/reviews/individual-reviews/tools-for-a-political-psychiatry. Accessed 8 October 2020.

Khazov, Sergei 2013. "Rainbow Russia." *Open Democracy*, 18 June. Available online: www.opendemocracy.net/en/odr/rainbow-russia. Accessed 5 October 2021.

Khazov-Cassia, Sergei 2013. "A Different Childhood." *Open Democracy*, 21 June. Available online: www.opendemocracy.net/en/odr/different-childhood. Accessed 5 October 2021.

Kinna, Ruth 2020a. "Review of *Luigi Galleani: The Most Dangerous Anarchist in America* by Antonio Senta." *Marx and Philosophy*, 12 March. Available online: https://marxandphilosophy.org.uk/reviews/17827_luigi-galleani-the-most-dangerous-anarchist-in-america-by-antonio-senta-reviewed-by-ruth-kinna/. Accessed 12 March 2020.

Kinna, Ruth 2020b. "Great Anarchists." Presentation given at the London Anarchist Book Fair, London, 17 October.

Kinna, Ruth and Clifford Harper 2020. *Great Anarchists: Pierre-Joseph Proudhon*. London: Dog Section Press.

Kirby, Dean 2022. "Putin Sends Mariupol Survivors to Remote Corners of Russia as Investigation Reveals Network of 66 Camps." *iNews*, 7 May. Available online: https://inews.co.uk/news/putin-mariupol-survivors-remote-corners-russia-investigation-network-camps-1615516. Accessed 7 May 2022.

Kishkovsky, Sophia 2009. "Chechnya's Favorite Russian: Leo Tolstoy." *The New York Times*, 28 December. Available online: www.nytimes.com/2009/12/29/arts/29iht-tolstoy.html. Accessed 8 October 2020.

Kitonga, Ndindi 2020. "Anti-Colonialism and Humanism." *New Politics*, vol. 17, issue 4. Available online: https://newpol.org/issue_post/anti-colonialism-and-humanism/. Accessed 10 July 2020.

Klikauer, Thomas 2013. *Managerialism: A Critique of an Ideology*. London: Palgrave Macmillan.

Klikauer, Thomas and Nadine Campbell 2020. "Review of *Anarchism, Organization and Management: Critical Perspectives for Students* by Martin Parker, Konstantin Stoborod and Thomas Swann (eds)." *Marx and Philosophy*, 13 July. Available online: https://marxandphilosophy.org.uk/reviews/18172_anarchism-organization-and-management-critical-perspectives-for-students-by-martin-parker-konstantin-stoborod-and-thomas-swann-eds-reviewed-by-thomas-klikauer-nadine-campbell/. Accessed 16 July 2020.

Knapp, Liza 1991. "Tolstoy on Musical Mimesis: Platonic Aesthetics and Erotics in 'The Kreutzer Sonata.'" *Tolstoy Studies Journal*, vol. 4. 25–42.

Knapp, Liza 2002. "The Development of Style and Theme in Tolstoy." *The Cambridge Companion to Tolstoy*. Ed. Donna Tussing Orwin. Cambridge: Cambridge University Press. 161–175.

Kobrin, Kirill 2020. "Sliding into Isolation: Russia and the World." *Open Democracy*, 23 December. Available online: www.opendemocracy.net/en/odr/russia-isolation-kobrin. Accessed 29 December 2020.

Kokobobo, Ani 2008. "Authoring Jesus: Novelistic Echoes in Tolstoy's Harmonization and Translation of the Four Gospels." *Tolstoy Studies Journal*, vol. 20. 1–13.

Kondakov, Alexander 2013. "Do Russians Give a Damn about Homosexuality?" *Open Democracy*, 20 June. Available online: www.opendemocracy.net/en/odr/do-russians-give-damn-about-homosexuality. Accessed 5 October 2021.

Kornblatt, Judith Deutsch 1992. *The Cossack Hero in Russian Literature: A Study in Cultural Mythology*. Madison, WI: University of Wisconsin Press.

Koshiw, Isobel 2022. "'Putin's Terror Affects Everyone': Anarchists Join Ukraine's War Effort." *Guardian*, 26 May. Available online: www.theguardian.com/world/2022/may/26/putin-anarchists-join-ukraine-war-effort. Accessed 27 May 2022.

Kropotkin, Peter 1991. *Russian Literature: Ideals and Realities*. Montréal: Black Rose Books.

Kropotkin, Peter 2009. *Mutual Aid: A Factor of Evolution*. London: Freedom Press.

Kropotkin, Peter 2012. *Ethics: Origin and Development*. Trans. Louis S. Friedland and Joseph R. Piroshnikoff. San Bernardino, CA: CreateSpace Independent Publishing Platform.

Kropotkin, Peter 2018. *Modern Science and Anarchy*. Ed. Iain McKay. Chico, CA: AK Press.

Kropotkin, Peter 2022. *The Curious One: Peter Kropotkin's Siberian Diaries*. Ed. Christopher Coquard, trans. Alexandra Agranovich. Montréal: Black Rose Books.

Kupfersmid, Joel 1995. "Does the Oedipus Complex Exist?" *Psychotherapy: Theory, Research, Practice, Training*, vol. 32, issue 4. 535–547.

Kusters, Wouter 2021. "Philosophy & Madness: A Discussion with Wouter Kusters on his New Book." *Mad in the UK*, 12 April. Available online: www.madintheuk.com/2021/04/philosophy-madness-a-discussion-with-wouter-kusters/. Accessed 15 April 2021.

Kyaw, Min Ye and Rebecca Ratcliffe 2022. "Myanmar's Junta Torching 'Village after Village' in Bid to Quell Opposition." *Guardian*, 29 January. Available online: www.theguardian.com/global-development/2022/jan/29/myanmars-junta-torching-village-after-village-in-bid-to-quell-opposition. Accessed 29 January 2022.

La Botz, Dan 2020. *Trotsky in Tijuana*. St. Petersburg, FL: Serge Books/BookLocker.

Lagalisse, Erica 2019. *Occult Features of Anarchism*. Oakland, CA: PM Press.

Lanzieri, Nicholas and Tom Hildebrant 2011. "Using Hegemonic Masculinity to Explain Gay Male Attraction to Muscular and Athletic Men." *Journal of Homosexuality*, vol. 58, issue 2. 275–293.

Lawrence, Tim 2020. "Covid-19 Has Hit Dance Culture Hard—but the Party Can Go On." *Guardian*, 21 September. Available online: www.theguardian.com/commentisfree/2020/jun/04/how-coronavirus-could-bridge-generational-divides-not-widen-them. Accessed 21 September 2020.

Lazar, Hillary 2021. "Love, Care, and Mutual Aid as Community Self-Defense. Life, Freedom, & Ethics: Kropotkin Now!" International Conference, 6 February. Available online: www.youtube.com/watch?v=zT5GvrzRLto. Accessed 13 February 2021.

LeBlanc, Ronald 1993. "Unpalatable Pleasures: Tolstoy, Food, and Sex." *Tolstoy Studies Journal*, vol. 6. 1–32.

LeBlanc, Ronald 2007. "Review Article: Daniel Rancour-Laferriere's *Russian Literature and Psychoanalysis*." *Tolstoy Studies Journal*, vol. 19. 119–122.

Lee, Josh 2021. "Queerpiphany Review: LGBTQ+ Bingewatch is Joyous—and Profound." *Guardian*, 11 November. Available online: www.theguardian.com/tv-and-radio/2021/nov/11/queerpiphany-review-munroe-bergdorf-tayce-mtv. Accessed 12 November 2021.

Leeder, Elaine 2021. "Sex, Politics and Anarchism: American Jewish Anarchist Women, 1920–1950." *The Commoner*, 20 October. Available online: www.thecommoner.org.uk/sex-politics-and-anarchism-american-jewish-anarchist-women-1920–1950/. Accessed 20 October 2021.

Le Guin, Ursula K. 1985. *Always Coming Home*. Berkeley, CA: University of California Press.

Leier, Mark 2006. *Bakunin: The Creative Passion*. New York: Thomas Dunne.

Lennard, Natasha 2020. "The Covid-19 Generation Divide between Millennials and Boomers Ignores the Real Problem." *Guardian*, 4 June. Available online: www.theguardian.com/commentisfree/2020/jun/04/how-coronavirus-could-bridge-generational-divides-not-widen-them. Accessed 5 June 2020.

Lepore, Jill 2021. "Burnout: Modern Affliction or Human Condition?" *The New Yorker*, 17 May. Available online: www.newyorker.com/magazine/2021/05/24/burnout-modern-affliction-or-human-condition. Accessed 3 June 2021.

Levinas, Emmanuel 1979. *Totality and Infinity: An Essay on Exteriority*. Trans. Alphonso Lingis. The Hague: Maartintus Nijhoff.

Lieven, Dominic 2000. *Empire: The Russian Empire and Its Rivals*. New Haven, CT: Yale University Press.

Lieven, Dominic 2012. "Tolstoy on War, Russia, and Empire." *Tolstoy on War*. Eds. Rick McPeak and Donna Tussing Orwin. Ithaca, NY: Cornell University Press. 12–25.

Lin, Kevin 2021. "Myanmar Workers and Unions on the Front Lines in Fight against Coup." *Labor Notes*, 26 February. Available online: https://labornotes.org/2021/02/myanmar-workers-and-unions-front-lines-fight-against-coup. Accessed 26 February 2021.

Lomnitz, Claudio 2014. *The Return of Comrade Ricardo Flores Magón*. New York: Zone Books.

Lönnqvist, Barbara 2007. "Tolstoy Rewriting the Caucasus." *Tolstoy Studies Journal*, vol. 19. 75–78.

Lopez, Barry 1998. "We Are Shaped by the Sound of Wind, the Slant of Sunlight." *High Country News*, 14 September. Available online: www.hcn.org/issues/138/barry-lopez-we-are-shaped-by-the-sound-of-wind-the-slant-of-sunlight. Accessed 31 December 2020.

Love, Jeff 2007. "Review of Гулин, А. В. Лев Толстой и пути русской истории." *Tolstoy Studies Journal*, vol. 19. 126–127.

Love, Jeff 2011. "The Roguish Tolstoy." *Tolstoy Studies Journal*, vol. 23. 34–43.

Love, Jeff 2012. "The Great Man in *War and Peace*." *Tolstoy on War*. Eds. Rick McPeak and Donna Tussing Orwin. Ithaca, NY: Cornell University Press. 85–97.

Lowe, Simon 2021. "One Hundred Years since a Hellish Vision of Technology Spawned that Fateful Word: Robot." *Guardian*, 10 January. Available online: www.theguardian.com/technology/2021/jan/10/art-meets-tech-to-mark-first-100-years-of-the-robot. Accessed 21 January 2021.

Ludwig, Emil 1927. "Mussolini as Napoleon's Pupil." *The New York Times*, 1 May. Available online: www.nytimes.com/1927/05/01/archives/mussolini-as-napoleons-pupil-the-corsicans-biographer-contrasts-the.html. Accessed 4 November 2019.

Lundskow, George 2020. "The Necessity of Prophetic Humanism in Progressive Social Change." *Erich Fromm's Critical Theory: Hope, Humanism, and the Future*. Eds. Kieran Durkin and Joan Braune. London: Bloomsbury Academic. 52–71.

Luxemburg, Rosa 1981. *Comrade and Lover: Rosa Luxemburg's Letters to Leo Jogiches*. Ed. and trans. Elżbieta Ettinger. Cambridge, MA: MIT Press.

MacLaughlin, Jim 2016. *Kropotkin and the Anarchist Intellectual Tradition*. London: Pluto.

McCall, Corey 2019. "Review: Verena Erlenbusch-Anderson, *Genealogies of Terrorism: Revolution, State Violence, Empire*." *Philosophy in Review*, vol. 39, issue 4. 173–176.

McGrattan, Ciara 2016. "The Hidden Histories of Queer Women of the Easter Rising." *GCN Ireland*, 22 March. Available online: https://gcn.ie/hidden-histories-queer-women-easter-rising/. Accessed 29 April 2022.

McHarg, Farquhar 2020. "Albert Einstein in Barcelona: 'My Name Is Albert Einstein and I Am also Revolutionary, an Anti-Authoritarian.'" *Libcom*, 12 November. Available online: http://libcom.org/history/albert-einstein-barcelona-my-name-albert-einstein-i-am-also-revolutionary-anti-authorita. Accessed 14 November 2020.

McKay, Iain 2017. "The State and Revolution: Theory and Practice." *Bloodstained: One Hundred Years of Leninist Counterrevolution*. Eds. Friends of Aron Baron. Chico, CA: AK Press. 62–117.

McLean, Hugh 2002. "Resurrection." *The Cambridge Companion to Tolstoy*. Ed. Donna Tussing Orwin. Cambridge: Cambridge University Press. 96–110.

McLean, Hugh 2008. "Review Article: *War and Peace*, Original Version." *Tolstoy Studies Journal*, vol. 20. 82–88.

McLaughlin, Paul 2002. *Mikhail Bakunin: The Philosophical Basis of his Anarchism*. New York: Algora Publishing.

McPeak, Rick 2012. "Tolstoy and Clausewitz: The Duel as a Microcosm of War." *Tolstoy on War*. Eds. Rick McPeak and Donna Tussing Orwin. Ithaca, NY: Cornell University Press. 111–122.

Makoii, Akhtar Mohammad 2021. "'I Wondered Whether a Bullet Had My Name on It': My Terrifying 24-Hour Journey Out of Afghanistan." *Guardian*, 11 December. Available online: www.theguardian.com/world/2021/dec/11/i-wondered-whether-a-bullet-had-my-name-on-it-my-terrifying-24-hour-journey-out-of-afghanistan. Accessed 12 December 2021.

Malatesta, Errico 2014. *The Method of Freedom: An Errico Malatesta Reader*. Ed. Davide Turcato. Oakland, CA: AK Press.

Malia, Martin 1961. *Alexander Herzen and the Birth of Russian Socialism*. New York: Universal Library.

Mälksoo, Maria 2022. "The Postcolonial Moment in Russia's War against Ukraine." *Journal of Genocide Research*. doi:10.1080/14623528.2022.2074947.

Mandelker, Amy 1990. "Feminist Criticism and *Anna Karenina*: A Review Article." *Tolstoy Studies Journal*, vol. 3. 82–103.

Marcuse, Herbert 1955. *Eros and Civilization: A Philosophical Inquiry into Freud*. Boston, MA: Beacon.

Marcuse, Herbert 1964. *One-Dimensional Man: Studies in the Ideology of Advanced Industrial Society*. Boston, MA: Beacon.

Marcuse, Herbert 1980. "Protosocialism and Late Capitalism: Toward a Theoretical Synthesis Based on Bahro's Analysis." Trans. Michel Vale *et al. International Journal of Politics*, vol. 10, issue 2/3. 25–48.

Marcuse, Herbert 2005. *Heideggerian Marxism*. Eds. Richard Wolin and John Abromeit. Lincoln, NE: University of Kansas Press.

Marshall, Lisa 2020. "We're Hard-Wired for Longing, New Study Suggests." *CU Boulder Today*, 11 May. Available online: www.colorado.edu/today/2020/05/11/were-hard-wired-longing-new-study-suggests. Accessed 25 June 2021.

Martin, Alexander M. 2012. "Moscow in 1812: Myths and Realities." *Tolstoy on War*. Eds. Rick McPeak and Donna Tussing Orwin. Ithaca, NY: Cornell University Press. 42–58.

Marx, Karl 1976. *Capital, Volume I: A Critique of Political Economy*. Trans. Ben Fowkes. London: Penguin Books.

Marx, Karl 1983. *The Portable Karl Marx*. Ed. Eugene Kamenka. New York: Penguin.

Massad, Joseph A. 2007. *Desiring Arabs*. Chicago, IL: University of Chicago Press.

Maude, Aylmer 1960. "Introduction." *The Kingdom of God Is Within You and Peace Essays*. Trans. Aylmer Maude. London: Oxford University Press.

Maude, Aylmer 1987a. *The Life of Tolstoy: The First Fifty Years*. Oxford: Oxford University Press.

Maude, Aylmer 1987b. *The Life of Tolstoy: Later Years*. Oxford: Oxford University Press.

Maximov, G. P. 1940. *The Guillotine at Work: The Leninist Counter-Revolution*. Chicago, IL: Globus Printing.

Mayer, Kenneth H. *et al.* 2021. "The Persistent and Evolving HIV Epidemic in American Men Who Have Sex with Men." *The Lancet*. https://doi.org/10.1016/S0140-6736(21)00321-4.

Mazurin, Boris 1993. "The Life and Labor Commune: A History and Some Reflections." *Memoirs of Peasant Tolstoyans in Soviet Russia*. Trans. William Edgerton. Bloomington, IN: Indiana University Press. 27–108.

Mbembe, Achille 2003. "Necropolitics." *Public Culture*, vol. 15, issue 1, 11–40.

Mbembe, Achille 2016. "The Society of Enmity." *Radical Philosophy Review*, vol. 200. Available online: www.radicalphilosophy.com/article/the-society-of-enmity. Accessed 16 July 2020.

Medzhibovskaya, Inessa 2004. "Dogmatism or Moral Logic? Simon Frank Confronts Tolstoy's Ethical Thought." *Tolstoy Studies Journal*, vol. 16. 18–29.

Medzhibovskaya, Inessa 2005. "Simon Frank Confronts Tolstoy's Ethical Thoughts (The Later Years." *Tolstoy Studies Journal*, vol. 17. 43–58.

Medzhibovskaya, Inessa 2008. *Tolstoy and the Religious Culture of his Time: A Biography of a Long Conversion, 1845–1887*. Lanham, MD: Lexington Books.

Medzhibovskaya, Inessa 2010. "Terror Un-Sublimated: Militant Monks, Revolution, and Tolstoy's Final Master Plots." *Tolstoy Studies Journal*, vol. 22. 17–38.

Melville, Herman 2001. *Moby Dick, or the Whale*. New York: Penguin.

Memmi, Albert 1991. *The Colonizer and the Colonized*. Boston, MA: Beacon Press.

Mendelsohn, Daniel 2021. "Ancient Greece's Army of Lovers." *The New Yorker*, 21 April. Available online: www.newyorker.com/magazine/2021/04/19/ancient-greeces-army-of-lovers. Accessed 14 July 2021.

Mergier, Anne Marie 2021. "Doble Holocausto para los Homosexuales." *Proceso*, 11 July. Available online: www.proceso.com.mx/reportajes/2021/7/11/doble-holocausto-para-los-homosexuales-267594.html. Accessed 23 July 2021.

Merz, Theo 2021. "Chechnya Opens Terror Inquiry into Gay Men Forcibly Returned from Moscow." *Guardian*, 8 February. Available online: www.theguardian.com/world/2021/feb/08/chechnya-opens-terror-inquiry-into-gay-men-forcibly-returned-from-moscow. Accessed 21 May 2022.

Messersmith-Glavin, Lara 2021. "Time under Tension: Lessons in Organizing from a Kettleball Gym." *Perspectives on Anarchist Theory*, vol. 32. 47–61.

Michel, Gary 2022. "Decolonize Russia." *The Atlantic*, 27 May. Available online: www.theatlantic.com/ideas/archive/2022/05/russia-putin-colonization-ukraine-chechnya/639428/. Accessed 27 May 2022.

Milivojevic, Dragan 1991. "Some Similarities and Differences between Tolstoy's Concepts of Identity and Vocation and their Parallels in Hinduism." *Tolstoy Studies Journal*, vol. 4. 97–103.

Milivojevic, Dragan 1993. "Tolstoy's Views on Buddhism." *Tolstoy Studies Journal*, vol. 3. 62–75.

Miller, Madeline 2012. *The Song of Achilles*. New York: Harper Collins.

Miri, Seyed Javad 2017. "Ali Shariati's Critique of Durkheim's Sociology of Religion." *Ali Shariati and the Future of Social Theory*. Eds. Dustin J. Byrd and Seyed Javad Miri. Chicago, IL: Haymarket Books. 85–97.

Moberg, Dennis J. 1999. "The Big Five and Organizational Virtue." *Business Ethics Quarterly*, vol. 9, issue 2. 245–272.

Mogutin, Yaroslav 1995. "Gay in the Gulag." *Index on Censorship*, vol. 24, issue 1. 66–69.

Mola, Mark 2016. "The Circassian Genocide." *Medium.com*, 16 May. Available online: https://medium.com/@markmola/the-circassian-genocide-e39aa41bbfdd. Accessed 9 November 2019.

Mole, Richard C. M. 2019. "Constructing Soviet and post-Soviet Sexualities." *Soviet and Post-Soviet Sexualities*. Ed. Richard C. M. Mole. London: Routledge. 1–15.

Mondloch, Chris 2013. "An Afghan Tragedy: The Pashtun Practice of Having Sex with Young Boys." *The Independent*, 29 October. Available online: www.independent.co.uk/voices/comment/afghan-tragedy-pashtun-practice-having-sex-young-boys-8911529.html. Accessed 8 July 2021.

Moore, Jason W. 2016. "The Rise of Cheap Nature." *Anthropocene or Capitalocene? Nature, History, and the Crisis of Capitalism*. Ed. Jason W. Moore. Oakland, CA: PM Press. 78–115.

Moran, Daniel 2001. "Clausewitz, Carl Philip Gottlieb von." *The Oxford Companion to Military History*. Ed. Richard Holmes. Oxford: Oxford University Press. 207–209.

Moreira, Marta 2020. "'Invertidos y Rompepatrias,' el libro que destapa la complicada relación de la izquierda con la homosexualidad." *Valencia Plaza*, 12 November. Available online: https://valenciaplaza.com/invertidos-y-rompepatrias-el-libro-que-destapa-la-complicada-relacion-de-la-izquierda-con-la-homosexualidad. Accessed 13 November 2020.

Morgachëv, Dimitry 1993. "My Life." *Memoirs of Peasant Tolstoyans in Soviet Russia*. Trans. William Edgerton. Bloomington, IN: Indiana University Press. 109–180.

Morson, Gary Saul Morson 2002. "*War and Peace*." *The Cambridge Companion to Tolstoy*. Ed. Donna Tussing Orwin. Cambridge: Cambridge University Press. 65–79.

Morson, Gary Saul Morson 2012. "Symposium of Quotations: Wit and Other Short Genres in *War and Peace*." *Tolstoy on War*. Eds. Rick McPeak and Donna Tussing Orwin. Ithaca, NY: Cornell University Press. 74–84.

Moyse, R. and J. Porter 2015. "The Experience of the Hidden Curriculum for Autistic Girls at Mainstream Primary Schools." *European Journal of Special Needs Education*, vol. 30, issue 2. 187–201.

Mureithi, Anita 2021. "Thank You, bell hooks." *Open Democracy*, 16 December. Available online: www.opendemocracy.net/en/thank-you-bell-hooks. Accessed 1 January 2022.

Murphy, Timothy F. 1984. "Freud Reconsidered: Bisexuality, Homosexuality, and Moral Judgement." *Journal of Homosexuality*, vol. 9, issue 2–3, 65–77.

Museu Marítim de Barcelona 2021. "Desire Flows Like the Sea: An LGTBIQ Look at Maritime Heritage." Available online: www.mmb.cat/en/exhibitions/desire-flows-like-the-sea/. Accessed 15 July 2021.

Nazaryan, Alexander 2013. "Blood and Tragedy: The Caucasus in the Literary Imagination." *The New Yorker.* Available online: www.newyorker.com/books/page-turner/blood-and-tragedy-the-caucasus-in-the-literary-imagination. Accessed 3 May 2019.

Nealon, Christopher 2020. "Introduction." *Sexual Hegemony: Statecraft, Sodomy, and Capital in the Rise of the World System.* Durham, NC: Duke University Press. 1–17.

Nelson, Elizabeth Hoffman 1998. "The Heyoka of the Sioux." *Fools and Jesters in Literature, Art, and History: A Bio-Bibliographical Sourcebook.* Westport, CT: Greenwood Press. 246–248.

Newlin, Thomas 2012. "'Swarm Life' and the Biology of *War and Peace.*" *Slavic Review*, vol. 71, issue 2. 359–384.

Newton, Huey P. 2009. *Revolutionary Suicide.* New York: Penguin.

Nietzsche, Friedrich 1974. *The Gay Science.* Trans. Walter Kaufmann. New York: Vintage Books.

Nietzsche, Friedrich 2002. *The Anti-Christ, Ecce Homo, Twilight of the Idols, and Other Writings.* Eds. Aaron Ridley and Judith Norman. Cambridge: Cambridge University Press.

O'Dowd, Niall 2022. "The Major Role of Gay Women in the 1916 Easter Rising." *Irish Central*, 30 April. Available online: www.irishcentral.com/opinion/niallodowd/gay-women-1916-easter-rising. Accessed 30 April 2022.

Okundaye, Jason 2021. "Ted Brown: The Man Who Held a Mass Kiss-In and Made History." *Guardian*, 8 April. Available online: www.theguardian.com/society/2021/apr/08/ted-brown-the-man-who-held-a-mass-kiss-in-and-made-history. Accessed 9 April 2021.

Olaya, Vicente 2021. "Zaragoza: La ciudad indefensa que derrotó al mayor ejército del mundo." *El País*, 27 April. Available online: https://elpais.com/babelia/2021-04-27/zaragoza-la-ciudad-indefensa-que-derroto-al-mayor-ejercito-del-mundo.html. Accessed 23 July 2021.

Oltermann, Philip and Shaun Walker 2020. "Chopin's Interest in Men Airbrushed from History, Programme Claims." *Guardian*, 30 November. Available online: www.theguardian.com/music/2020/nov/25/chopins-interest-in-men-airbrushed-from-history-programme-claims. Accessed 30 November 2020.

Oosterhuis, Harry 2010. "The 'Jews' of the Antifascist Left: Homosexuality and Socialist Resistance to Nazism." *Journal of Homosexuality*, vol. 29, issue 2–3. 227–257.

Orend, Brian 2008. "War." *Stanford Encyclopedia of Philosophy.* Ed. Edward N. Zalta. Available online: https://plato.stanford.edu/archives/fall2008/entries/war. Accessed 11 April 2020.

Orwin, Donna Tussing 1988. "Roundtable: Richard F. Gustafson, *Leo Tolstoy. Resident and Stranger.*" *Tolstoy Studies Journal*, vol. 1. 18–21.

Orwin, Donna Tussing 1993. *Tolstoy's Art and Thought, 1847–1880.* Princeton, NJ: Princeton University Press.

Orwin, Donna Tussing 2002a. "Introduction: Tolstoy as Artist and Public Figure." *The Cambridge Companion to Tolstoy.* Ed. Donna Tussing Orwin. Cambridge: Cambridge University Press. 49–62.

Orwin, Donna Tussing 2002b. "Chronology." *The Cambridge Companion to Tolstoy.* Ed. Donna Tussing Orwin. Cambridge: Cambridge University Press. 1–47.

Orwin, Donna Tussing 2002c. "Courage in Tolstoy." *The Cambridge Companion to Tolstoy.* Ed. Donna Tussing Orwin. Cambridge: Cambridge University Press. 222–236.

Orwin, Donna Tussing 2002d. "Editor's Preface." *The Cambridge Companion to Tolstoy.* Ed. Donna Tussing Orwin. Cambridge: Cambridge University Press. xii–xiii.

Orwin, Donna Tussing 2012a. "Introduction." *Tolstoy on War.* Eds. Rick McPeak and Donna Tussing Orwin. Ithaca, NY: Cornell University Press. 1–11.

Orwin, Donna Tussing 2012b. "*War and Peace* from the Military Point of View." *Tolstoy on War.* Eds. Rick McPeak and Donna Tussing Orwin. Ithaca, NY: Cornell University Press. 98–110.

Orwin, Donna Tussing 2012c. "The Awful Poetry of War: Tolstoy's *Borodino*." *Tolstoy on War*. Eds. Rick McPeak and Donna Tussing Orwin. Ithaca, NY: Cornell University Press. 123–139.

Osgood, Kelsey 2016. "Life at One of England's Last Tolstoyan Communes." *The New Yorker*, 6 January. Available online: www.newyorker.com/books/page-turner/life-at-one-of-englands-last-tolstoyan-communes. Accessed 26 October 2020.

Pachankis, John E. *et al.* 2020. "Sex, Status, Competition, and Exclusion: Intraminority Stress from Within the Gay Community and Gay and Bisexual Men's Mental Health." *Journal of Personality and Social Psychology*, vol. 119, issue 3. 713–740.

Parini, Jay 1990. *The Last Station: A Novel of Tolstoy's Final Year*. New York: Anchor Books.

Parker, Martin *et al.* (eds). 2020. *Anarchism, Organization and Management: Critical Perspectives for Students*. London: Routledge.

Pasternak, Boris 2010. *Doctor Zhivago*. Trans. Richard Pevear and Larissa Volokhonsky. New York: Vintage.

Pateman, Barry 2017. "Cries in the Wilderness: Alexander Berkman and Russian Prisoner Aid." *Bloodstained: One Hundred Years of Leninist Counterrevolution*. Eds. Friends of Aron Baron. Chico, CA: AK Press. 243–258.

Pelikan, Jaroslavl 1985. *Jesus: His Life Throughout the Centuries*. New Haven, CT: Yale University Press.

Percy, William A. 1990a. "Fascism." *The Encyclopedia of Homosexuality*. Ed. Wayne R. Dynes. New York: Garland Press. 387–390.

Percy, William A. 1990b. "Goethe." *The Encyclopedia of Homosexuality*. Ed. Wayne R. Dynes. New York: Garland Press. 483–484.

Percy, William A. 1990c. "Symposia." *The Encyclopedia of Homosexuality*. Ed. Wayne R. Dynes. New York: Garland Press. 1272–1274.

Peterson, Dale E. 2004. "Cossacks in Spain: Tolstoyan Resonances in *For Whom the Bell Tolls*." *Tolstoy Studies Journal*, vol. 16. 33–41.

Pevear, Richard 2009. "Introduction." *Lev Tolstoy's Hadji Murat*. Trans. Richard Pevear and Larissa Volokhonsky. New York: Vintage. vii–xiii.

Phelps, Christopher 2017. "The Sexuality of Malcolm X." *Journal of American Studies*, vol. 51, issue 3. 659–690.

Pietikainen, Petteri 2007. *The Alchemists of Human Nature*. London: Routledge.

Plato 360 BCE. "Phaedrus." Trans. Benjamin Jowett. Available online: http://classics.mit.edu/Plato/phaedrus.html. Accessed 28 November 2020.

Plato 2015. *Great Dialogues of Plato*. Trans. W. H. D. Rouse. New York: Penguin.

Plokhy, Serhii 2015. *The Gates of Europe: A History of Ukraine*. New York: Basic Books.

Polanyi, Karl 2014. *The Great Transformation: The Political and Economic Origins of Our Time*. Boston, MA: Beacon Press.

Polosina, Anna 2008. "Leo Tolstoy and the *Encyclopédistes*." *Tolstoy Studies Journal*, vol. 20. 53–61.

Poole, Randall A. 2010. "'Russia's First Modern Man': Tolstoy, Kant, and Russian Religious Thought." *Tolstoy Studies Journal*, vol. 22. 99–117.

Proudhon, Pierre-Joseph 2011. *Property Is Theft! A Pierre-Joseph Proudhon Reader*. Ed. Iain McKay. Chico, CA: AK Press.

Pushkin, Alexander 1998. "Two Poems." Trans. Michael Green. *The Columbia Anthology of Gay Literature*. Ed. Byrne R. S. Fone. New York: Columbia University Press. 458.

Racy, Gustavo 2020. "Review of *Aspects of the New Right-Wing Extremism* by Theodor W. Adorno." *Marx and Philosophy*, 17 September. Available online: https://marxandphilosophy.org.uk/reviews/18335_aspects-of-the-new-right-wing-extremism-by-theodor-w-adorno-reviewed-by-gustavo-racy/. Accessed 17 September 2020.

Ramnath, Maia 2015. "No Gods, No Masters, No Brahmins: An Anarchist Inquiry on Caste, Race, and Indigeneity in India." *No Gods, No Masters, No Peripheries: Global Anarchisms*. Eds. Raymond Craib and Barry Maxwell. Oakland, CA: PM Press. 44–79.

Rancour-Laferriere, Daniel 1985. *Signs of the Flesh: An Essay on the Evolution of Hominid Sexuality*. Berlin: Mouton de Gruyter.

Rancour-Laferriere, Daniel 1988. *The Mind of Stalin*. Ann Arbor, MI: Ardis Publishers.

Rancour-Laferriere, Daniel 1989. "Helene as Pre-Oedipal Self-Object." *Tolstoy Studies Journal*, vol. 2. 41–52.

Rancour-Laferriere, Daniel 1995. *The Slave Soul of Russia: Moral Masochism and the Cult of Suffering*. New York: New York University Press.

Rancour-Laferriere, Daniel 1998. *Tolstoy on the Couch: Misogyny, Masochism, and the Absent Mother*. New York: New York University Press.

Rapp, John A. 2012. *Daoism and Anarchism: Critiques of State Autonomy in Ancient and Modern China*. London: Continuum.

Reid, Tim 2002. "Kandahar Comes out of the Closet." *The Times*, 12 January. 16.

Reis, Shmuel P. *et al.* 2019. "The Holocaust, Medicine, and Becoming a Physician: The Crucial Role of Education." *Israel Journal of Health Policy Research*, vol. 8. Available online: https://ijhpr.biomedcentral.com/articles/10.1186/s13584-019-0327-3. Accessed 12 November 2020.

Reitz, Charles 2019. *Ecology and Revolution: Herbert Marcuse and the Challenge of a New World System Today*. Routledge: New York.

Remley, William L. 2018. *Jean-Paul Sartre's Anarchist Philosophy*. London: Bloomsbury.

Roberts, Larry-bob 2010. *The International Homosexual Conspiracy*. San Francisco, CA: Manic D Press.

Robinson, Kim Stanley 2017. *Red Mars*. New York: Del Rey.

Roddenberry, Gene *et al.* 1990. "The Best of Both Worlds, Part II." *Star Trek, The Next Generation*, Season 4. California: Paramount Pictures.

Roelcke, Volker *et al.* 2021. "Announcing the *Lancet* Commission on Medicine and the Holocaust: Historical Evidence, Implications for Today, Teaching for Tomorrow." *The Lancet*, vol. 397, issue 10277, 862–864. https://doi.org/10.1016/S0140-6736(21)00157-4.

Rogers, Philip 2005. "The Sufferings of Young Olenin: Tolstoy's Werther." *Tolstoy Studies Journal*, vol. 17. 59–70.

Rousseau, Jean-Jacques 1996. "Discourse on the Origin and Foundations of Inequality among Men." *Modern Political Thought*. Ed. David Wootton. Indianapolis, IN: Hackett. 404–463.

Rubin, Gayle S. 1984. "Thinking Sex: Notes for a Radical Theory of the Politics of Sexuality." *Pleasure and Danger: Exploring Female Sexuality*. Ed. Carole S. Vance. Boston, MA: Routledge. 143–178.

Rule, Philip C. S. J. 1988. "Roundtable: Richard F. Gustafson, *Leo Tolstoy. Resident and Stranger*." *Tolstoy Studies Journal*, vol. 1. 21–23.

Ruthsatz, Joanne *et al.* 2015. "Molecular Genetic Evidence for Shared Etiology of Autism and Prodigy." *Human Heredity*, vol. 79. 53–59.

Said, Edward 1978. *Orientalism*. New York: Pantheon Books.

Salem, Nour 2020. "Sarah Hegazi in Syria." *Syria Untold*, 20 October. Available online: https://syriauntold.com/2020/10/20/sarah-hegazi-in-syria/. Accessed 31 October 2020.

Salter, Michael 2019. "The Problem with a Fight Against Toxic Masculinity." *The Atlantic*, 27 February. Available online: www.theatlantic.com/health/archive/2019/02/toxic-masculinity-history/583411. Accessed 15 September 2021.

Samet, Elizabeth D. 2012. "The Disobediences of *War and Peace*." *Tolstoy on War*. Eds. Rick McPeak and Donna Tussing Orwin. Ithaca, NY: Cornell University Press. 160–174.

Sartre, Jean-Paul 1983. *Cahiers pour une morale*. Paris: Gallimard.

Schama, Simon 2016. "What Tolstoy's 'War and Peace' Can Teach Us." *Financial Times*, 8 January. Available online: www.ft.com/content/8a003e2c-b497-11e5-8358-9a82b43f6b2f. Accessed 28 October 2019.

Schiffman, Richard 2016. "Psilocybin: A Journey beyond the Fear of Death?" *Scientific American*, 1 December. Available online: www.scientificamerican.com/article/psilocybin-a-journey-beyond-the-fear-of-death. Accessed 20 September 2021.

Schild, Maarten 1990. "Sa'di." *The Encyclopedia of Homosexuality*. Ed. Wayne R. Dynes. New York: Garland Press. 1142–1143.

Schneider, Tobias and Theresa Lütkefend 2019. "Nowhere to Hide: The Logic of Chemical Weapons Use in Syria." *Global Public Policy Institute*. Available online: www.gppi.net/2019/02/17/the-logic-of-chemical-weapons-use-in-syria. Accessed 29 September 2019.

Schopenhauer, Arthur 1851. "On Women." Available online: www.theabsolute.net/misogyny/onwomen.html. Accessed 26 December 2019.

Scott, James C. 1998. *Seeing Like a State: How Certain Schemes to Improve the Human Condition Have Failed*. New Haven, CT: Yale University Press.

Shafer, David A. 2005. *The Paris Commune: French Politics, Culture, and Society at the Crossroads of the Revolutionary Tradition and Revolutionary Socialism*. New York: Palgrave Macmillan.

Shakespeare, William 2020. *Henry* V. Eds. Barbara A. Mowat and Paul Werstine. New York: Simon & Schuster.

Shakhidzhanian, Vladimir and Svetlana Reiter 2013. "Kill or Cure?" *Open Democracy*, 19 June. Available online: www.opendemocracy.net/en/odr/kill-or-cure. Accessed 5 October 2021.

Shantz, Jeff and Dana W. Williams 2014. *Anarchy and Society: Reflections on Anarchist Sociology*. Chicago, IL: Haymarket Books.

Shaw, Devine Zane 2020. "Review of *Critiquing Brahmanism: A Collection of Essays* by K. Murali (Ajith)." *Marx and Philosophy*, 9 December. Available online: https://marxandphilosophy.org.uk/reviews/18560_critiquing-brahmanism-a-collection-of-essays-by-k-murali-ajith-reviewed-by-devin-zane-shaw/. Accessed 9 December 2020.

Shcherbakov, Viktor 1997. "Archival Research: An Unknown Source of *War and Peace* (*My Notes* by Freemason P. Ia. Titov)." *Tolstoy Studies Journal*, vol. 9. 66–83.

Shelley, Mary 2003. *Frankenstein, or the Modern Prometheus*. London: Penguin.

Shestov, Lev 1969. "The Good in the Teaching of Tolstoy and Nietzsche." *Dostoevsky, Tolstoy and Nietzsche*. Ed. Bernard Martin. Athens, OH: Ohio University Press. 1–140.

Shively, Charley 1990a. "Anarchism." *The Encyclopedia of Homosexuality*. Ed. Wayne R. Dynes. New York: Garland Press. 51–52.

Shively, Charley 1990b. "Hafiz." *The Encyclopedia of Homosexuality*. Ed. Wayne R. Dynes. New York: Garland Press. 515–516.

Shkurenok, Natalia 2022. "Why Aren't More Russians Protesting War in Ukraine? We Asked an Expert." *Open Democracy*, 24 January. Available online: https://beta.opendemocracy.net/en/odr/sergei-davidis-anti-war-movement-russia/. Accessed 30 January 2022.

Shlapentokh, Dmitry 2019. "Marx, the 'Asiatic Mode of Production,' and 'Oriental Despotism' as 'True' Socialism." *Comparative Sociology*, 18. 489–521.

Shul'ts, Sergei 2013. "Hemingway and Tolstoy: 'The Snows of Kilimanjaro' and 'Death of Ivan Il'ich.'" *Tolstoy Studies Journal*, vol. 25. 82–89.

Siegel, Lee 2005. "The Tower of Babel." *The Nation*, 17 November. Available online: www.thenation.com/article/archive/tower-babel/. Accessed 15 July 2021.

Singer, Peter 1999. *A Darwinian Left: Politics, Evolution, and Cooperation*. New Haven, CT: Yale University Press.

Sizova, I. I. 2008. "Review of *Leo Tolstoy and Russian Peasant Sectarian Writers: Selected Correspondence*." *Tolstoy Studies Journal*, vol. 20. 105–106.

Sloane, David A. 1991. "Pushkin's Legacy in *Anna Karenina*." *Tolstoy Studies Journal*, vol. 4. 1–24.

Sloane, David A. 2005. "Review Article: *The Overcoming of History in War and Peace*." *Tolstoy Studies Journal*, vol. 17. 104–108.

Sloane, David A. *et al.* 1997. "Critical Reflections on Kathryn B. Feuer's *Tolstoy and the Genesis of War and Peace*." *Tolstoy Studies Journal*, vol. 9. 59–65.

Smith, David Norman 2020. "Anti-Authoritarian Marxism." *Erich Fromm's Critical Theory: Hope, Humanism, and the Future*. Eds. Kieran Durkin and Joan Braune. London: Bloomsbury Academic. 131–165.

Smith, Leonard 2001. "Mutinies." *The Oxford Companion to Military History*. Ed. Richard Holmes. Oxford: Oxford University Press. 613–616.

Smith, Paul Julian 1993. "'The Captive's Tale': Race, Text, Gender." *Quixotic Desire: Psychoanalytic Perspectives on Cervantes*. Eds. Ruth Anthony El Saffar and Diana de Armas Wilson. Ithaca, NY: Cornell University Press. 227–235.

Smolski, Andrew *et al.* 2022. "Case Studies in the Sociology of Absence and Emergence: Anarcho-Populism in Russia and Mexico." *Theory in Action*, vol. 15, issue 1. 1–24.

Snyder, Timothy 2022. "The War in Ukraine Has Unleashed a New Word." *New York Times*, 22 April. Available online: www.nytimes.com/2022/04/22/magazine/ruscism-ukraine-russia-war.html. Accessed 14 May 2022.

Sokoloski, Richard 1997. "Tolstoy's *The Death of Ivan Ilych*: First and Final Chapter." *Tolstoy Studies Journal*, vol. 9. 49–58.

Sokurov, Alexander 2002. *Russian Ark*. Seville: Seville Pictures.

Solomon, Sheldon *et al.* 2015. *The Worm at the Core: On the Role of Death in Life*. London: Penguin.

Sorel, Georges 2004. *Reflections on Violence*. Trans. T. E. Hulme and J. Roth. Mineola, NY: Dover.

Sorokin, Vladimir 2022. "Vladimir Putin Sits Atop a Crumbling Pyramid of Power." *Guardian*, 27 February. Available online: www.theguardian.com/commentisfree/2022/feb/27/vladimir-putin-russia-ukraine-power. Accessed 10 April 2022.

Spiegel, Leo A. 1978. "Moral Masochism." *The Psychoanalytic Quarterly*, vol. 47, issue 2. 209–236.

Stamenova, Alina 2020. "Why Miners in Ukraine's Longest City Are Holding an Underground Strike." *Open Democracy*, 17 September. Available online: www.opendemocracy.net/en/odr/why-miners-ukraines-longest-city-are-holding-underground-strike. Accessed 4 October 2020.

Staples, Louis 2022. "Evil Twinks and Gay Gangsters: Why We Need to Remember History's Horrid Homosexuals." *Guardian*, 24 May. Available online: www.theguardian.com/tv-and-radio/2022/may/24/bad-gays-podcast-interview-alexander-the-great-ronnie-kray. Accessed 25 May 2022.

Sternhell, Zeev 1994. *The Birth of Fascist Ideology: From Cultural Rebellion to Political Revolution*. Trans. David Maisel. Princeton, NJ: Princeton University Press.

Stites, Richard 1989. *Revolutionary Dreams: Utopian Vision and Experimental Life in the Russian Revolution*. Oxford: Oxford University Press.

Stites, Richard 1990. *The Women's Liberation Movement in Russia: Feminism, Nihilism, and Bolshevism, 1860–1930*. Princeton, NJ: Princeton University Press.

Stroganov, M. V. 2014. "Tolstoy and Napoleon." *Tolstoy Studies Journal*, vol. 26. 55–61.

Struve, Pëtr 1994. "The Intelligentsia and Revolution." *Vekhi: Landmarks*. Trans. Marshall E. Shatz and Judith E. Zimmerman. New York: Routledge. 115–129.

Subrat, Piro 2019. *Invertidos y Rompepatrias: Marxismo, anarquismo y desobediencia sexual y de género en el Estado español (1868–1982).* Madrid: Editorial Imperdible.

Taggart, Andrew 2020. "If Work Dominated Your Every Moment, Would Life Be Worth Living?" *Open Democracy*, 6 February. Available online: www.opendemocracy.net/en/transformation/if-work-dominated-your-every-moment-would-life-be-worth-living/. Accessed 16 February 2020.

Takhar, Opinderjit Kaur 2011. "Egalitarian Hermeneutics: From the *Bani* of Guru Nank: His Attitudes towards Caste and Females." *Understanding Sikhism*, vol. 13, issue 1–2. 42–51.

Tarasulo, Yitzhak Yankel 1983. "*The Napoleonic Invasion of 1812 and the Political and Social Crisis in Russia.*" PhD dissertation, Yale University.

Tatum, Megan 2021. "Outcry over Persecution of Health Workers in Myanmar." *The Lancet*, vol. 397, issue 10285. 1609.

Tavis, Anna 1990. "Comrade Lenin or Count Leo Tolstoy? Reflections after Some Memorable Meetings at Harrogate." *Tolstoy Studies Journal*, vol. 3. 104–108.

Taylor, Ella 2019. "Saint Petersburg Fiddles, Moscow Burns." *Criterion*, 27 June. Available online: www.criterion.com/current/posts/6463-war-and-peace-saint-petersburg-fiddles-moscow-burns. Accessed 11 December 2020.

Teneromo, Isaak 1912. *Departure of a Grand Old Man.* Russian Empire: P. Thiman and F. Reinhardt.

Tennyson, Lord, Alfred 2017. "The Charge of the Light Brigade" (1854). Available online: www.poetryfoundation.org/poems/45319/the-charge-of-the-light-brigade. Accessed 28 October 2019.

Terras, Victor 1988. "Roundtable: Richard F. Gustafson, *Leo Tolstoy. Resident and Stranger.*" *Tolstoy Studies Journal*, vol. 1. 13–15.

The New Arab 2022. "Coptic Pope Laments Ukraine War in Orthodox Easter Address, Stops Short of Condemning Russia." *The New Arab*, 24 April. Available online: https://english.alaraby.co.uk/news/coptic-pope-laments-ukraine-war-during-easter-address. Accessed 24 April 2022.

Thompson, Gabriel 2020. "'The Sun Is Hot and You Can't Breathe in a Mask'—Life as an Undocumented Farmworker." *Guardian*, 28 May. Available online: www.theguardian.com/us-news/2020/may/28/undocumented-farmworker-us-immigration-california. Accessed 28 May 2020.

Thompson, Michael J. 2020. "Erich Fromm and the Ontology of Social Relations." *Erich Fromm's Critical Theory: Hope, Humanism, and the Future.* Eds. Kieran Durkin and Joan Braune. London: Bloomsbury Academic. 23–42.

Tillich, Paul 2000. *The Courage to Be.* 2nd ed. New Haven, CT: Yale University Press.

Tolstaia, S. A. 2010. *The Diaries of Sophia Tolstoy.* Trans. Cathy Porter. New York: HarperCollins.

Tolstaya, Sofiya Andreevna 2014a. "Song without Words." *The Kreutzer Sonata Variations.* Ed. and trans. Michael R. Katz. New Haven, CT: Yale University Press. 165–254.

Tolstaya, Sofiya Andreevna 2014b. "Whose Fault?" *The Kreutzer Sonata Variations.* Ed. and trans. Michael R. Katz. New Haven, CT: Yale University Press. 71–164.

Tolstoy, Leo 1886. *What I Believe.* Trans. Constantine Popoff. New York: William S. Gottsberger.

Tolstoy, Leo 1900. "Thou Shalt Not Kill." Available online: http://dwardmac.pitzer.edu/Anarchist_Archives/bright/tolstoy/notkill.html. Accessed 11 October 2020.

Tolstoy, Leo 1942. *What Then Must We Do?*Oxford: Oxford University Press.

Tolstoy, Leo 1960. *The Kingdom of God Is Within You and Peace Essays.* Trans. Aylmer Maude. London: Oxford University Press.

Tolstoy, Leo 1982. *The Raid and Other Stories*. Trans. Louise and Aylmer Maude. Oxford: University of Oxford.

Tolstoy, Leo 1985. *Tolstoy's Diaries*. Ed. and translated by R. F. Christian. London: Flamingo.

Tolstoy, Leo 1987. *A Confession and Other Religious Writings*. Trans. Jane Kentish. London: Penguin Books.

Tolstoy, Leo 2004. *Resurrection*. Trans. Louise Maude. Mineola, NY: Dover.

Tolstoy, Leo 2005. *Master and Man and Other Stories*. Trans. Ronald Wilks and Paul Foote. London: Penguin.

Tolstoy, Leo 2006a. *The Cossacks and Other Stories*. Trans. David McDuff and Paul Foote. London: Penguin Books.

Tolstoy, Leo 2006b. *Childhood*. Trans. C. J. Hogworth. Chapel Hill, NC: Project Gutenberg.

Tolstoy, Leo 2009a. *Father Sergius*. Trans. Louise and Aylmer Maude. Chapel Hill, NC: Project Gutenberg.

Tolstoy, Leo 2009b. *Hadji Murat*. Trans. Richard Pevear and Larissa Volokhonsky. New York: Vintage.

Tolstoy, Leo 2010. *War and Peace*. Trans. Louise and Aylmer Maude. Oxford: Oxford University Press.

Tolstoy, Leo 2012. *The Death of Ivan Ilych and Other Stories*. Trans. Aylmer Maude and J. D. Duff. New York: Signet Classics.

Tolstoy, Leo 2017. *The Decembrists*. Ed. Taylor Anderson. San Bernardino, CA: CreateSpace Independent Publishing Platform.

Tolstoy, Leo 2018. *Anna Karenina*. Trans. Constance Garnett. San Bernardino, CA: CreateSpace Independent Publishing Platform.

Tolstoy, Leo 2019. *The Power of Darkness*. Trans. Louise and Aylmer Maude. Mineola, NY: Dover.

Triandis, Harry C. 2001. "Individualism-Collectivism and Personality." *Journal of Personality*, vol. 69, issue 6. 907–924.

Troianovski, Anton 2022. "Atrocities in Ukraine War Have Deep Roots in Russian Military." *New York Times*, 17 April. Available online: www.nytimes.com/2022/04/17/world/europe/ukraine-war-russia-atrocities.html. Accessed 16 May 2022.

Trotsky, Leon 1951. "Tolstoy, Poet and Rebel." Trans. John G. Wright. Available online: www.marxists.org/archive/trotsky/1908/09/tolstoy.htm. Accessed 14 May 2022.

Tucker, Kenneth 1991. "How New Are New Social Movements?" *Theory, Culture, and Society*, vol. 8, issue 2. 75–98.

Turgenev, Ivan 1878a. "Дурак." Available online: https://ilibrary.ru/text/1378/p.12/index.html. Accessed 18 February 2021.

Turgenev, Ivan 1878b. "Лазурное Царство." Available online: https://rvb.ru/turgenev/01text/vol_10/02senilia/0243.htm. Accessed 20 February 2021.

Ulam, Adam 1973. *Stalin: The Man and His Era*. New York: Viking.

Ungurianu, Dan 2012. "The Use of Historical Sources in *War and Peace*." *Tolstoy on War*. Eds. Rick McPeak and Donna Tussing Orwin. Ithaca, NY: Cornell University Press. 26–41.

University of East Anglia 2015. "Research Examines Relationship between Autism and Creativity: New Research Has Found that People with High Levels of Autistic Traits Are More Likely to Produce Unusually Creative Ideas." *ScienceDaily*, 13 August. Available online: www.sciencedaily.com/releases/2015/08/150813222253.htm. Accessed 24 February 2021.

Venturi, Franco 1960. *Roots of Revolution: A History of the Populist and Socialist Movements in Nineteenth Century Russia*. Trans. Francis Haskell. New York: The Universal Library.

Vergara, Camila 2020. "Populism as Plebeian Politics: Inequality, Domination, and Popular Empowerment." *The Journal of Political Philosophy*, vol. 28, issue 2. 222–246.

Vinitsky, Ilya 2007. "Behind the Door: A Few Remarks Concerning the Direction of Prince Andrei's Gaze." *Tolstoy Studies Journal*, vol. 19. 80–86.

Voline 1975. *The Unknown Revolution*. Montréal: Black Rose Books.

Wachtel, Andrew 2002. "History and Autobiography in Tolstoy." *The Cambridge Companion to Tolstoy*. Ed. Donna Tussing Orwin. Cambridge: Cambridge University Press. 176–190.

Walicki, Andrzej 1979. *A History of Russian Thought from the Enlightenment to Marxism*. Trans. Hilda Andrew-Rusiecka. Stanford, CA: Stanford University Press.

Walicki, Andrzej 1991. *Russia, Poland, and Universal Regeneration: Studies on Russian and Polish Thought of the Romantic Epoch*. London: University of Notre Dame Press.

Walker, Shaun 2021. "Hungary's Viktor Orbán Will Hold Referendum on Anti-LGBT Law." *Guardian*, 21 July. Available online: www.theguardian.com/world/2021/jul/21/hungarys-viktor-orban-will-hold-referendum-on-anti-lbgt-law. Accessed 26 July 2021.

Waltz, Kenneth N. 2001. *Man, the State, and War: A Theoretical Analysis*. New York: Columbia University Press.

Warfield, Liam *et al.* (eds) 2021. *Queercore: How to Punk a Revolution*. Oakland, CA: PM Press.

Welch, David A. 2012. "Tolstoy the International Relations Theorist." *Tolstoy on War*. Eds. Rick McPeak and Donna Tussing Orwin. Ithaca, NY: Cornell University Press. 175–189.

Wesson, Robert G. 1962. "The Soviet Communes." *Soviet Studies*, vol. 13, issue 4. 341–336.

Wexler, Alice 1989. *Emma Goldman in Exile: From the Russian Revolution to Spanish Civil War*. Boston, MA: Beacon Press.

Wible, Pamela 2018. "What I've Learned from My Tally of 757 Doctor Suicides." *Washington Post*, 13 January. Available online: www.washingtonpost.com/national/health-science/what-ive-learned-from-my-tally-of-757-doctor-suicides/2018/01/12/b0ea9126-eb50–11e7–9f92-10a2203f6c8d_story.html. Accessed 16 February 2020.

Wilkerson, Isabel 2020. "America's 'Untouchables': The Silent Power of the Caste System." *Guardian*, 28 July. Available online: www.theguardian.com/world/2020/jul/28/untouchables-caste-system-us-race-martin-luther-king-india. Accessed 2 August 2020.

Williams, Christine *et al.* 1999. "Sexuality in the Workplace: Organizational Control, Sexual Harassment, and the Pursuit of Pleasure." *Annual Review of Sociology*, vol. 25. 73–93.

Williams, Wesley 2002. "Aspects of the Creed of Imam Ahmad Ibn Hanbal: A Study of Anthropomorphism in Early Islamic Discourse." *International Journal of Middle East Studies*, vol. 34, issue. 3. 441–463.

Williams, Zoe 2021. "Trauma, Trust and Triumph: Psychiatrist Bessel van der Kolk on How to Recover from our Deepest Pain." *Guardian*, 20 September. Available online: www.theguardian.com/society/2021/sep/20/trauma-trust-and-triumph-psychiatrist-bessel-van-der-kolk-on-how-to-recover-from-our-deepest-pain. Accessed 20 September 2021.

Williamson, Victoria *et al.* 2021. "Moral Injury: The Effect on Mental Health and Implications for Treatment." *The Lancet Psychiatry*, vol. 8, issue 6. 453–455.

Willsher, Kim 2020. "French Reporter Who Joined Police Exposes Racism and Violence." *Guardian*, 3 September. Available online: www.theguardian.com/world/2020/sep/03/french-reporter-who-joined-police-exposes-racism-and-violence-valentin-gendrot. Accessed 1 November 2020.

Wilson, David 2011. "Health Promotion of the Infant and Family." *Wong's Nursing Care of Infants and Children*. Eds. Marilyn J. Hockenberry and David Wilson. 9th ed. St. Louis, MO: Elsevier. 464–520.

Wilson, Jennifer 2014. "(Drag)ging Tolstoy into Queer Theory: On the Cross-Dressing Motif in *War and Peace*." *Tolstoy Studies Journal*, vol. 26. 29–38.

Wilson, Jennifer 2021. "Among the Rank and File." *The Nation*, 5 April. Available online: www.thenation.com/article/culture/gogol-nose-other-stories. Accessed 10 April 2021.

Wittfogel, Karl 1957. *Oriental Despotism: A Comparative Study of Total Power*. New Haven, CT: Yale University Press.

Yalom, Irvin D. 1980. *Existential Psychotherapy*. New York: Basic Books.

Yarmolinsky, Avrahm 1962. *Road to Revolution*. New York: Collier Books.

Yousef, Leel 2020. "Strategies for Rebellion: A Queer Reading of the Syrian Revolution." *Syria Untold*, 6 October. Available online: https://syriauntold.com/2020/10/06/strategies-for-rebellion-a-queer-reading-of-the-syrian-revolution/. Accessed 28 October 2020.

Yusufji, Salim (ed.) 2017. *Ambedkar: The Attendant Details*. New Delhi: Navayana.

Yuzich, Yuriy 2018. "'Glory to Ukraine!' Who and When Was the Slogan Created?" *Історична правда*, 4 October. Available online: www.istpravda.com.ua/eng/articles/2018/10/4/153036/. Accessed 19 March 2022.

Zakaria, Rafia 2021. "*The Right to Sex* by Amia Srinivasan Review—The Politics of Sexual Attraction." Available online: www.theguardian.com/books/2021/aug/19/the-right-to-sex-by-amia-srinivasan-review-the-politics-of-sexual-attraction. Accessed 20 August 2021.

Zatat, Narjas 2021. "Malcolm X: Muslim and Misunderstood, a Pioneering Force of the US Civil Rights Movement." *The New Arab*, 21 February. Available online: https://english.alaraby.co.uk/english/indepth/2021/2/21/malcolm-x-misunderstood-pioneer-of-us-civil-rights-movement. Accessed 22 February 2021.

Ziarek, Ewa Płonowska 2001. *An Ethics of Dissensus: Postmodernity, Feminism, and the Politics of Radical Democracy*. Stanford, CA: Stanford University Press.

Zolotov, Andrei 2011. "100 Years after Excommunication, Church Cannot Look Kindly Upon Tolstoy." *Christianity Today*, 1 March. Available online: www.christianitytoday.com/ct/2001/marchweb-only/3–5-44.0.html. Accessed 20 March 2019.

Zorin, Andrei 2020. *Critical Lives: Leo Tolstoy*. London: Reaktion Books.

INDEX

For Product Safety Concerns and Information please contact our EU
representative GPSR@taylorandfrancis.com
Taylor & Francis Verlag GmbH, Kaufingerstraße 24, 80331 München, Germany

www.ingramcontent.com/pod-product-compliance
Ingram Content Group UK Ltd.
Pitfield, Milton Keynes, MK11 3LW, UK
UKHW020149200926
475702UK00016B/2621
* 9 7 8 1 0 3 2 3 4 2 5 5 9 *